NUTRITION
CHEMISTRY AND BIOLOGY
SECOND EDITION

CRC SERIES IN MODERN NUTRITION
Edited by Ira Wolinsky and James F. Hickson, Jr.

Published Titles

Manganese in Health and Disease, Dorothy J. Klimis-Zacas

Nutrition and AIDS: Effects and Treatments, Ronald R. Watson

Nutrition Care for HIV-Positive Persons: A Manual for Individuals and Their Caregivers, Saroj M. Bahl and James F. Hickson, Jr.

Calcium and Phosphorus in Health and Disease, John J.B. Anderson and Sanford C. Garner

Edited by Ira Wolinsky

Published Titles

Practical Handbook of Nutrition in Clinical Practice, Donald F. Kirby and Stanley J. Dudrick

Handbook of Dairy Foods and Nutrition, Gregory D. Miller, Judith K. Jarvis, and Lois D. McBean

Advanced Nutrition: Macronutrients, Carolyn D. Berdanier

Childhood Nutrition, Fima Lifschitz

Nutrition and Health: Topics and Controversies, Felix Bronner

Nutrition and Cancer Prevention, Ronald R. Watson and Siraj I. Mufti

Nutritional Concerns of Women, Second Edition, Ira Wolinsky and Dorothy J. Klimis-Zacas

Nutrients and Gene Expression: Clinical Aspects, Carolyn D. Berdanier

Antioxidants and Disease Prevention, Harinda S. Garewal

Advanced Nutrition: Micronutrients, Carolyn D. Berdanier

Nutrition and Women's Cancers, Barbara Pence and Dale M. Dunn

Nutrients and Foods in AIDS, Ronald R. Watson

Nutrition: Chemistry and Biology, Second Edition, Julian E. Spallholz, L. Mallory Boylan, and Judy A. Driskell

Melatonin in the Promotion of Health, Ronald R. Watson

Nutritional and Environmental Influences on the Eye, Allen Taylor

Laboratory Tests for the Assessment of Nutritional Status, Second Edition, H.E. Sauberlich

Advanced Human Nutrition, Robert E.C. Wildman and Denis M. Medeiros

Handbook of Dairy Foods and Nutrition, Second Edition, Gregory D. Miller, Judith K. Jarvis, and Lois D. McBean

Nutrition in Space Flight and Weightlessness Models, Helen W. Lane and Dale A. Schoeller

Eating Disorders in Women and Children: Prevention, Stress Management, and Treatment, Jacalyn J. Robert-McComb

Childhood Obesity: Prevention and Treatment, Jana Pařízková and Andrew Hills

Alcohol and Coffee Use in the Aging, Ronald R. Watson

Handbook of Nutrition in the Aged, Third Edition, Ronald R. Watson

Vegetables, Fruits, and Herbs in Health Promotion, Ronald R. Watson

Nutrition and AIDS, Second Edition, Ronald R. Watson

Advances in Isotope Methods for the Analysis of Trace Elements in Man, Nicola Lowe and Malcolm Jackson

Nutritional Anemias, Usha Ramakrishnan

Handbook of Nutraceuticals and Functional Foods, Robert E. C. Wildman

The Mediterranean Diet: Constituents and Health Promotion, Antonia-Leda Matalas, Antonis Zampelas, Vassilis Stavrinos, and Ira Wolinsky

Vegetarian Nutrition, Joan Sabaté

Nutrient–Gene Interactions in Health and Disease, Naïma Moustaïd-Moussa and Carolyn D. Berdanier

Micronutrients and HIV Infection, Henrik Friis

Tryptophan: Biochemicals and Health Implications, Herschel Sidransky

Nutritional Aspects and Clinical Management of Chronic Disorders and Diseases, Felix Bronner

Forthcoming Titles

Handbook of Nutraceuticals and Nutritional Supplements and Pharmaceuticals, Robert E. C. Wildman

Insulin and Oligofructose: Functional Food Ingredients, Marcel B. Roberfroid

Julian E. Spallholz
L. Mallory Boylan
and Judy A. Driskell

NUTRITION
CHEMISTRY AND BIOLOGY

SECOND EDITION

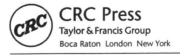

CRC Press
Taylor & Francis Group
Boca Raton London New York

CRC Press is an imprint of the
Taylor & Francis Group, an **informa** business

CRC Press
Taylor & Francis Group
6000 Broken Sound Parkway NW, Suite 300
Boca Raton, FL 33487-2742

First issued in paperback 2019

© 1999 by Taylor & Francis Group, LLC
CRC Press is an imprint of Taylor & Francis Group, an Informa business

No claim to original U.S. Government works

ISBN-13: 978-0-8493-8504-9 (hbk)
ISBN-13: 978-0-367-40020-0 (pbk)

Library of Congress Cataloging-in-Publication Data

Nutrition: chemistry and biology / Julian E. Spallholz, L. Mallory
Boylan, Judy A. Driskell. — 2nd ed.
    p. cm. — (CRC series in modern nutrition)
    Includes bibliographical references and index.
    ISBN 0-8493-8504-0 (alk. paper)
    1. Nutrition. 2. Metabolism. I. Spallholz, Julian E.
II. Boylan, Lee Mallory, 1951- . III. Driskell, Judy A. (Judy
Anne) IV. Series: Modern nutrition (Boca Raton, Fla.)
QP141.S59 1998
572'.4—dc21
                                98-34621
                                CIP

Library of Congress Card Number 98-34621

Visit the Taylor & Francis Web site at
http://www.taylorandfrancis.com

and the CRC Press Web site at
http://www.crcpress.com

About the Authors

Julian E. Spallholz, PhD, received his BS and MS degrees from Colorado State University in Ft. Collins, in biological sciences and biochemistry in 1965 and 1968, respectively. From 1968 to 1971, he was a graduate student in the Department of Biochemistry–Biophysics at the University of Hawaii, John A. Burns School of Medicine, Honolulu, where he received his doctoral degree in 1971. After graduation (1971–1978), Dr. Spallholz was a postdoctoral research fellow at Colorado State University, instructor of biochemistry at the University of Colorado Dental School, Denver, and research chemist with the Veterans Administration's Medical Research Program at Long Beach, California. In 1978, Dr. Spallholz was research professor of chemistry at the State University of New York at Albany and joined the faculty at Texas Tech University in Lubbock. Dr. Spallholz is presently Professor of Nutrition and Adjunct Professor of Chemistry and Biochemistry. He has served as Director of the Institute for Nutritional Sciences and the Nutrition Department at Texas Tech. He founded and served as Editor-in-Chief of the *Journal of Nutritional Immunology* (1989–1996). His research interests are in the nutritional and toxic aspects of selenium and its compounds.

L. Mallory Boylan, PhD, RD, LD, received her BS and MS degrees in nutrition from the University of Alabama at Tuscaloosa in 1975 and 1978, respectively. Following graduate school she worked several years as a clinical dietitian, specializing in medical nutrition therapy prior to continuing her education at Virginia Tech at Blacksburg. She obtained her doctoral degree in human nutrition in 1986. Since receiving her doctoral degree she has taught medical nutrition therapy and vitamins at Texas Tech University in Lubbock and served as Director of the American Dietetic Association Approved Didactic Program in Dietetics there. Dr. Boylan has been active in the Texas Dietetic Association and at the national level where she is a member of The American Dietetic Association Scholarship Committee and has been panel Chair of the Didactic Program Review Committee of the Division of Education Accreditation Approval of the Council on Education. Dr. Boylan was promoted to Associate Professor of Nutrition in 1992. Her research is in the area of obesity and the roles of vitamin E and selenium in health and disease.

Judy Anne Driskell, PhD, RD, received her BS degree in biology in 1965 from the University of Southern Mississippi and her MS and PhD degrees from Purdue University in Indiana in 1967 and 1970, respectively. She has served in research/teaching and extension positions at Auburn University, Florida State University, Virginia Polytechnic Institute and State University, and is presently at the University of Nebraska. She also has served as the Nutrition Scientist for the U.S. Department of Agriculture/Cooperative State Research Service in Washington, D.C. Dr. Driskell is a member of numerous professional organizations including the American Society for Nutritional Sciences, the Institute of Food Technologists, and the American Dietetic Association. In 1993 she received the Professional Scientist Award of the Food Science and Human Nutrition Section of the Southern Association of Agricultural Scientists. In addition, she was the 1987 recipient of the Borden Award for Research in Applied Fundamental Knowledge of Human Nutrition. Dr. Driskell recently co-edited the CRC books *Sports Nutrition: Minerals and Electrolytes* and *Sports Nutrition: Vitamins and Trace Elements*. Dr. Driskell is presently Professor of Nutritional Science and Dietetics. Her research interests center around vitamin metabolism and requirements.

Series Preface

The CRC Series in Modern Nutrition is dedicated to providing the widest possible coverage of topics in nutrition. Nutrition is an interdisciplinary, interprofessional field par excellence. It is noted by its broad range and diversity. We trust the titles and authorship in this series will reflect that range and diversity.

Published for a broad audience, the volumes in the CRC Series in Modern Nutrition are designed to explain, review, and explore present knowledge and recent trends, developments, and advances in nutrition. As such, they will appeal to professionals as well as the educated layman. The format for the series will vary with the needs of the author and the topic, including, but not limited to, edited volumes, monographs, handbooks, and texts.

Contributors from any bona fide area of nutrition, including the controversial, are welcome.

I welcome the timely contribution of the book *Nutrition: Chemistry and Biology, 2nd Edition,* by my colleagues Julian E. Spallholz, L. Mallory Boylan, and Judy A. Driskell.

Ira Wolinsky, Ph.D.
University of Houston
Series Editor

Contents

Chapter 1
The Elements of Life... 1

Macronutrients: The Energy Nutrients

Chapter 2
Carbohydrates 9

Chapter 3
Lipids 23

Chapter 4
Proteins 41

Micronutrients: The Catalysts

Chapter 5
Vitamins 55

Chapter 6
Minerals 117

The Most Important Nutrient

Chapter 7
Water 167

Bioavailability of Nutrients

Chapter 8
Nutrient Digestion 173

Chapter 9
Nutrient Absorption 185

Cellular Metabolism

Chapter 10
Body Energy 201

Chapter 11
Components of Cells 209

Energy Utilization

Chapter 12
Catabolic Pathways 219

Chapter 13
Anabolic Pathways 241

Chapter 14
Nucleic Acids, Genes, and Protein Synthesis 253

Metabolic Aspects

Chapter 15
Free Radicals, Lipid Peroxidation, and the Antioxidants 265

Chapter 16
Digestive and Metabolic Interactions Between Medications and
Nutrients/Foods 277

Chapter 17
Nutrient Metabolism and Dietary Recommendations 287

Appendices and Index

Appendix A
Review of Chemistry and Biology Concepts of Importance in Nutrition 307

Appendix B
Photosynthesis and Energy Transfer 321

Appendix C
References 331

Index 335

Preface

The manuscript for *Nutrition: Chemistry and Biology* originated with a collection of teaching notes that were used to teach advanced nutrition. The material in the first edition accompanying the text fulfilled the perceived need of students at Texas Tech University for a one-semester advanced nutrition course with prerequisites of introductory nutrition, anatomy, and one semester of biochemistry.

Nutrition: Chemistry and Biology, 2nd Edition, is much expanded with new and updated information on food sources of nutrients, effects of cooking, new approved carbohydrate and fat substitutes, applications of nutritional therapy, and the newest dietary recommendations. The chapters have been rearranged from the first edition to accommodate this new information and previous information that has been updated. I am particularly pleased to have had the assistance of my new co-authors, Dr. L. Mallory Boylan and Dr. Judy Driskell, in advising me on the revision and contributing most of the new material. This new edition should serve students even better.

The study of nutrition draws upon many sciences and specialties which continue to evolve. Nutritional practice and understanding remains a chemical science. The near complete nutritional human requirements of enteral nutritional formulas and the new Food and Drug Administration's approval of Olestra are examples of nutritional applications of chemistry. As Lavoisier once stated, "La vie est une function of chemique"; and so it remains.

In conclusion, the authors thank the editorial and production staff of CRC Press for their patience during the text's revision and for their efforts in providing you, the student, with a textbook that the authors hope you will enjoy and that will aid you in learning about the science and practice of nutrition. If you gain any nutritional insights not previously held, all the effort in bringing you this revised edition will have been worthwhile.

CHAPTER **1**

The Elements of Life

PERIODIC ARRANGEMENT OF ELEMENTS AND
THE ORGANIC CLUSTER

The periodic table (Figure 1.1) contains 111 elements. Only 90 of these elements occur naturally in the environment, and still fewer elements comprise the living world. Scientists have long sought means to predict, interpret, detect, and measure quantitatively the elements necessary for life. The discovery of life's elements, contained by the totality of present knowledge, suggests that life has evolved from the less biologically complex to the more biologically complex. From bacteria to higher vertebrates and humans, nature has repeatedly selected for all life forms a basic group of only six elements. These six elements, the organic cluster (Figure 1.2), include the first element of the periodic table (see Figure 1.1), hydrogen, then carbon, nitrogen, oxygen, phosphorus, and sulfur. These six relatively small elements universally comprise most of the structural organization of the nutrients: proteins, carbohydrates, lipids, and vitamins. In addition, they make up most of the structural forms of the nucleic acids, deoxyribonucleic (DNA), and ribonucleic acids (RNA), and all the metabolic intermediates of metabolism.

The primordial selection of these six elements, which comprise the total organic bulk of all living matter, appears to have been made on the basis not only of physical size but also on chemical reactivity and the requirement to form intramolecular covalent bonds. Proteins, lipids, and carbohydrates are composed principally of monomers, small molecular units of carbon, oxygen, hydrogen, and nitrogen. The ability of carbon to form —C—C— bonds, extended carbon chains, and cyclic carbon compounds with an occasional mix of nitrogen and sulfur permitted the formation of the myriad of organic compounds. Silicon, located just below carbon in the periodic table, is also capable of forming extended chains. Chains of silicon, however, alternate with oxygen (—O—Si—O—Si—O), forming silicones. Such molecules were not biologically selected over carbon, for what would have been a much different type of macromolecular world.

1

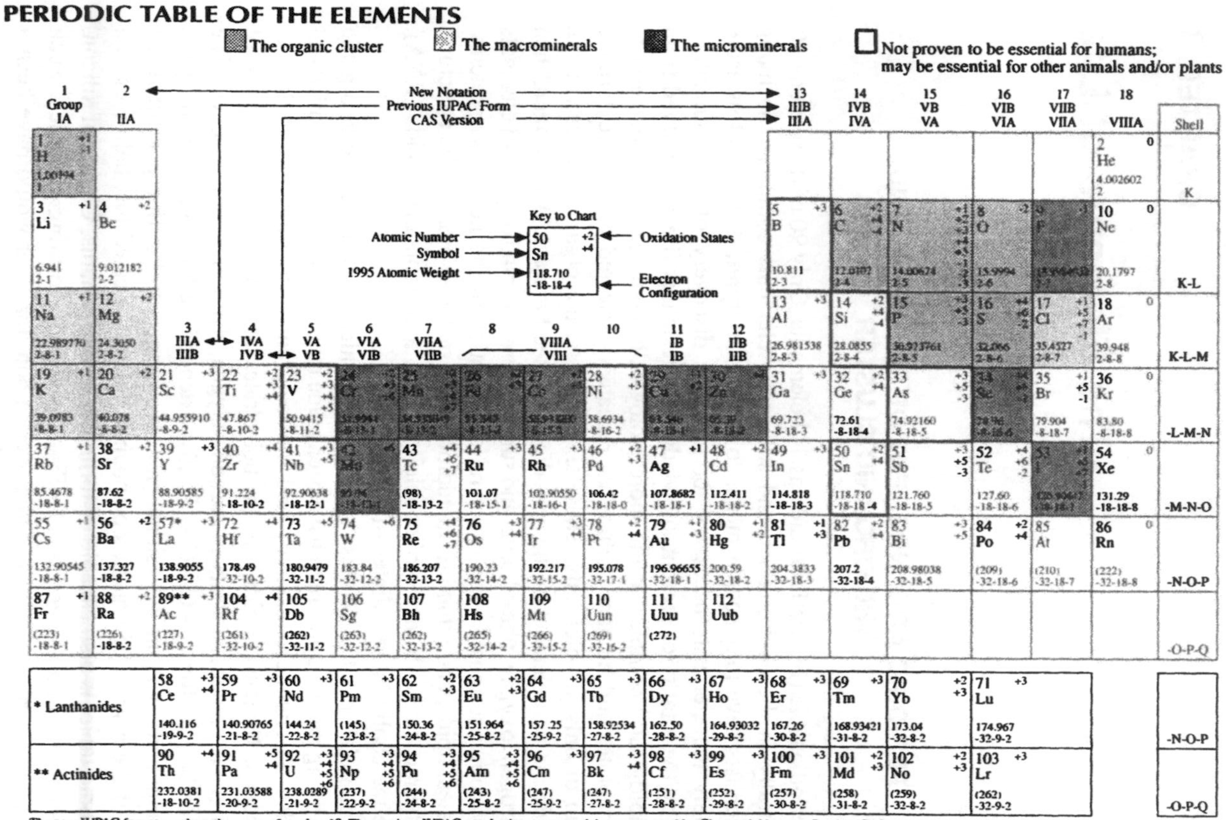

PERIODIC TABLE OF THE ELEMENTS

The organic cluster The macrominerals The microminerals Not proven to be essential for humans; may be essential for other animals and/or plants

New Notation
Previous IUPAC Form
CAS Version

Key to Chart

- Atomic Number — 50
- Symbol — Sn
- 1995 Atomic Weight — 118.710
- Oxidation States — +2 +4
- Electron Configuration — -18-18-4

The new IUPAC format numbers the groups from 1 to 18. The previous IUPAC numbering system and the system used by Chemical Abstracts Service (CAS) are also shown. For radioactive elements that do not occur in nature, the mass number of the most stable isotope is given in parentheses.

References

1. G. J. Leigh, Editor, *Nomenclature of Inorganic Chemistry*, Blackwell Scientific Publications, Oxford. 1990.
2. *Chemical and Engineering News*, 63(5), 27, 1985.
3. Atomic Weights of the Elements, 1995. *Pure & Appl. Chem.*, 68, 2339, 1996.

Figure 1.1 Periodic table of the elements.

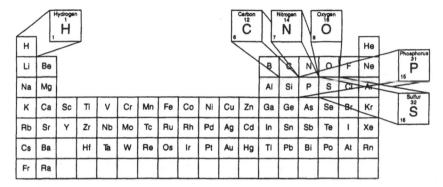

Figure 1.2 Organic cluster.

The elements of the organic cluster appear also to have been selected because of their abundance in the primordial atmosphere at the time the first molecules, probably amino acids, were found in the primordial soup. Evidence does suggest that the composition of the primordial atmosphere was probably much different from our present atmosphere in that it contained no oxygen but was comprised mostly of methane (CH_4), ammonia (NH_3), and smaller amounts of carbon monoxide (CO). Such gaseous mixtures saturated with water vapor, when subjected to electric discharge in the laboratory, result in the synthesis of small organic molecules resembling amino acids. The primordial atmosphere, as it is believed to have existed, together with the addition of sulfur as hydrogen sulfide (H_2S) and driven by intense ultraviolet radiation through an ozone-free atmosphere, provided conditions suitable for the synthesis of the first biological organic molecules.

DISTRIBUTION OF ELEMENTS IN THE UNIVERSE, ON EARTH, AND IN THE HUMAN BODY

While the true origin of the organic molecules still remains open to conjecture, the association of the elemental composition of the human body to that of the universe, the primordial atmosphere, the earth's crust, and seawater remains fascinating to contemplate. The universe is composed of approximately 91% hydrogen and 8.7% helium. All of the other 88 naturally occurring elements make up the remaining 0.3% of the universe and can be viewed within the periodic table as being derived from hydrogen and helium. There is within the periodic table a general inverse relationship between elemental abundance and atomic number. In different words, the larger the atomic number, generally, the rarer the element is in the universe, land, and sea. After H and He, we find four elements of the organic cluster, C, N, O, and S, to be relatively abundant in the universe. In the earth's crust and atmosphere, we also find H, C, N, and O to be abundant. The composition of seawater closely approximates the elemental composition of the human body. People are composed of approximately 88.5% H and O. Salt water is 99% H and O, and only 1% of seawater includes all the other elements listed in Table 1.1.

Table 1.1 Approximate Elemental Composition (Percent Total Number Atoms)[a]

Human	Universe	Today's Atmosphere	Primordial Atmosphere	Earth's Crust	Seawater	Seawater (ppm)	
H 63	**H** 91	**N** 78.1	**H**	**O** 47	**H** 66	Br 65	La 0.0003
O 25.5	He 8.7	**O** 20.9	**C** CH$_4$(?)	Si[b] 28	**O** 33	Sr 13	Ye 0.0003
C 9.5	**O** 0.057	Ar 0.934	**N** NH$_4$(?)	Al 7.9	Cl[b] 0.33	B[b] 4.6	Ni[b] 0.0001
N 1.4	**N** 0.042	**C** 0.009	**O** CO(?)	Fe[b] 4.5	Na[b] 0.28	Si[b] 4.0	Sc 0.00004
Ca[b] 0.31	**C** 0.021		**S** H$_2$S(?)	Ca[b] 3.5	Mg[b] 0.33	F 1.4	Hg 0.00003
P 0.22	Si[b] 0.003			Na[b] 2.5	**S** 0.17	**N** 0.7	Au 0.000006
Cl[b] 0.03	Ne 0.003			K[b] 2.5	Ca[b] 0.006	Al 0.5	Ra ⎫
K[b] 0.06	Mg[b] 0.002			Mg[b] 2.2	K[b] 0.006	Ru 0.2	Cd ⎬ Trace
S 0.05	Fe[b] 0.002			Ti 0.46	**C** 0.0014	Li 0.1	Cr[b] ⎭
Na[b] 0.03	**S** 0.001			**H** 0.22	Br 0.0005	**P** 0.1	Co[b]
Mg[b] 0.01				**C** 0.19		Ba 0.05	Sn
		Exclusive of water vapor	Exclusive of water vapor			I[b] 0.05	and others
<0.01[c]	<0.01[c]	<0.10[c]		<0.10[c]	<0.10[c]	As 0.02	
						Fe[b] 0.02	
						Mn[b] 0.01	
						Cu[b] 0.01	
						Zn[b] 0.005	
						Pb 0.004	
						Se[b] 0.004	
						Cs 0.002	
						U 0.002	
						Mo[b] 0.0005	
						Th 0.0005	
						Ce 0.0004	
						Ag 0.0003	
						V[b] 0.0003	

[a] Elements set in bold are of the organic cluster.
[b] Essential mineral.
[c] All other elements.

ELEMENTAL REQUIREMENTS OF MICROORGANISMS, PLANTS, ANIMALS, AND HUMANS

Bacteria, plants, animals, and humans require, in addition to the organic elements, various amounts and types of other elements, collectively referred to as minerals. Reexamination of Table 1.1 reveals that all major elements of the universe, with the exception of the inert gases helium (He) and neon (Ne), are included in plant and/or animal life. With the exception of Al, Ti, and Br, all major elements of the earth's crust and seawater include those elements needed by bacteria, plants, animals, and humans.

As life forms increase in complexity from the simplest single cells of the amoebae and bacteria to the more complex plants and animals, there is a general increase in the number of required elements that comprise less than 0.1% and often less than 0.01% of our environment. The latter elements are the micro- and ultramicro- (trace) elements, elements required by life forms in very minute amounts. The elemental requirements of many bacteria, plants, and humans are given in Table 1.2. The required elements for bacteria, plants, and humans as representative of the vertebrates, shows 15 elements in common to all life forms. With few exceptions, bacteria and plants have similar known elemental requirements, with the elemental requirements of humans being the most extensive.

The biological complexity of life changes the requirements and the ways in which the need for the elements of the organic cluster (C, H, O, N, S, P) can be met. Bacterial requirements for the elements of the organic cluster are met by simple common salts, i.e., ammonium sulfate (NH_4SO_4) and an organic carbon source, i.e., glucose. Plants fulfill their need for the elements of the organic cluster from atmospheric CO_2 and the remaining elements from soils (H_2O, NH_4SO_4, NH_4PO_4). Animals and humans rely solely on the organic molecules — carbohydrates, lipids, proteins, and vitamins produced by bacteria and plant and animal foods — to fulfill their needs for the elements of the organic cluster. Macro-, micro-, and ultramicro-(trace) elements are provided to humans by foods from both plant and animal origin. A review of chemistry and biology concepts of importance in nutrition is given in Appendix A.

Table 1.2 Elements Required by Bacteria, Plants, and Humans[a]

Bacteria	Source of Elements	Plants	Source of Elements	Humans	Source of Elements
H	H_2O	H	H_2O	H	H_2O, protein
O		O		O	Carbohydrates, lipids
C	HCO_3^-, glucose, citrate	C	CO_2	C	Carbohydrates, lipids, protein
N	NH_3, NH_4^+	N	NH_3, NH_4^+	N	Protein
Ca		Ca		Ca	
P	PO_4^{-2}	P	PO_4^{-2}	P	PO_4^{-2}
S	SO_4^{-2}	S	SO_4^{-2}	S	Amino acids, vitamins
K		K		K	
Cl		Cl		Cl	
Na		—		Na	
Mg		Mg		Mg	
Fe	Salts	Fe	Salts	Fe	Salts
Zn		Zn		Zn	
Cu		Cu		Cu	
Se[b]		—		Se	Se-amino acids
Mn		Mn		Mn	
—		—		I	
Mo		Mo		Mo	
—		—		Cr[b]	
—		—		Co	Vitamin B_{12}
—		B[b]		B[b]	
—		Ni[b]		Ni[b]	
—		—		F[b]	
—		Si[b]		Si[b]	
—		—		Sn[b]	?
—		V[b]		V[b]	
W[b]		As[b]		As[b]	
—		—		—	

[a] Listed by decreasing amounts in humans. The requirements for elements by bacteria, plants, animals, and humans are similar, but the nutritional source of the elements becomes increasingly more complex for animals and humans than for bacteria and plants.

[b] May or may not have a biological function in all species within each class heading.

Macronutrients:
The Energy Nutrients

CHAPTER 2

Carbohydrates

The word *carbohydrate* has been compounded from the description of this group of organic molecules, the "carbon hydrates," whose carbon compounds are extensively hydrated. The carbohydrates are either polyhydroxyaldehydes or polyhydroxyketones. Dietarily, carbohydrates provide approximately 50% of the caloric needs of Americans. Being derived from plants, vegetables, and cereal grains, a greater proportion of the caloric needs of people in developing countries are met by the carbohydrates.

MONOSACCHARIDES

Carbohydrates are grouped according to the number of carbon atoms per molecule, such as the trioses (three-carbon unit), the pentoses (five-carbon unit), and the hexoses (six-carbon unit). Nutritionally, the most important carbohydrates are the hexoses.

Glucose

The most important hexose metabolically is the monosaccharide, D-glucose. D-glucose is commonly referred to as blood glucose or blood sugar. Glucose comes in two epimeric forms, α-D-glucose and β-D-glucose (Figure 2.1). Glucose is found in each disaccharide as well as being found in all polysaccharides including glycogen, the major storage form of carbohydrate in the body. While glucose is the most important metabolic carbohydrate, glucose, galactose, fructose, and other monosaccharides are infrequent dietary carbohydrate constituents. Insignificant amounts of glucose are naturally consumed in diets.

Fructose and Galactose

The sweetest carbohydrate is fructose which is found in fruits, honey, and many syrups. Many people consume fructose which is added to carbonated beverages or

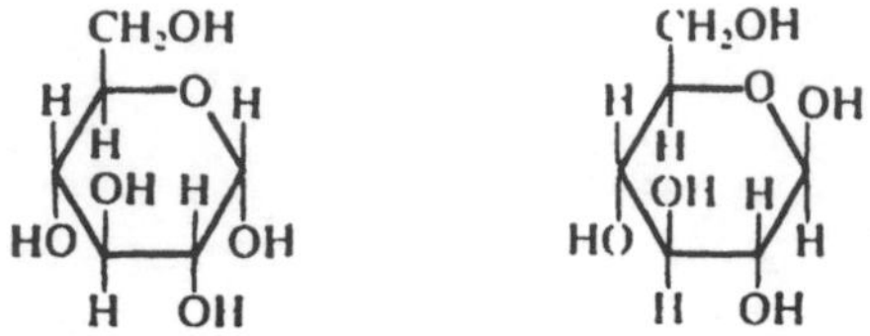

CH₂OH

α-D-glucose

C'H₂OH

β-D-glucose

Figure 2.1   Structure of glucose.

products sweetened with high-fructose corn syrup. The third important monosaccharide is galactose, found as a constituent of lactose. Galactose, like glucose, is seldom found free in foods. In a rare condition called galactosemia, the body lacks the enzyme galactose-1-phosphate transferase, so that galactose cannot be metabolized for energy. In the absence of this enzyme toxic metabolites of galactose may accumulate. Thus if galactose or lactose is consumed, vomiting, weight loss, and cirrhosis of the liver may occur along with mental retardation, cataracts, and even death.

DISACCHARIDES

The disaccharides are the more common sources of calories in the diet of most Americans than are the monosaccharides. Sucrose, table sugar, and lactose, milk sugar, are the most widely consumed disaccharides, being more abundant in the diet than the third disaccharide, maltose or malt sugar. Each of the disaccharides consists of one monomeric unit of glucose plus one molecule of either fructose, galactose, or glucose (Figure 2.2).

Sucrose

Sucrose is a very sweet tasting carbohydrate that is the most widely used food additive in the American diet. Although found primarily as an extensively used food additive in the American diet, smaller amounts of sucrose are naturally found in a few foods. Because sucrose is sweet and inexpensive, processed foods often contain proportionately large amounts of sucrose. Sugar cane and sugar beets are the sources of the sucrose which is added to foods, with small amounts of sucrose being found naturally in fruits, vegetables, and grains. Many people consume 20 to 30% of their calories as sucrose, but it is generally best to limit sucrose to 10% or less of caloric intake. Sucrose, especially in sticky foods which remain in the mouth for a long period of time, promotes the development of dental caries. Other health effects of sucrose are controversial and less definitive. It is difficult to discern if sucrose causes hyperactivity or obesity or if it is other dietary factors which are displaced in the diet due to the high sucrose consumption. For example, is a high sucrose-containing food replacing fruits, vegetables, or whole grain foods normally found in the diet and is the high sucrose food also high in fat? In some people consumption of high amounts of sucrose will result in elevated blood triglyceride levels and cardiovascular

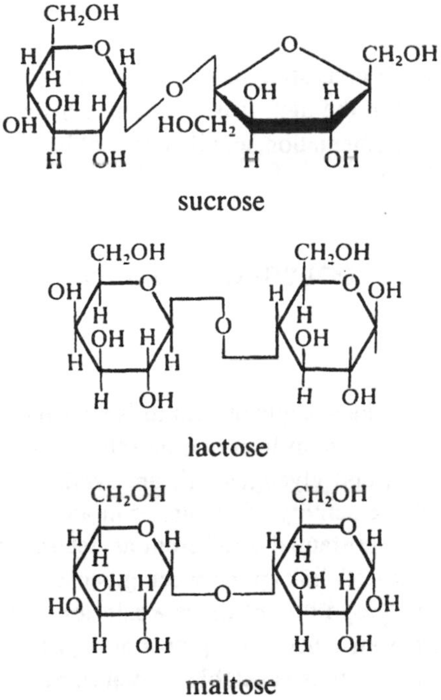

Figure 2.2 Structures of the disaccharides.

disease risk can be higher for these individuals. Nevertheless, the association between a high consumption of sucrose in the diet and cardiovascular disease is minimal. While sucrose consumption does not cause diabetes mellitus *per se,* people with diabetes mellitus must dietarily control the amount of sucrose and other carbohydrates consumed in order to maintain normoglycemia.

Lactose

While lactose is less prevalent in the diets of most adults than is sucrose, it is the major, if not the only, carbohydrate in the diet of nursing infants and infants fed most commercial infant formulas. Infants after birth normally produce large amounts of intestinal lactase, the enzyme which hydrolyzes lactose into glucose and galactose, which are absorbed and metabolized for energy. Intestinal lactase synthesis generally declines in the elderly, to a point where about 20% of Caucasians and 50 to 80% of Hispanics, African-Americans, and native American Indians develop lactose intolerance. If lactose exceeds the body's ability to digest it, then the undigested lactose can be fermented by the bacteria of the lower bowel producing fermented acids and gases, carbon dioxide, or methane. The lactose also osmotically pulls water into the intestine which may cause cramping and a watery acidic diarrhea. Lactose intolerance may also occur temporarily after any infection which may also cause diarrhea or in some individuals, malnutrition.

Maltose

Maltose, a disaccharide consisting of two molecules of glucose is not naturally found to any great extent in the diet. It is found as a hydrolysis product of starch, in the malting process of fermentation, and it is present in corn syrups, another major carbohydrate food additive.

POLYSACCHARIDES

Starch

Three homopolysaccharides of glucose comprise the major dietary carbohydrates and the major carbohydrate store of liver and muscle. These three homopolysaccharides are starch, cellulose, and glycogen. All are synthesized from glucose, made either by the photosynthetic activity of plants, or in animal and human tissues. All three polysaccharides are substantially different as determined by the composition of their glycosidic (R—O—R) linkage between glucose subunits. The polysaccharide providing the largest proportion of dietary calories is starch.

Starch is assembled from glucose by plants as a principal energy store of the cereal grains (wheat) and tuberous vegetables (potato). Starch contains two types of glucose bonding (Figure 2.3). The bond providing the extended glucose polymer in the starch molecule is the α-(1→4) glycoside. A second glycoside, the α-(1→6) glycoside, provides for branching and termination of the linear arrays of α-(1→4) glycoside chains of glucose. Polymers of glucose in α-(1→4) linear chains are amylose. Amylose with α-(1→6) glycosidic branching is amylopectin. Digestive enzymes specific for α-(1→4) glycosides and α-(1→6) glycosides in the mouth and small intestine rapidly degrade the starch polymer to polysaccharides, fragments of

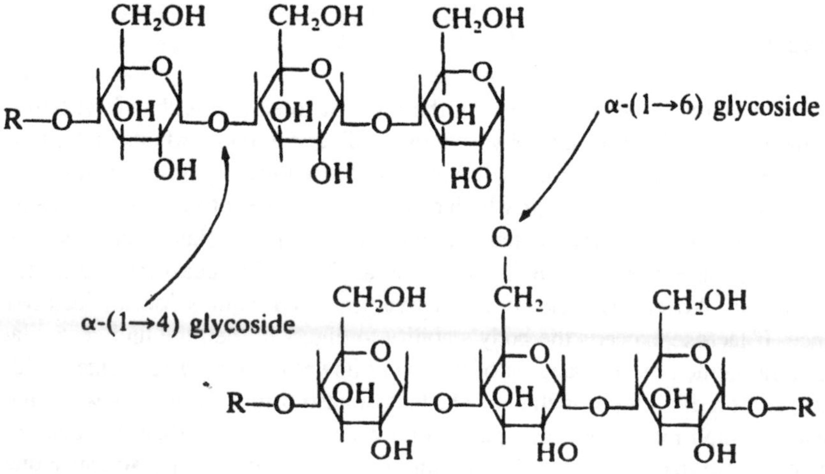

Figure 2.3 Structure of starch.

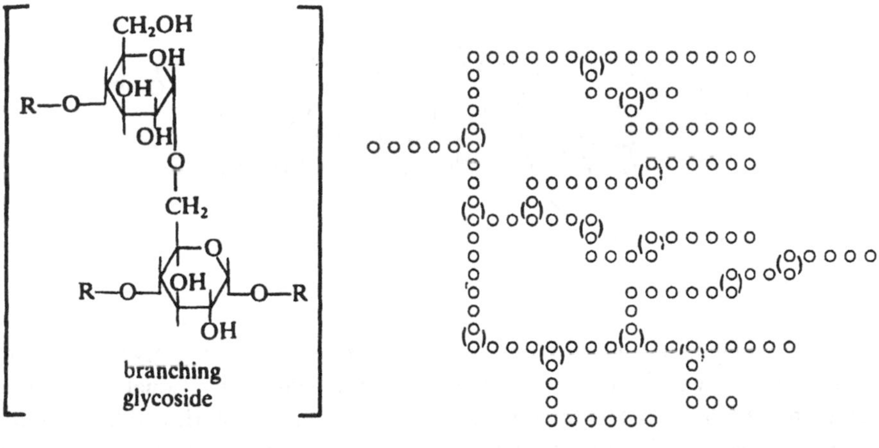

Figure 2.4 Structure of glycogen.

starch containing terminal α-(1→6) glycoside residues that cannot be degraded further by the α-(1→4) maltoglycosidase, to dextrins, maltose, and ultimately to the monosaccharide glucose. Dextrins are further degraded to maltose, isomaltose, and glucose by the enzyme α-(1→6) isomaltoglycosidase, isomaltase; and α-(1→4) glycosidase, maltase.

Glycogen

Polysaccharides stored in the liver and in muscle are glycogen. Glycogen (Figure 2.4) is structurally very similar to starch, containing both the α-(1→4) and α-(1→6) glycosides linking the glucose units. The difference between starch and glycogen is that glycogen is more highly branched, as it contains a proportionately higher amount of α-(1→6) glycosides than does starch. The larger amount of branching provides for the rapid hydrolysis of glycogen to glucose to provide energy for muscular contraction and for the elevation of blood glucose from the liver.

Some people are unable to metabolize glycogen normally due to a variety of enzyme abnormalities referred to as hepatic glycogen storage disease (GSD). In type II GSD the individual lacks amylo-1,6-glucosidase, which is the debranching enzyme. As glycogen hydrolysis cannot proceed normally beyond the α-(1→6) branching, signs and symptoms such as hypoglycemia, muscle weakness, myopathy, hepatomegaly, and failure to thrive may occur.

Cellulose

The third polysaccharide of glucose is the most abundant of all organic molecules in the biosphere. It is cellulose (Figure 2.5). One need only view a pristine forest to contemplate the vast amounts of cellulose present in wood fiber. The cell walls of trees and other plants are composed mainly of cellulose. This polysaccharide is

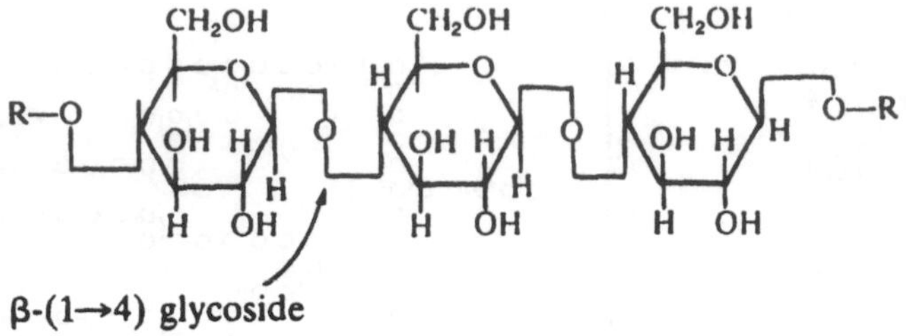

β-(1→4) glycoside

Figure 2.5 Structure of cellulose.

similar in composition to amylose, but instead of the α-(1→4) glycosidic bond, cellulose possesses a β-(1→4) glycoside between glucose units. Equal quantities of starch and cellulose contain the same caloric value, but the calories within cellulose are largely unavailable to monogastric animals including humans because they do not possess a β-(1→4) glycosidase and consequently the glucose cannot be released from its polymer structure. β-(1→4) glycosidases are synthesized by many bacteria, and in the human gastrointestinal tract some small amount of glucose may be released from cellulose to the extent that β-(1→4) glycosidases are present. Ruminants (cattle, sheep) derive calories from cellulose because of the extensive hydrolytic action of the β-(1→4) glycosides produced by bacteria and other microflora of the rumen.

Dietary Fiber

Hemicelluloses, pectins, gums, and mucilages are heteropolysaccharides: polysaccharides composed of the monosaccharides glucose, galactose, pentoses, uronic acid, and so on. These carbohydrates, present in plants, together with cellulose and lignin, constitute what is called dietary fiber. Dietary fiber is not subject to a universally accepted definition. Different types of fiber have been defined and classified by the solubility of the fiber in acid or alkali solutions or as the carbohydrate not subject to human digestive enzymes. The author's preferred definition of dietary fiber is: *that portion of dietary carbohydrate and lignin unabsorbed following digestion by human or bacterial enzyme activity.* Glucose and similar monosaccharides from starch, cellulose, and most other components of dietary fiber possess the same caloric values following intestinal absorption, irrespective of the source of hydrolytic enzymes.

Fiber is also classified based upon the water solubility of its components. The insoluble components of fiber include cellulose and lignin. Such insoluble fiber is in some vegetables, grains and especially in brans. A high intake of dietary insoluble fiber with adequate water will increase fecal weight and move the intestinal contents of the diet more rapidly through the intestines. A high dietary intake of fiber may decrease the risk of constipation, diverticulosis, and colon cancer. Soluble fiber such as is found in fruits, legumes, barley, oats, and psyllium, a fiber laxative, may slow gastric emptying and in some individuals lessen the glycemic effect of carbohydrates, lowering the circulating levels of blood cholesterol.

While most Americans do not consume the recommended 20 to 35 g of fiber per day, there are possible negative effects from a very high high-fiber diet. As bacteria in the colon ferment fiber, water, gas, and short chain fatty acids are produced. This fermentation can cause gas or flatus and bloating with loose stools in some people. This problem is reduced if dietary fiber intake is increased gradually. A bulky high-fiber diet may cause early satiety and lessen consumption of food. This is an advantage for many people but may have negative effects on people who are not in good nutritional status, the elderly, and young children.

DIETARY FIBER: A GENERIC TERM

Fiber is a generic term with a different meaning when used by a botanist (microfibrils), a cereal chemist (cellulose), or an animal nutritionist (indigestible feed matter). To the human nutritionist, fiber is that cell wall plant material (carbohydrates and lignin) which remains mostly undigested by the enzymes of the human gastrointestinal tract. The principal source of dietary fiber is the structural component of plant cell walls; the polymers of cellulose, hemicelluloses, and pectins; all carbohydrates. Lignin, the noncarbohydrate polymer of cell walls, is highly insoluble and is the "woody" component of plant cell walls (Table 2.1).

Table 2.1 Dietary Fiber Components

Major Component	Chemical Composition	Colonic Function	Nutritional/Clinical Effects
Cellulose	Homopolyglycan β-(1→4) glycosides	Nondigestible, partially fermentable, imbibes water, laxative	Dilution of colonic excretory metabolites; prevents diverticulitis
Hemicellulose	Heteropolyglycan (250 known polymers) β-(1→4) xyloside backbone; several side chains or arabinose or glucuronic acid residues	Partially fermentable, imbibes water, laxative	Dilution of colonic excretory metabolites; prevent diverticulitis; may weakly bind minerals
Pectins	Heteropolysaccharides, major component β-(1→4) linkage of galacturonic acid, uronic acid, and methyluronic side chains	Gel formation, antidiarrhetic	May reduce blood cholesterol; increased fecal steroid and lipid excretion; may have increases in Ca^{2+} and Mg^{2+} excretion proportionate to uronic acid content
Lignin	Noncarbohydrate polymers of phenylpropanes; derived from coumaryl, coniferyl, and sinapyl alcohols	Antioxidant phenols; almost chemically inert to digestion or fermentation	May bind bile acids and some cations; provides fecal bulk

Also included under the generic term "fiber" are the nonstructural components of plants consisting of polysaccharides not found within the plant cell wall and other noncarbohydrate materials. Plant substances within this group include the gums, mucilages, and storage and chemically modified polysaccharides. Polysaccharides of the cell wall of seaweed and algae are distinctive in that xylans, mannans, and cellulose analogs, often containing sulfates, replace the normal cellulose in cell walls. Some people even argue that gums, mucilages, and so on are not fibrous and should not be included within the definition of fiber. Such distinctions make it difficult to find a universally acceptable definition for dietary fiber.

CHEMISTRY OF DIETARY FIBER

Cellulose

Cellulose, β-(1$\rightarrow$4) homoglycan (Figure 2.5), is the highly insoluble main structural component of the plant cell wall. It is the major organic hydrocarbon found in nature and the principal fibrous component of plant cells. Because cellulose is an unbranched linear polymer it can be densely packed into a microfibrillar structure within the plant's cell wall. Cellulose remains mostly indigestible by monogastric animals and humans because of the lack of synthesis of β-(1$\rightarrow$4) glucosidase (cellulose). Cellulose, however, is readily digested by the microflora of polygastric animals. Cellulose, like cooked starch, can imbibe water, increasing fecal weight. Cellulose may also bind bile acids, increasing the excretion of these cholesterol metabolites, thereby lowering serum cholesterol.

Hemicellulose

The hemicelluloses (unrelated to cellulose) comprise a diverse group of heteropolysaccharides. Unlike cellulose, which contains no branching, hemicelluloses are highly branched. The main homopolymer chain consists mainly of β-(1$\rightarrow$4) linked xylose, mannose, and galactosides. From the primary chain are found branches of arabinose, galactose, and 4-O-methylglucuronic acid. Hemicelluloses are those plant cell wall polysaccharides isolated from the extraction of plant cells with dilute sodium hydroxide (Figure 2.6).

Pectins

Pectins are derived from intracellular and plant cell wall materials. Fruits and vegetables contain a proportionately high dry weight content of pectins. The pectins are chemically complete hetero- and homopolysaccharides whose principal polymer is D-galacturonic acid (Figure 2.6). Many other carbohydrates, including arabinose, galactose, fructose, and so on, are found in the hydrolyzates of pectins, which form the side-chain linkages from the major polymer. Some of the carbohydrates, like

(1) Cellulose:

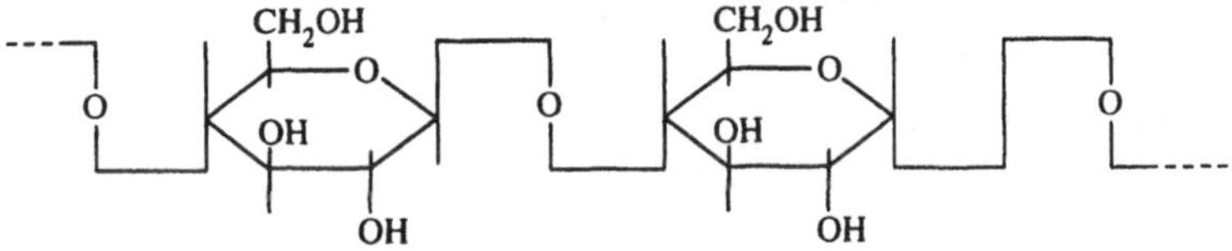

MW 50,000 to 2.5 million β-(1 → 4) glycosides

(2) Hemicellulose (xylans): β-(1 → 4) xylose

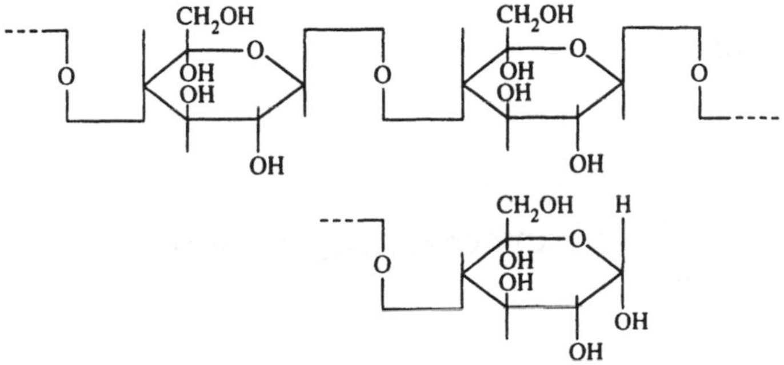

(3) Pectins: β-(1 → 4) galacturonic acid

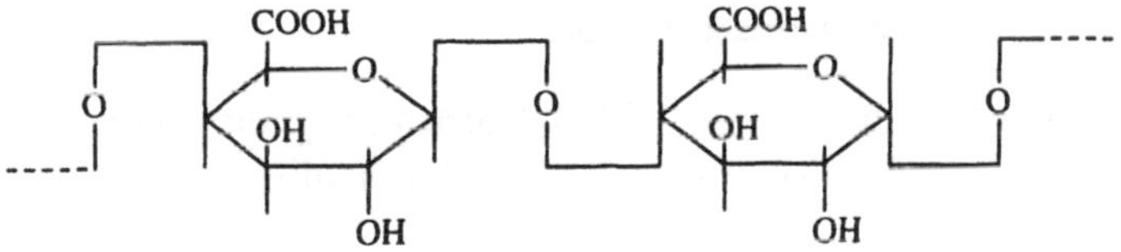

(4) Lignin: varied aromatic noncarbohydrate polymer

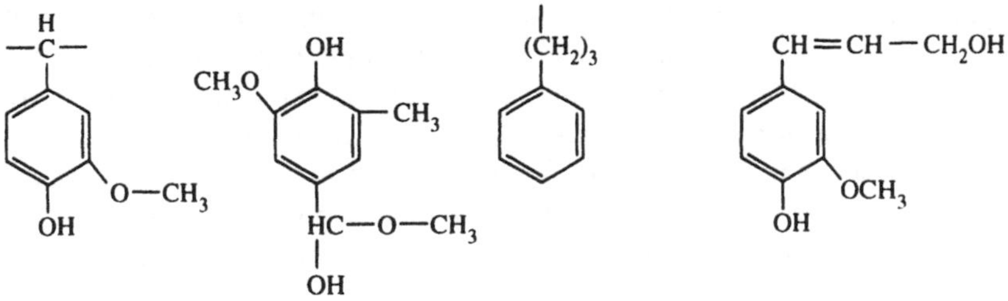

coniferyl

phenylpropyl
monomeric
precursor

coniferyl alcohol
monomic precursor

Figure 2.6 Structures of cellulose, hemicellulose, pectins, lignin.

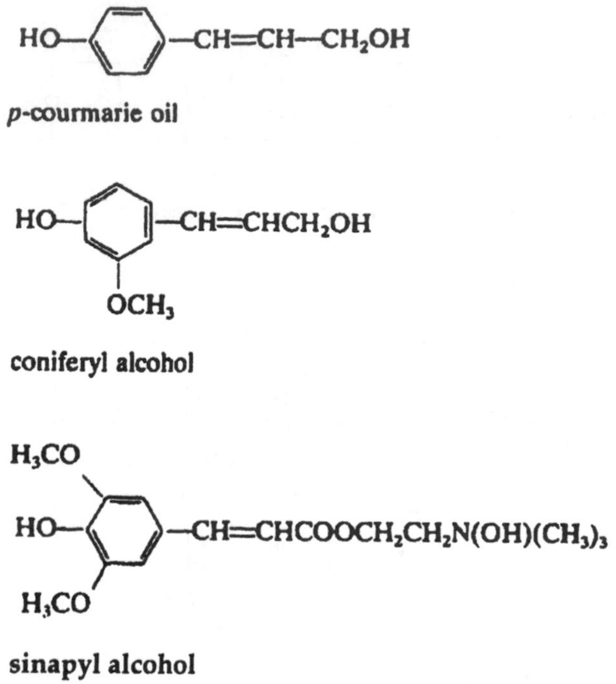

HO—⟨ ⟩—CH=CH—CH$_2$OH

p-courmarie oil

HO—⟨ ⟩—CH=CHCH$_2$OH
|
OCH$_3$

coniferyl alcohol

H$_3$CO
\
HO—⟨ ⟩—CH=CHCOOCH$_2$CH$_2$N(OH)(CH$_3$)$_3$
/
H$_3$CO

sinapyl alcohol

Figure 2.7 Structures of three major aromatic alcohols.

xylose and fructose, may be O-methylated (-OCH$_3$). Structurally, the pectins within plants chelate calcium ions, which contributes to their insolubility.

Lignin

Lignin is a term referring to the noncarbohydrate aromatic polymers of the plant cell wall. It constitutes the "woody" material usually obtained from maturing plants. Lignin is a complex, highly variable polymer of 40 or more phenylpropanoids. Since lignin is variable in structure, no specific chemical structure can be assigned. Three major aromatic alcohols — coumaryl, coniferyl, and sinapyl alcohol — are the major monomers contributing to the final lignin polymer (Figure 2.7). Lignin is highly insoluble and resistant to digestive enzymes and fermentation reactions.

Gums, Mucilages, and Algal Polysaccharides

Gums (resins) are polysaccharides synthesized by plants in response to, and at the site of, an injury. Mucilages are polysaccharides produced by secretory cells of plants to prevent excessive transpiration. Algal polysaccharides are composed of mannans, xylose, and other carbohydrate polymers which serve functionally to replace the cellulose found in the cell walls of other plants. These carbohydrates, comprising a small proportion of the total carbohydrate portion of the diet, are often included in classifications of dietary fiber.

NUTRITIONAL PROPERTIES OF DIETARY FIBER

Dietary fiber, such as the fiber from vegetables and bran, chemically purified cellulose, gums and mucilages, and so on, each possess one or more important nutritional properties based on its inherent chemical composition. In general, the nutritional properties that various fibers possess are fermentability, contributions to the bulk density of fecal material, ability to imbibe water, and their general capacity to bind minerals. Collectively, the chemical composition of dietary fiber affects the physiology and microbiology of the gastrointestinal tract and the digestive process through fermentation, production of flatus, and changes in intraluminal pressures.

FERMENTATION

A major contribution to the ever-changing composition of the intestinal content of the gut is fiber. The composition of the fiber interacts with and changes the microfloral population, resulting in the fermentation of some fibrous components primarily in the ascending colon of the large intestine. Here, fiber of vegetable origin, and to a lesser degree fiber from bran, are fermented by bacteria under nearly anaerobic conditions. The fermentation products are notably gases: some hydrogen, carbon dioxide, and methane. These gases are voided either through the pulmonary system or are passed as flatus. Additional fermentation products include the formation of some alcohols and volatile fatty acids: commonly acetic, proprionic, and butyric acids. Absorption of these fermentation products is a source of available calories. During fermentation, fecal weight is increased by the rapid increase in the mass of the bacterial population which can constitute as much as 40 to 50% of the fecal dry weight. Lignin is not fermented as it passes through the gastrointestinal tract.

HYDRATION

Fiber and polysaccharides in general have the capacity to imbibe and hold water within the fiber's structural matrix. The amount of water imbibed by fiber is dependent on its structure and solubility, which are determined in part by the number of hydrophilic moieties — hydroxyl, carboxyl, sulfoxyl, and carbonyls — which permit the hydration of fiber to occur. Generally, vegetable fibers have a greater capacity to hold water, gram for gram, than do bran or lignin. Because vegetable fibers are highly fermentable, the actual ability of dietary fiber to become hydrated and retain water, contributing to fecal bulk throughout digestion, may be quite different. Fecal bulking agents used in pharmaceutical preparations are often combinations of cellulose and vegetable fibers.

METAL BINDING

Fiber, because of its carboxylic-containing carbohydrates, has the ability to bind various nutritional and toxic cations — Ca^{2+}, Zn^{2+}, (toxic) Cd^{2+}, Hg^{2+}, and so on —

thereby preventing absorption. Most vegetable fibers and fiber-containing residues of uronic acids function like weak cation-exchange resins, binding these minerals. Persons with adequate mineral nutriture do not seem to be affected adversely by high-fiber diets. However, persons eating high-fiber diets and having a marginal intake of certain minerals, such as zinc, may be in jeopardy of establishing a chronic mineral deficiency.

In addition to binding cations and preventing the absorption of minerals, fiber may bind organic molecules, notably the bile acids. Although controversial, fiber, particularly pectins and lignins, appears to be hypocholesteremic by lowering the ileal reabsorption of bile acids, which have been chemically modified by the bacterial flora of the gastrointestinal tract. The effects of fiber binding the bile acids are complex and vary considerably within and between individuals as changes in dietary practices occur.

IMPORTANCE OF FIBER AS A NUTRIENT

Present-day nutritional interest in the role of dietary fiber in the prevention of disease was renewed in the early 1970s by a British surgeon, D. Burkett. Its importance in the diet is seen by many nutritionists and by the public at large to be so important that it could be a seventh nutrient class.

The list of diseases that fiber is claimed to prevent or ameliorate is extensive, but there is no definitive proof. Diseases of the colon — diverticulosis, constipation, appendicitis, hemorrhoids, ulcers, precancerous polyps, and cancer — are believed by some people to be reduced or prevented by a high dietary fiber intake. Fiber's importance in reducing these diseases is thought to be derived from fiber bulk, hydration, binding of bile acids, fermentation of short-chain fatty acids, increased fecal transit time, and dilution of fecal mutagens and carcinogens. Metabolic diseases for which fiber has been deemed preventative include obesity, diabetes, heart diseases, hypertension, vascular diseases of various types, embolisms, gallstones, and senile osteoporosis in addition to others. Endocrine diseases, hiatal hernias, Crohn's disease, and dental caries are also thought to be ameliorated by dietary fiber. The physical, chemical, and metabolic mechanisms whereby dietary fiber may affect these diseases remains largely speculative. Clearly, dietary fiber affects dietary practices and the physiology of the gastrointestinal tract by providing fecal bulk, altering fecal transit time and intestinal physiology and microbiology. In addition, dietary fiber can provide a feeling of satiety, reducing the caloric density of the diet. Whether or not dietary fiber is truly a nutrient class and significantly affects the health of people to which such claims have been attributed remains to be decided by additional research and deliberation.

FIBER AND CHOLESTEROL

In 1961, A. Keys and co-workers reported that pectins in the human diet lowered levels of serum cholesterol. *In vitro* studies of D. Kritechevsky and J. Story in 1974 provided evidence that nonnutritive fiber (cellophane and cellulose) did not bind the bile acids taurocholate or glycocholate but that some nutritive fibers did bind the bile acids. These and other studies provided evidence for the hypothesis that a lower serum cholesterol, hypocholesteremia, could be produced by increasing the amounts of dietary fiber, thereby increasing the fecal excretion of these bile salts and decreasing serum cholesterol through a reduction in bile acid reabsorption.

Not all fiber components have been shown to be effective in reducing serum cholesterol levels. Fiber components most consistent in lowering total serum cholesterol in various animal and human experiments include pectin, guar, and other gums — those fiber components that are viscous and imbibe water. Wheat bran and nonnutritive fiber apparently do not bind bile acid salts *in vivo,* as total fecal excretion in humans remains unaffected. In contrast, oat bran fed to human subjects over an 11-day period lowered total serum cholesterol approximately 25%. LDL cholesterol was reduced, whereas HDL cholesterol and VLDL cholesterol remained unchanged. It is apparent that the bile acid binding resins, such as cholestyramine and probably lignin, are hypocholesteremic by facilitating excretion of bile acids, thereby preventing intestinal reabsorption. Less apparent is the experimental effect of other components of fiber in reducing serum cholesterol. While fecal excretion of bile acids may be slightly enhanced by the dietary addition of pectin, guar and other gums, legumes and oat bran (similar to the mechanism of cholestyramine), clofibrate, nicotinic acid and analogs, these fiber components also have a hypolipidemic effect by reducing hepatic lipogenesis. These and other complex physiological and metabolic factors confound the exact mechanism as to how soluble fiber is hypocholesteremic. As reduction in serum cholesterol is considered a positive factor in the overall risk reduction of atherosclerosis and heart disease, the effects of dietary fiber and individual fiber components as hypercholesteremic agents are likely to be further investigated.

FIBER AND COLON CANCER

Investigations of human colon (large bowel) cancer and fiber ingestion were rekindled in 1956 by T. L. Cleave, and later by D. P. Burkett in 1971, in epidemiological studies of Africans. Numerous epidemiological investigations (about 70%) have been able to confirm an inverse correlation between ingestion of diets high in fiber content and the incidence of colon cancer. This inverse correlation is most strongly associated with consumption of cereal fiber and is less strongly associated with the consumption of vegetable fibers. There has been little or no correlation with consumption of legume and fruit fibers. In controlled human studies that have investigated the effects of fiber in reducing the incidence of colon cancer with the consumption of vegetable fiber, conclusive evidence for the ameliorating effect of fiber on colon cancer has not been found. The effect of vegetable fiber in protecting against colon cancer may be because of the higher consumption of certain vitamins, such as vitamins E, A, β-carotene, and other retinoids found in plants.

Highly controllable experimentation with animals and fiber suggest that fiber from wheat, corn, soybean, and oat bran may even enhance the appearance of some chemically induced colon cancer. Other animal experiments with different brans have shown either limited protection against colon cancer or no experimental effect at all. To the extent that fiber may be effective in the prevention of colon cancer, the effects observed are probably related in some manner to reduced exposure to mutagens and carcinogens by fecal dilution and increased bowel transit time, a modified intestinal microflora, binding and excretion of fecal mutagens and carcinogens, or a combination of two or more of these factors.

Bile acid and metal binding to dietary fiber may reduce the facilitation of mutagenic substances in colon cancer induction, while fermentation of fiber is known to produce additional amounts of butyric acid, an anticarcinogen, and lower intestinal pH by production of butyric and other short-chain fatty acids. The role of both nonfermentable and fermentable dietary fiber in the prevention of colon cancer, if significant at all, still remains to be deciphered experimentally.

CHAPTER 3

Lipids

Lipid is a generic word for a diverse group of organic compounds. Chemically, the lipids are defined as *those organic compounds that are insoluble in water, but are generally soluble in one or a mixture of several organic solvents.* Many organic solvents are able to dissolve lipid compounds because both are nonpolar. Table 3.1 lists the polarity and boiling points of some commonly used organic solvents that can be compared to water, which is extensively hydrogen bonded and polar.

LIPID CLASSIFICATION

Lipids, as heterogeneous as they are, are usually classified as being either simple or compound lipids (Table 3.2). That classification is maintained here with only a few modifications. The primary emphasis for the lipids, as it was for the carbohydrates, is to focus attention on the most important dietary lipids. Dietary lipids of significant importance include the fatty acids, the triglycerides, cholesterol and esters of cholesterol, and the fat-soluble vitamins. Discussion of the fat-soluble vitamins is deferred to the nutrient section on "Vitamins."

The extreme diversity of lipid compounds, both in structure and function, makes any classification of these molecules almost unsatisfactory. As a collection of molecular diversity, however, most of the lipids are formed from a small number of identifiable biological molecules which comprise the building blocks of this group of compounds. All of the important lipid nutrients that yield either calories or are essential are comprised of fatty acids or fatty acids esterified to glycerol. If phosphatidic acid is included, all phosphatidyl derivatives are then included as derivatives of fatty acids and glycerol. Isoprene, another small lipid molecule, is a five-carbon compound derived from acetyl coenzyme A (see Chapter 5). Isoprene molecules can be thought of as the "glucose" or "amino acid" of the lipid compounds. From isoprene, "polylipids" are synthesized by plants, animals, and humans, giving rise to β-carotene and vitamin A, plant sterols, cholesterol and bile acids, all the adreno-

Table 3.1   Properties of Some Solvents

Solvent	Polarity, E	Boiling Point (°C)
Nonlipid (hydrophilic)		
Water, H_2O	80	100
Ethanol, CH_3CH_2OH	24	79
Acetone, $CH_3\overset{\underset{\parallel}{O}}{C}CH_3$	21	57
Lipid (hydrophobic)		
Chloroform, CH_3Cl	4.8	61
Ether, $(CH_3CH_2)_2O$	4.3	35
n-Hexane, $CH_3(CH_2)_4CH_3$	1.9	37

corticosteroids, sex hormones, vitamins D, E, and K, and related compounds such as ubiquinone, Coenzyme Q. Classifying all the lipids or viewing them as a heterogeneous group of molecules formed from primarily fatty acids, glycerol, or units of isoprene simplifies one's perspective of this large array of diverse molecules. As nature fashioned it, simple units continue to unfold biological diversity.

FATTY ACIDS

Much can be learned about the nutritionally important lipids — their metabolism, structure, and function — by understanding the properties of the saturated and

Table 3.2   Classification of the Lipids

Simple lipids	
Fatty acids:	C_2 to C_{24}, saturated and unsaturated
Monoglycerides:	monoacylglycerol
Diglycerides:	diacylglycerol
Triglycerides:	triacylglycerol
Cholesterol:	cholesterol esters
Bile acids:	cholic acid, taurocholic acid, glycoholic acid, etc.
Vitamin A:	vitamin A esters
Waxes:	esters of alcohols
Prostaglandins:	hormones of the essential fatty acids
Compound lipids: derivatives of phosphatidic acid	
Phosphatidylcholine (lecithin)	
Phosphatidylethanolamine	
Phosphatidylserine	
Phosphatidylinositol	
Sphingolipids	
Plasmologens	
Other lipids	
Glycolipids	
Liproproteins	
Adrenocorticotropins	
Androgens	
Estrogens	
Chylomicrons, HDLs, LDLs, VLDLs	

unsaturated fatty acids. Saturated fatty acids of dietary importance are composed of straight-chain monocarboxylic acids, $CH_3CH_2CH_2(CH_2)_nCOOH$. The simplest fatty acid of dietary importance is acetic acid, CH_3COOH. A dilute solution of acetic acid is known as vinegar. Fatty acids are extended by the addition of methylene (—CH_2—) groups between the terminal methyl and carboxylic acid moieties. The carbon range of saturated fatty acids is from C_2 to C_{24}, with the predominant nutritional fatty acids being of even carbon numbers, C_{14}, C_{16}, C_{18}.

Examination of the properties of the saturated monocarboxylic fatty acids (Table 3.3) reveals that the smaller (C_2 to C_5) fatty acids have appreciable solubility in water and do not strictly adhere to the definition given for lipids. In these few fatty acids, the carboxylic acid moiety dominates chemically over the hydrocarbon portion of the molecule. Intermediate-sized fatty acids (C_6 to C_{11}) are oils, and higher-molecular-weight fatty acids are solids at room temperature. In these larger fatty acids, the hydrocarbon portion of the molecule chemically dominates the carboxylic acid moiety. This dominance by the hydrocarbon portion of the molecule in these higher-molecular-weight fatty acids is measurable as increasing melting points.

Even-numbered fatty acids have higher melting points than those of the preceding odd-numbered fatty acids. Nutritionally, the even-numbered fatty acids, beginning with acetic acid, predominate in the diet. The majority of saturated monocarboxylic fatty acids in the diet are the C_{14}, C_{16}, and C_{18} even-numbered fatty acids. These three fatty acids — myristic, palmitic, and stearic, respectively — comprise a large proportion of the saturated fatty acids found in plant oils and animal fats (Table 3.3).

Table 3.3 Saturated Fatty Acids

Name	Carbon Atoms	Molecular Weight	Solubility (g/100 ml H_2O)[a]	Melting Point (°C)
Acetic (ethanoic)	C_2:0	60	x	16.6
Proprionic	C_3:0	74	x	−22.0
Butyric	C_4:0	88	5.6	−7.9
Pentanoic	C_5:0	102	3.7	−59.0
Caproic	C_6:0	116	0.4	−9.5
Heptanoic	C_7:0	130	0.24	−10.0
Caprylic	C_8:0	144	0.25	16.0
Pelargonic	C_9:0	158	vsl	12.0
Capric	C_{10}:0	172	sl	31.5
Undecylic	C_{11}:0	186	i	29.3
Lauric	C_{12}:0	200	i	40.0
Tridecylic	C_{13}:0	214	i	51.0
Myristic	C_{14}:0	228	i	58.0
Pentadecylic	C_{15}:0	232	i	—
Palmitic	C_{16}:0	256	i	64.0
Margaric	C_{17}:0	270	i	61.0
Stearic	C_{18}:0	284	i	69.0
Nondecylic	C_{19}:0	298	i	—
Arachilic	C_{20}:0	312	i	76.3
Behenic	C_{22}:0	340	i	80.7
Lignoceric	C_{24}:0	369	i	81.0

[a] vsl, very slightly soluble; sl, slightly soluble; i, insoluble.

H   H   H
—C═C—   —C═C—
                                                          H

cis configuration   trans configuration

Figure 3.1 *Cis* and *trans* configurations of unsaturated fatty acids.

A second type of fatty acid, the monocarboxylic monounsaturated and mono-carboxylic polyunsaturated fatty acids, contain one or more carbon–carbon double bonds (see Figure 3.1). Double bonds in fatty acids are distinguished by a suffix in the abbreviated formula. Stearic acid is a fully saturated fatty acid with a full complement of hydrogen atoms. Its formula is $C_{18}:0$ (Table 3.3) and no double bonds are in its structure. Oleic acid is a common C_{18} monounsaturated fatty acid. Its formula is $C_{18}:1$, designating that one double bond exists in the molecule. Since the double bond could occur in any one of 16 different positions in the aliphatic carbon chain, the position of the double bond in the molecule is usually parenthetically noted in some manner in the formula, as, for example, $C_{18}:1(9)$ or $C_{18}:1^{\Delta 9}$. These formulas tells us that the double bond exists in oleic acid between the number 9 and 10 carbon atoms of the fatty acid counting from the C_1, the carboxylic acid carbon atom. This same IUPAC (International Union of Pure and Applied Chemists) nomen-clature is followed for the polyunsaturated fatty acids, with the number and position of each double bond explicitly noted. Another way of numbering the unsaturated fatty acids is the omega nomenclature system. The omega nomenclature begins by numbering the terminal methyl carbon of the fatty acid chain as carbon number 1, just the opposite of the IUPAC system. Thus, linoleic and linolenic acids are omega-6 fatty acids. Oleic acid is therefore an omega-9 fatty acid, the number designating the position of the first double bond from the methyl group of the fatty acid.

Table 3.4 reveals that the addition of a single double bond to an otherwise identical saturated fatty acid lowers the melting point. The addition of more double bonds (more unsaturation) results in still further lowering of the melting point of fatty acids of comparable or larger carbon chain length. The addition of double

Table 3.4 Some Unsaturated Fatty Acids

Name	Carbon Atoms	Molecular Weight	Solubility[a]	Melting Point (°C)
Acrylic[1]	$C_3:1$	72	x	12.3
Methacrylic[1]	$C_4:1$	86	s	16.0
Oleic	$C_{18}:1^{\Delta 9}$	282	i	14.0
Eleomargaric	$C_{17}:2^{\Delta 9,13}$	280	i	48.0
Linoleic	$C_{18}:2^{\Delta 9,12}$	280	i	−5.0
Linolenic	$C_{18}:3^{\Delta 9,12,15}$	278	i	−11.0
Arachidonic	$C_{20}:4^{\Delta 5,8,11,14}$	304	i	−49.5

[a] g/100 ml H_2O; s, soluble; i, insoluble.
[1] not dietary fatty acids.

bonds not only results in lower melting points but in unsaturated fatty acids becoming oils, as compared to similar saturated fatty acids being solids at room temperature.

Monounsaturated fatty acids may exist in two different isomeric forms, as determined by the orientation of the hydrogen atoms about the carbon–carbon double bond. If both hydrogen atoms are positioned on one side of the carbon–carbon bond, a monounsaturated fatty acid would be in the *cis* configuration (Figure 3.1). If one H is positioned on one side of the carbon–carbon double bond and the other H is positioned on the opposite side, a monocarboxylic unsaturated fatty acid would be in the *trans* configuration (Figure 3.1). With few exceptions, naturally occurring mono- and polyunsaturated fatty acids are found to exist in the *cis* configuration. When heated to high temperatures, mono- and polyunsaturated fatty acids of triglycerides are partially hydrogenated by the addition of hydrogen to the carbon–carbon double bonds to form some *trans* fatty acids. The American diet therefore contains *trans* fatty acids formed in corn oil margarines, and shortenings in foods cooked at high temperatures in fats and oils.

It is estimated that stick margarines formed of partially hydrogenated vegetable oils may contain up to 36% of the total fatty acids in the *trans* isomeric form. It follows that processed snack foods using margarine, shortenings, or cooked in partially hydrogenated vegetable oils will also contain *trans* fatty acids. The average per capita consumption of *trans* fatty acids in the American diet is estimated to be 12 g per day: 5 g per day from animal fats and 7 g per day from margarine and shortening. *Trans* fatty acids appear to be absorbed and metabolized similarly to *cis* fatty acids and yield energy, although their metabolism may be slightly slowed. The *trans* fatty acids appear in all lipid fractions of the body, and concern has been expressed about the long-term safety of *trans* fatty acid consumption. There are presently some correlated associations between *trans* fatty acid consumption and cancer of the colon or breast, atherosclerosis, or heart disease. Thus the chemical and physical characteristics of the fatty acids can thus be summarized as follows:

1. Fatty acids are weak organic monocarboxylic acids with hydrocarbon chains which are most often acyclic and unbranched.
2. Fatty acids contain a polar (hydrophilic) carboxylic acid and a nonpolar (hydrophobic) hydrocarbon whose carbon chain length determines some of the physical properties of the fatty acid.
3. Dietary fatty acids are most often even-carbon chain lengths, C_{12}, C_{14}, C_{16}, C_{18}, C_{20}.
4. Fatty acids may be saturated or unsaturated and the unsaturated fatty acids may exist in either the *cis* or *trans* isomeric forms, with the *cis* form predominant in nature. Carbon–carbon double bonds are usually not found between the carboxylic moiety C_1 and C_9 of the hydrocarbon chain, i.e., beyond omega-9.

MONO-, DI-, AND TRIGLYCERIDES

Human and animal diets contain very few "free" unbound fatty acids. With the exceptions of acetic acid from bacterial fermentation and the presence of other short-chain fatty acids in milk, dietary fatty acids exist bound to a water-soluble triose,

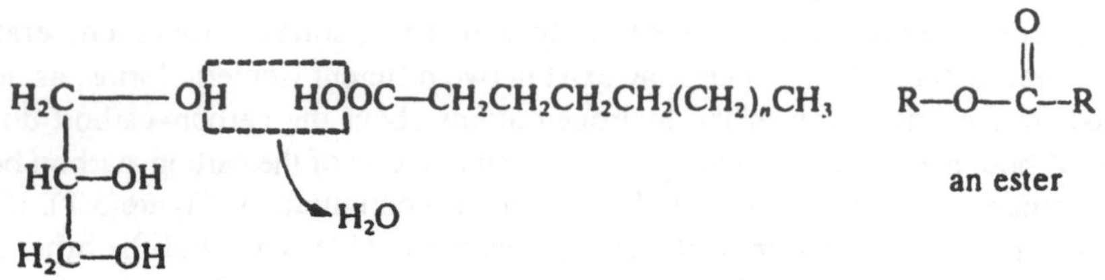

$$H_2C\text{——}OH \qquad HOOC\text{—}CH_2CH_2CH_2CH_2(CH_2)_nCH_3 \qquad R\text{—}O\text{—}\overset{\displaystyle O}{\overset{\|}{C}}\text{--}R$$

$$HC\text{—}OH$$

$$H_2C\text{—}OH \qquad \qquad \searrow H_2O$$

an ester

Figure 3.2 Structure of a monoglyceride.

glycerol. Fatty acids combine with glycerol, forming the neutral lipids. The linkage between glycerol and the fatty acid is an ester bond formed by the elimination of a molecule of water from the hydrogen of glycerol and the hydroxyl of the carboxylic acid moiety of the fatty acid forming a monoglyceride shown in Figure 3.2.

Esterification of additional fatty acids to the monoglyceride results in the formation of a diglyceride and triglyceride, Figure 3.3. The triglyceride is a n .utral lipid. It is the major caloric lipid in the diet and is commonly referred to as animal fat and vegetable oil. Fats and oils are the major storage forms of lipids (depot fat) and energy of the body. The dietary contribution of triglycerides, animal fats, and vegetable oils to the total caloric intake of the average American is 34%.

Triglycerides, fats and oils, contain fatty acids of variable carbon chain length, e.g., mixed triglycerides, and various degrees of saturation or unsaturation (Table 3.5). The glycerol portion of the triglyceride contributes little to the physical characteristics of the glycerides. It is, rather, the characteristics of the individual fatty acids that determine whether the triglyceride will be a fat or an oil. Fats are triglycerides which are primarily of animal origin and contain a greater proportion of long-chain saturated fatty acids esterified to glycerol. The major saturated fatty acids found in animal fat are palmitic (C_{16}:0) acid, followed by lesser amounts of stearic (C_{18}:0) acid. Fats contain more oleic (C_{18}:1) acid than palmitic or stearic acid, but contain much less polyunsaturated fatty acids than do most oils at room temperature because of their greater content of the monounsaturated fatty acid, oleic (C_{18}:1) acid, and the polyunsaturated fatty acids linoleic (C_{18}:2) acid and linolenic (C_{18}:3) acid. Linoleic and linolenic are two of the polyunsaturated fatty acids (PUFA). The composition of some common fats and oils is shown in Table 3.5.

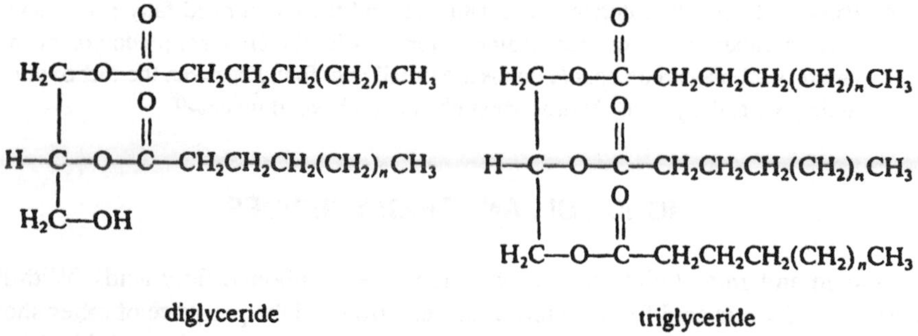

diglyceride

triglyceride

Figure 3.3 Structure of a diglyceride and triglyceride.

Table 3.5 Fatty Acid Composition of Fats and Oils (Percent Fatty Acids)[a]

Name	Saturated FA $(C_4:0-C_{14}:0)$	$(C_{16}:0-C_{18}:0)$	$(C_{18}:1)$	PUFA	Melt. Pt. °C
Fats					
Butter	21.6	38.4	25.1	3.7	25
Tallow	4.7	43.5	36.0	4.3	40
Lard	2.0	36.7	40.9	11.4	30
Poultry	2.4	30.2	39.2	17.6	25
Menhaden (fish)	9.0	22.8	15.5	28.5	−5
Oils					
Coconut	74.2	11.2	5.7	1.8	25
Olive	0	13.8	71.5	8.9	−6
Peanut	0.1	11.8	45.6	31.0	3
Soybean	0.3	14.0	22.8	57.6	−16
Corn	0	12.4	24.6	58.1	−20
Sunflower	0.1	9.9	21.7	66.7	−17

Adapted from G. J. Brisson, *Lipids in Human Nutrition* (Englewood, N.J.: Jack K. Burgess, Inc., 1981).
[a] The higher content of saturated fatty acids in animal fats and much higher content of unsaturated and PUFA in oils are very apparent and contrast sharply with one another. Coconut oil is the exception among the plant oils in having a high proportion of saturated shorter-chain fatty acids. At room temperature coconut oil is a solid.

Among mammals, the fatty acid content of depot fat is subject to slight variation and is influenced only slightly by diet. The total fat content of milk is under genetic control and contains a higher proportion of the shorter-chain fatty acids, but qualitatively the lipids of milk can be influenced by the diet of the mother. A comparison of human depot fat and milk fat with beef depot and milk fat is given in Table 3.6. The data reveal similarity between the fatty acid composition between human and beef depot fat and greater diversity in the fatty acids of milk. Beef milk fat has a higher proportion of short-chain fatty acids than does human milk and a lower content of oleic acid, exhibiting an overall tendency toward greater lipid saturation.

CHOLESTEROL AND DERIVATIVES

Usually classified as a simple lipid, cholesterol (Figure 3.4) is the most widely distributed sterol in animal and human tissues. Present in the diet from the ingestion of only animal foods, cholesterol esters are hydrolyzed and absorbed as chylomicrons and circulate with the lipoproteins. Cholesterol is also actively synthesized from acetyl-CoA and isoprene by the liver, intestinal epithelium, adrenal glands, and skin. Cholesterol is present in tissues as cholesterol esters in plasma, adrenals, intestinal epithelium, and liver and as free cholesterol in the central and peripheral nervous systems.

From cholesterol, specialized body tissues and intestinal bacteria synthesize many derivatives of cholesterol — sterols and steroids — some of which are metabolically active as hormones or hormone-like compounds (Figure 3.5). From the adrenal are synthesized the adrenocorticoids; from the ovaries and testes, the estro-

Table 3.6 Approximate Composition of Depot and Milk Fats
(Percent Fatty Acids)[a]

	Human Depot Fat[b]		Human Milk Fat[a]	Beef Depot Fat[b]	Beef Milk Fat[a]
C_4:0	—		—	—	17
C_6:0	—		—	—	6
C_8:0	—		—	—	2
C_{10}:0	—		1	—	4
C_{12}:0	—	1	3	—	4
C_{14}:0	3	5	6	7	13
C_{16}:0	23	26	30	29	27
C_{18}:0	6	5	7	21	8
C_{16}:1	5		—	—	—
C_{18}:1	50		41	41	17
C_{18}:2	10		12	3	2

[a] Adapted from G. J. Brisson, Lipids in Human Nutrition (Englewood,
N.J.: Jack K. Burgess, Inc., 1981).
[b] Compiled from other sources.

gens and androgens; and from the skin, 7-dehydrocholesterol and vitamin D. The
liver synthesizes the bile acids, which are converted in the gastrointestinal tract into
bile salts which assist with lipid digestion and absorption. The microflora of the
intestinal tract convert cholesterol into unabsorbed excretory products, the neutral
sterols.

PHOSPHATIDIC ACID AND DERIVATIVES

Addition of phosphoric acid forming a phosphoester of any α,β-diglyceride
provides the principal phospholipid nucleus, phosphatidic acid (Figure 3.6), precursor to a large variety of compound lipids collectively named phospholipids.

Phospholipids

Dietary compound lipids are essential in the diet only to the extent that they
provide calories, the mineral phosphorus, and esterified essential fatty acids. Phos-

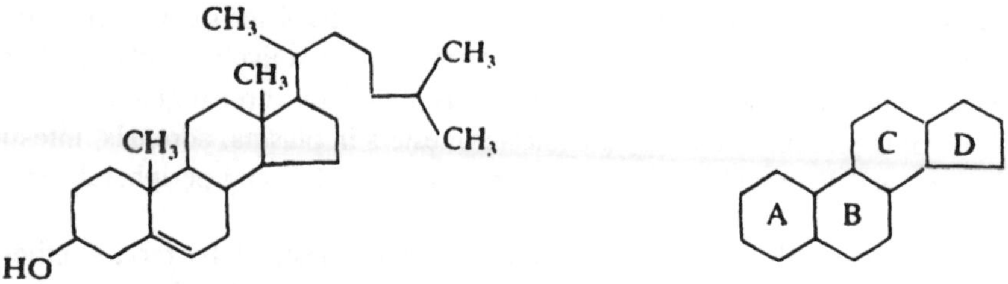

cholesterol   steroid nucleus

Figure 3.4 Structure of cholesterol.

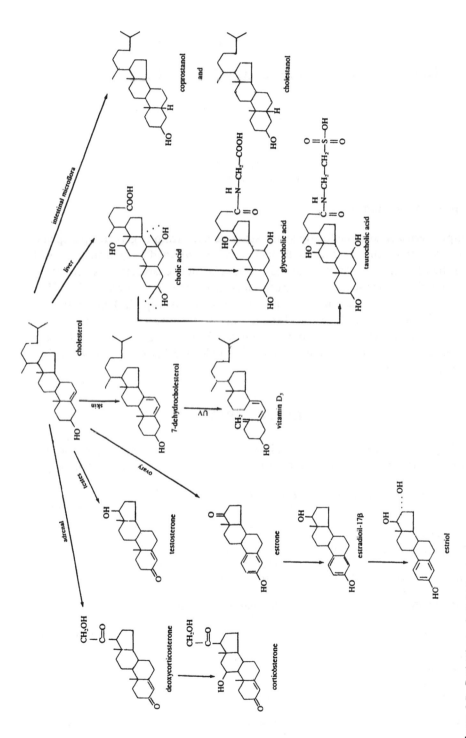

Figure 3.5 Derivatives of cholesterol.

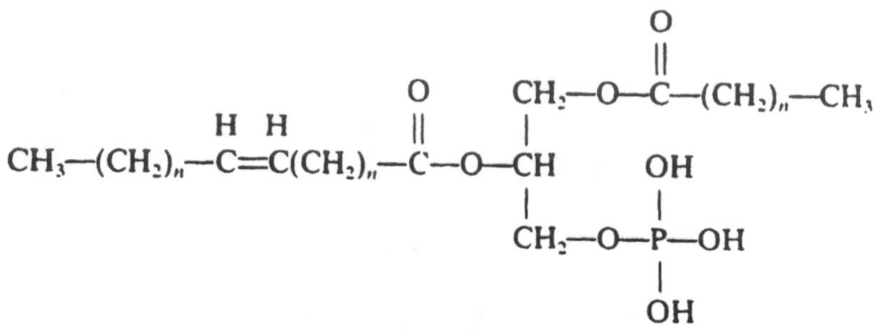

$$CH_3-(CH_2)_n-C\overset{H}{=}\overset{H}{C}(CH_2)_n-\overset{O}{\overset{\|}{C}}-O-CH \quad \begin{array}{c} CH_2-O-\overset{O}{\overset{\|}{C}}-(CH_2)_n-CH_3 \\ OH \\ CH_2-O-P-OH \\ OH \end{array}$$

L-phosphatidic acid
(diacylglycerolphosphate)

Figure 3.6 Phosphatidic acid.

pholipid derivatives are cellularly synthesized *de novo* from α-glycerol phosphate, fatty acids, and some other molecule which, when esterified to phosphatidic acid, gives the phospholipids their name and special chemical characteristics. Generally, phospholipids comprise the major structural component of membranes (65 to 85%) where, because of their amphipathic (hydrophobic–hydrophilic) property they chemically mediate the transition between the more lipid characteristics of the membrane and its aqueous environment. Table 3.7 lists some of the characteristics and functions of the more important phospholipids, and Figure 3.7 provides their chemical structures.

GLYCOLIPIDS

Conjugates of carbohydrates — glucose, galactose, N-acetylglucosamine, and N-acetylneuraminic acid with sphingosine (or dihydrosphingosine) — are all gly-

Table 3.7   Characteristics of the Phospholipids and Glycolipids

Lipid	Major Function
Phospholipids	
Phosphatidylcholine (lecithin)	Major membrane lipid of most cells
Phosphatidylethanolamine (cephalin)	Major membrane lipid of most cells
Phosphatidylserine (cephalin-like)	Bacterial phospholipid
Phosphatidylinositol (inositide)	Major brain phospholipid
Phosphatidylglycerol	Bacterial phospholipid
Diphosphatidylglycerol (cardiolipin)	Heart lipid, concentrated in mitochondria
Plasmalogens	Membrane components of heart, brain, liver, and muscles
Sphingomyelin	Insulates nerve axon
Glycolipids	
Ceramide	Major brain glycolipid
Cerebroside	Provides the different blood types; brain and nerve glycolipids
Ganglioside (hexosamine)	Cell surface glycolipids, found in nerve endings

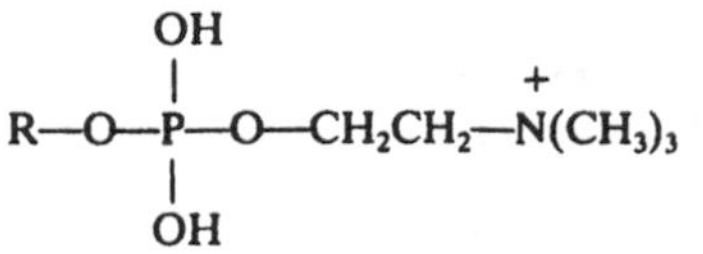

OH
|
R—O—P—O—CH₂CH₂—⁺N(CH₃)₃
|
OH

phosphatidylcholine (lecithin)

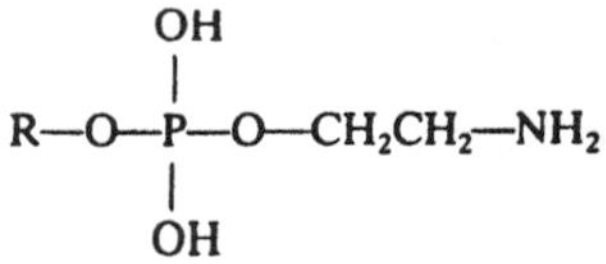

OH
|
R—O—P—O—CH₂CH₂—NH₂
|
OH

phosphatidylethanolamine (cephalin)

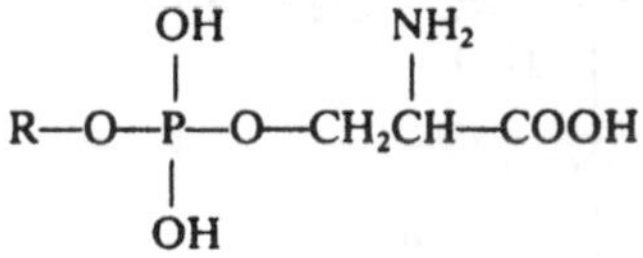

OH   NH₂
| |
R—O—P—O—CH₂CH—COOH
|
OH

phosphatidylserine (cephalin-like)

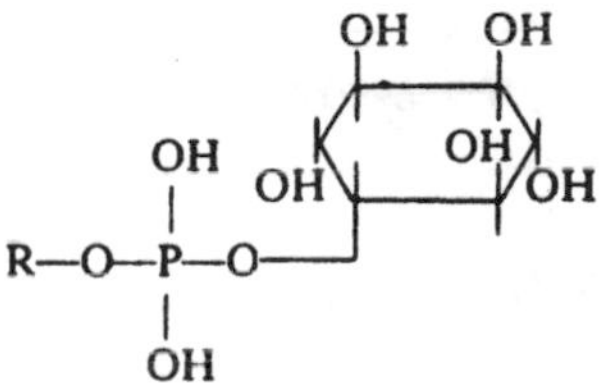

OH
|
R—O—P—O—
|
OH

phosphatidylinositol

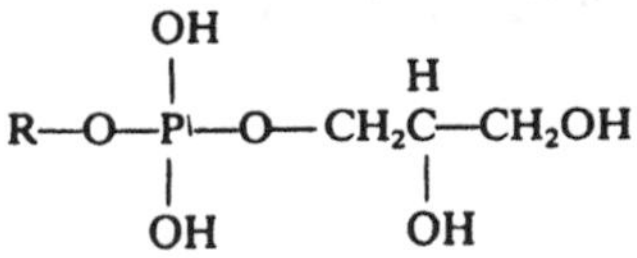

OH   H
| |
R—O—P⎮—O—CH₂C—CH₂OH
| |
OH   OH

phosphatidylglycerol

OH   OH
| H |
R—O—P—O—CH₂C—CH₂—O—P—OH
| | |
OH   OH   OH

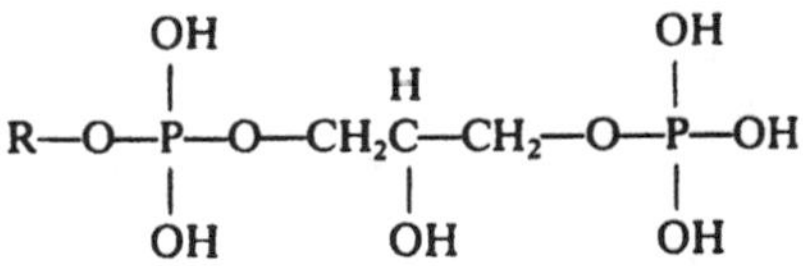

diphosphatidylglycerol (cardiolipin)

R = 1,2-diacylglycerol, the remaining portion of L-phosphatidic acid

Figure 3.7 Chemistry of the phospholipids and glycolipids.

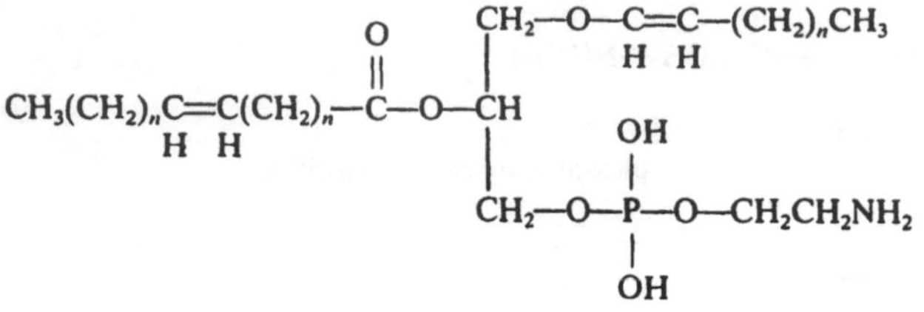

$$CH_3(CH_2)_n \underset{\text{H H}}{C=C}(CH_2)_n - \overset{\overset{\displaystyle O}{\|}}{C} - O - CH \begin{matrix} CH_2 - O - \underset{\text{H H}}{C=C} - (CH_2)_n CH_3 \\ \\ OH \\ | \\ CH_2 - O - \underset{\underset{\displaystyle OH}{|}}{\overset{}{P}} - O - CH_2CH_2NH_2 \end{matrix}$$

a plasmalogen

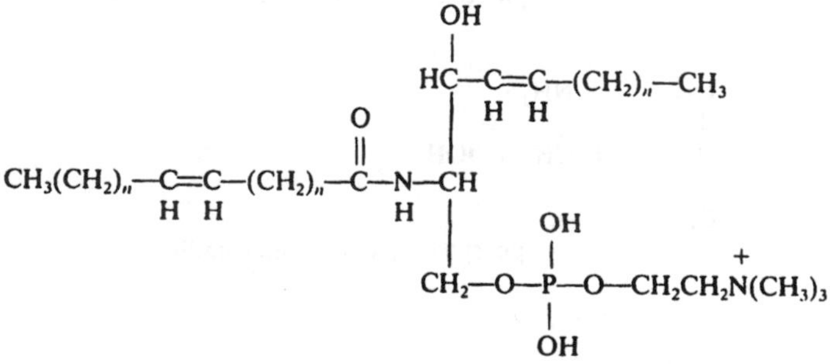

$$CH_3(CH_2)_n - \underset{\text{H H}}{C=C} - (CH_2)_n - \overset{\overset{\displaystyle O}{\|}}{C} - \underset{\underset{\displaystyle H}{|}}{N} - CH \begin{matrix} OH \\ | \\ HC - \underset{\text{H H}}{C=C} - (CH_2)_n - CH_3 \\ \\ OH \\ | \\ CH_2 - O - \underset{\underset{\displaystyle OH}{|}}{\overset{}{P}} - O - CH_2CH_2N(CH_3)_3^+ \end{matrix}$$

sphingomyelin

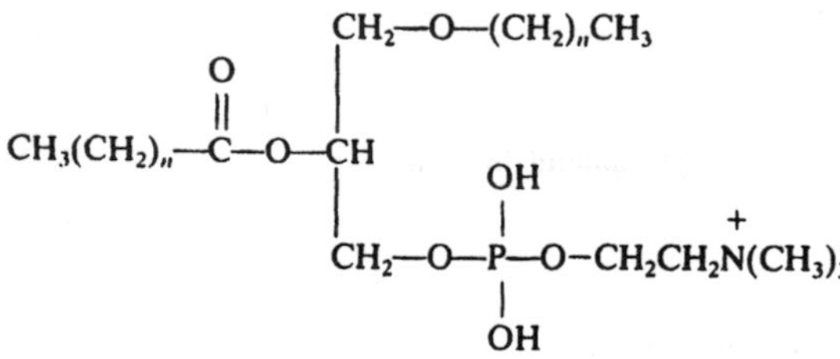

$$CH_3(CH_2)_n - \overset{\overset{\displaystyle O}{\|}}{C} - O - CH \begin{matrix} CH_2 - O - (CH_2)_n CH_3 \\ \\ OH \\ | \\ CH_2 - O - \underset{\underset{\displaystyle OH}{|}}{\overset{}{P}} - O - CH_2CH_2N(CH_3)_3^+ \end{matrix}$$

alkylphospholipid

$$CH_3 - (CH_2)_{14} - \overset{\overset{\displaystyle O}{\|}}{C} - \underset{\underset{\displaystyle H}{|}}{N} - CH \begin{matrix} OH \\ | \\ HC - \underset{\text{H H}}{C=C} - (CH_2)_{12} - CH_3 \\ \\ CH_2 - OH \end{matrix}$$

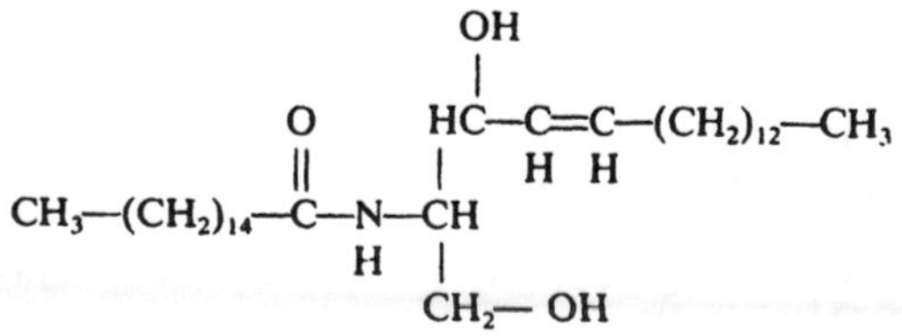

ceramide

Figure 3.7 *Continued.*

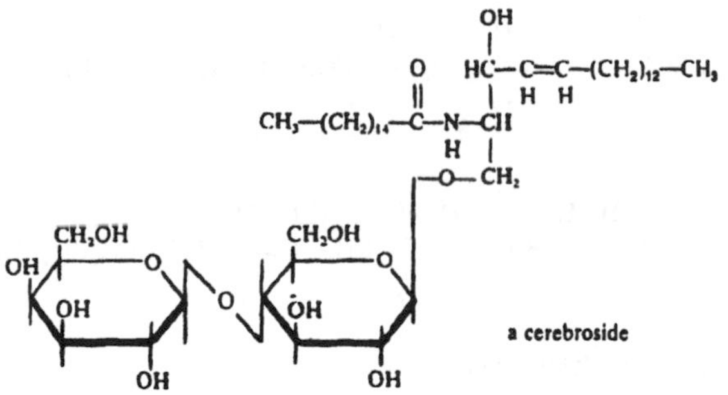

a cerebroside

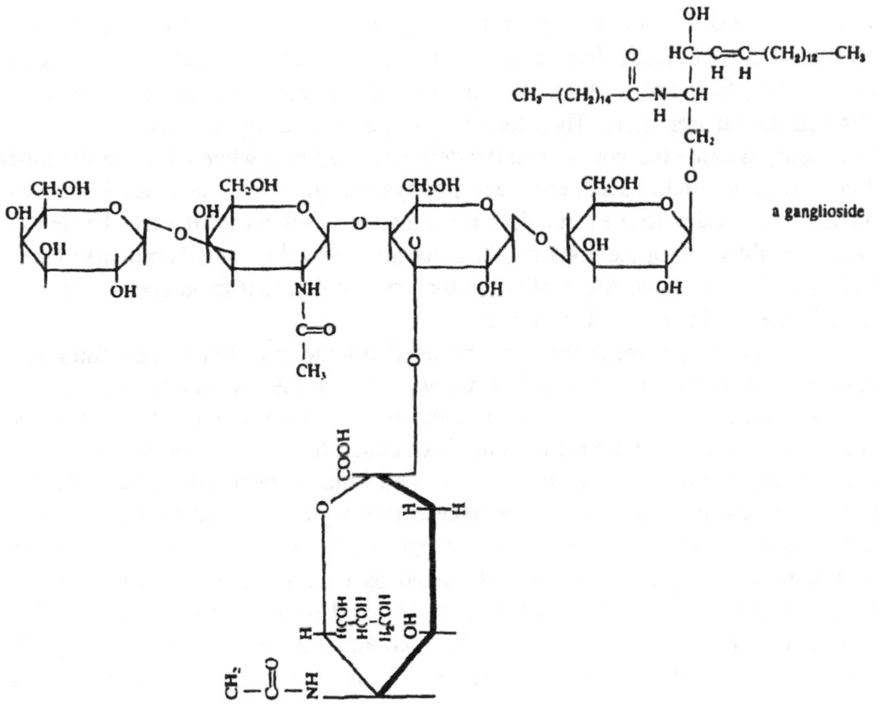

a ganglioside

Figure 3.7 *Continued.*

colipids. Ceramide is the common component of all glycolipids. To ceramide is affixed a carbohydrate moiety, forming cerebrosides and gangliosides (Figure 3.7). The glycolipids are common membrane components of the central nervous system and peripheral nerve tissues (Table 3.7).

THE ESSENTIAL FATTY ACIDS: PRECURSORS OF THE PROSTAGLANDINS

The requirement for the essential fatty acids in the diets of rats was first demonstrated in 1929 by George and Mildred Burr, who found that a rigid exclusion of

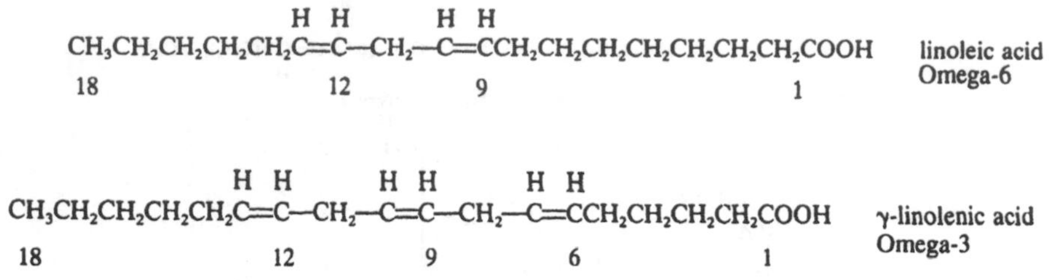

$$\underset{18}{CH_3CH_2CH_2CH_2CH_2}\overset{H\ H}{\underset{12}{C=C}}-CH_2-\overset{H\ H}{\underset{9}{C=C}}CH_2CH_2CH_2CH_2CH_2CH_2CH_2\underset{1}{COOH} \qquad \text{linoleic acid} \atop \text{Omega-6}$$

$$\underset{18}{CH_3CH_2CH_2CH_2CH_2}\overset{H\ H}{\underset{12}{C=C}}-CH_2-\overset{H\ H}{\underset{9}{C=C}}-CH_2-\overset{H\ H}{\underset{6}{C=C}}CH_2CH_2CH_2CH_2\underset{1}{COOH} \qquad \text{γ-linolenic acid} \atop \text{Omega-3}$$

Figure 3.8 Essential fatty acids.

fat from rats caused caudal necrosis, loss of body weight, and early death in the animals. Inclusion of three drops of fat daily or 2% fatty acids to the diet of the rats prevented the deficiency disease. A year later, these authors described the effects of various oils, fats, and fatty acids in preventing the observed deficiency disease in rats fed the fat-free diets. They found that coconut oil, hydrogenated coconut oil, and methylstearate did not prevent the deficiency disease when added to the fat-free diet of rats, but that linseed, corn, and poppyseed oil, as well as methyllinolate and oleate, when added to the same diet, prevented the deficiency disease. These experiments established for the first time the quantitative need for small amounts of dietary lipid and demonstrated the qualitative dietary requirement for a specific fatty acid (i.e., linoleic acid) in the diet of rats.

The concept and recognition of the need for the essential dietary fatty acid(s) has now been firmly established. The dietary need for the essential fatty acids (EFAs) is met by ingestion of linoleic and linolenic acids. Whereas animals and humans are able to synthesize and elongate many fatty acids *de novo* (the principal product is palmitic acid) and oxidize them to mono- and biunsaturated fatty acids (dienes) up to C_9, animals and humans lack the necessary enzymes to oxidize these fatty acids further and introduce double bonds into fatty acids beyond C_9. It is for this reason that oleic acid ($C_{18}:2^{\Delta 6,9}$) can be synthesized by cells in the endoplasmic reticulum from palmitic acid, but linoleic acid ($C_{18}:2^{\Delta 9,12}$) and γ-linolenic acid ($C_{18}:3^{\Delta 6,9,12}$) with unsaturation beyond C_9 cannot be synthesized and must be obtained dietarily. These essential fatty acids are shown in Figure 3.8. Since *only plants* have the enzymes capable of inserting $^{\Delta 12}$Omega-6 and $^{\Delta 15}$Omega-3 double bonds into C_{18} fatty acids, plant oils containing esterified linoleic acid and linolenic acids should be components of an adequate diet.

SYNTHESIS OF EICOSATRIENOIC, EICOSATETRAENOIC, AND EICOSAPENTAENOIC ACIDS

The essential fatty acid linoleic ($C_{18}:2^{\Delta 9,12}$) acid can be oxidized by enzymes of the endoplasmic reticulum of mammalian liver cells to γ-linolenic acid ($C_{18}:^{\Delta 6,9,12}$). This essential fatty acid, γ-linolenic acid, is elongated by addition of two carbons (acetyl-CoA) and oxidized to form eicosatetraenoic acid, ($C_{20}:4^{\Delta 5,8,11,14}$); better known as arachidonic acid. Arachidonic acid is then esterified and made a component

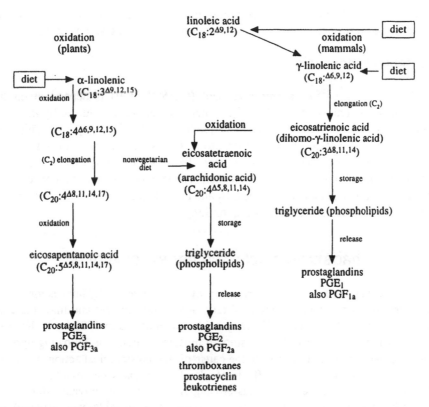

Figure 3.9 Route of synthesis.

of membrane phospholipids. In addition to its function in membrane structure, arachidonic acid serves as a pool of immediate precursor for the prostaglandins, a variety of hormone-like molecules (Figure 3.9).

Eicosatrienoic Acid

The synthesis of eicosatrienoic acid, first in a series of C_{20} polyunsaturated fatty acids, is formed by oxidation of linoleic ($C_{18}:2^{\Delta 9,12}$) to γ-linolenic acid ($C_{18}:3^{\Delta 6,9,12}$) by the enzymes of the endoplasmic reticulum of mammalian liver cells. This essential fatty acid, γ-linolenic (as opposed to α-linolenic acid; $C_{18}:3^{\Delta 9,12,15}$), is elongated by the addition of two carbon atoms (an acetyl-CoA) to form dihomo-γ-linolenic acid ($C_{20}:3^{\Delta 8,11,14}$). This PUFA, also known as eicosatrienoic acid, is stored as a phospholipid within cell membranes, where it serves as a precursor to a group of compounds within the family of prostaglandins designated E_1.

Eicosatetraenoic Acid

Oxidation of eicosatrienoic acid ($C_{20}:3^{\Delta 8,11,14}$) by the endoplasmic reticulum produces the $C_{20}:4$ PUFA, eicosatetraenoic acid ($C_{20}:4^{\Delta 5,8,11,14}$), better known as arachidonic acid. This PUFA is also stored within the phospholipid fraction of cell membranes, where it resides as a precursor to the family of prostaglandins designated E_2.

Eicosapentaenoic Acid

The synthesis of eicosapentaenoic acid (C_{20}:$5^{\Delta 5,8,11,14,17}$) is dependent on the precursor α-linolenic acid (C_{18}:$3^{\Delta 9,12,15}$). Alpha-linolenic acid, oxidized by the same endoplasmic reticulum enzymes, is converted to a C_{18}:$4^{\Delta 6,9,12,15}$ fatty acid. This fatty acid is further elongated by two carbon atoms (acetyl-CoA) and oxidized to form eicosapentaenoic acid. This longer polyene, like the other C_{20} PUFAs, is stored within the phospholipid fraction of all membranes, where it may be converted to the family of prostaglandins designated E_3 and thromboxanes. The route of synthesis of all these fatty acids is shown in Figure 3.9.

PROSTANOIC ACID AND PROSTAGLANDINS

The prostaglandins are a diverse array of hydroxylated C_{20} fatty acids which originate from the dietary C_{18} essential fatty acids, linoleic acid and linolenic acid. The discovery of this group of C_{20} fatty acids was initiated in 1930 by R. Kurzrok and C. Lieb, whose observations of smooth muscle contractions following application of semen prompted a search for the cause of the physiological action. U. S. von Euler, having observed similar effects of glandular extracts on smooth muscle in 1935, named the affective compounds prostaglandins, after the prostate gland. Subsequently, these first fatty acid compounds, some quite unstable, were isolated and structurally identified in 1962 by S. Bergstrom and colleagues. Recognition that the prostaglandins were derived from the essential fatty acids came in 1964, the association having been made by S. Bergstrom. These remarkable intuitive discoveries have led researchers to discover an array of C_{20}-derived fatty acids, almost all of which are hydroxylated and include the prostaglandins, thromboxanes, and prostacyclins (Figure 3.10).

Prostaglandins, synthesized by most cells, are made in response to mechanical, chemical, immunological, or inflammatory insults. They may not be hormones *per se*, but certainly they appear to modulate hormonal responses. As molecules with specific and potent pharmacologic effects, they are under intensive investigation by pharmaceutical companies and independent researchers for physiologic application in the treatment of diseases.

Among the noted biochemical and physiological responses to prostaglandins are induction of cyclic AMP and subsequent effects; vasoconstriction and vasodilation and their consequences for maintenance of blood pressure; inhibition of platelet cell aggregation; induction of erythema; increased vascular permeability; edema; and inflammatory responses.

While a detailed description of the entire chemistry of the prostaglandins would exceed the intent of this introductory chapter, it should be noted that the parent molecule of the prostaglandins is prostanoic acid (C_{20}:O; Figure 3.10), formed upon

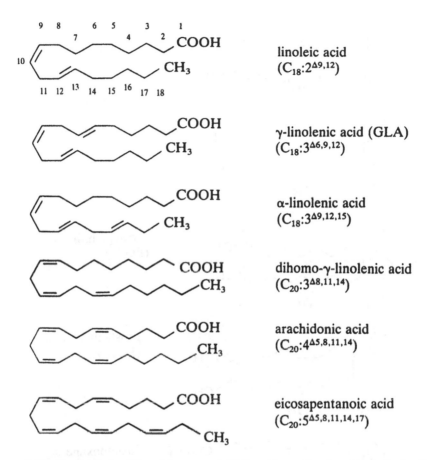

Figure 3.10 Structural chemistry of the essential fatty acids, prostanoic acid, prostaglandins, and derivatives.

oxidation of C_8 and C_{12} by the enzyme prostaglandin synthase, forming a five-membered ring of carbons 8, 9, 10, 11, and 12. In this manner the prostaglandins of the PGE_1, PGE_2, and PGE_3 and other series are derived from eicosanoids: eico-satrienoic, eicosatetraenoic (arachidonic), and eicosapentaenoic acids. Further chemical modifications to either the mono-, di-, or triene fatty acid side chains (hydroxylations or ketal formation) or to the C_{8-12} ring (hydroxylations and/or ketal formations) results in the synthesis of a chemically different prostaglandin. Insertion of an oxygen into the C_{8-12} ring produces the family of thromboxanes; addition of a second oxygen ring produces the family of prostacyclins, and side-chain epoxidation of arachidonic acid leads to the leukotrienes. Representative structures of all these families of prostaglandins are given in Figure 3.10.

Presently, there are more than 100 known prostaglandins, isomers, and derivatives, with more likely to be discovered in the future.

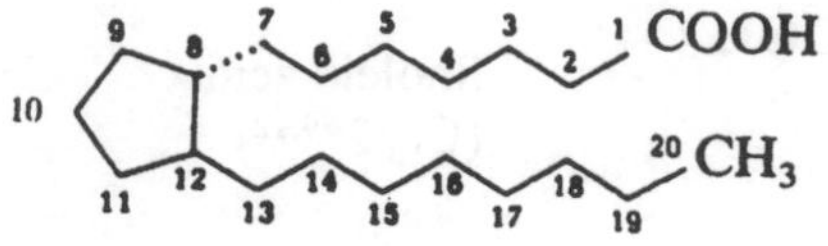

prostanoic acid
($C_{20}:0$)

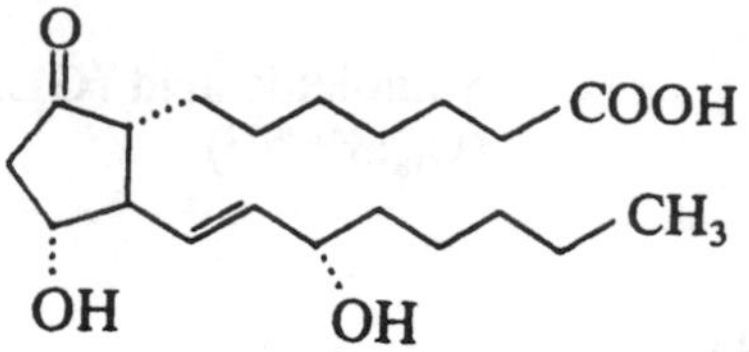

prostaglandin E_1
(PGE_1)

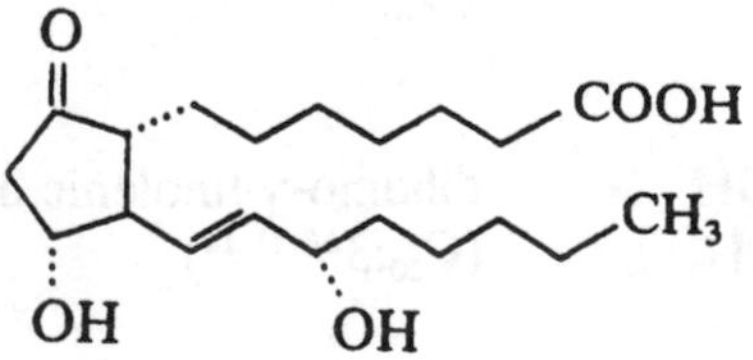

prostaglandin E_2
(PGE_2)

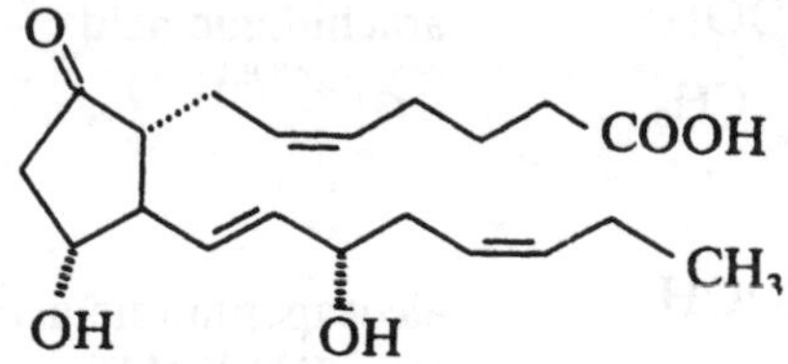

prostaglandin E_3
(PGE_3)

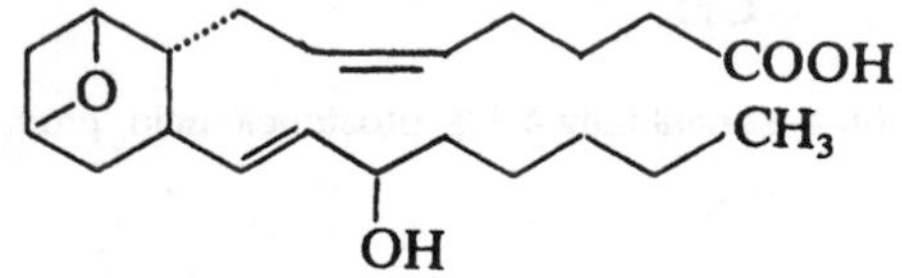

thromboxane A_2
(TXA_2)

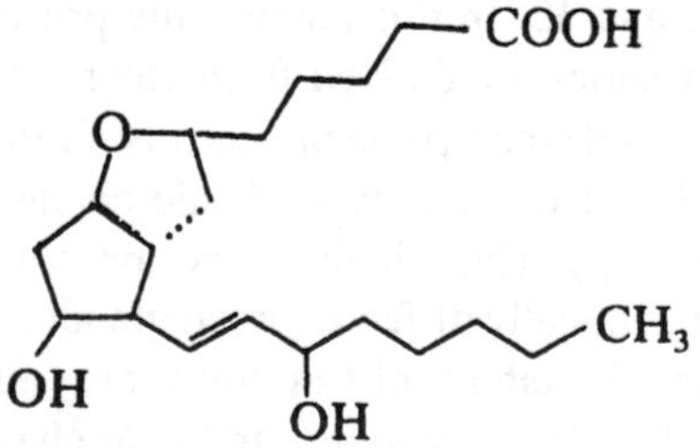

prostacyclin
(PGI_2)

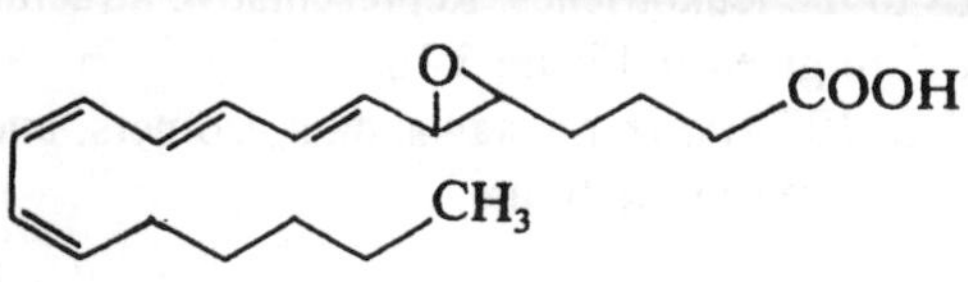

leukotriene A
(LTA)

Figure 3.10 *Continued.*

CHAPTER 4

Proteins

The dietarily essential nitrogen-containing class of foods is called proteins. Like carbohydrates and lipids, proteins also contain carbon, hydrogen, and oxygen. Proteins contain about 16% nitrogen by weight. Proteins, derived from the Greek word *proteus* means "first." Proteins were the first substances to be recognized as a vital part of living tissue. Proteins are essential nutritionally, with about half of the dry weight of most animal cells being protein.

AMINO ACIDS: THE BUILDING BLOCKS OF PROTEIN

All proteins are assembled from their basic units, the amino acids. Each cell uses amino acids to synthesize its own variety of proteins. Amino acids or organic compounds of a similar nature were probably first formed in that primordial soup at the beginning of biological time. About 20 to 22 amino acids are commonly found in most proteins. All the amino acids except proline and hydroxyproline (which are really imino acids) are α-amino carboxylic acids. They contain a basic amino group and an acidic carboxyl group attached to the α-carbon. They differ from each other by the remainder of the molecule (R). With the exception of glycine, all amino acids assembled into protein in animals and humans are L-amino acids (Figure 4.1). Glycine does not exist as either the D- or L-isomer, because it does not possess an (asymmetric) chiral carbon center as do all other amino acids found in protein and in biological fluids. Amino acids of the D-isomer are found in bacteria and racemic mixtures of synthetically made amino acids, but they are not incorporated into animal or human protein. The D-amino acids must undergo isomerization and be converted to the L-isomer of the amino acid before being incorporated into protein.

AMINO ACID CLASSIFICATION BY STRUCTURE

Amino acids can be and have been classified in several ways. The classification used here is one based on the structural similarities of amino acids. The structural

NH₂
|
CH₂
no asymmetric ___ |
center   COOH

glycine

COOH
|↙
H₂N—CH
|
R

L-amino acid

chiral
'asymmetric'
centers

HOOC
|
HC—NH₂
|
R

D-amino acid

Figure 4.1 Asymmetry in amino acids.

divisions include the aliphatic, acidic, basic, aromatic, sulfur-containing, selenium-containing, and secondary amino acids. The structures of 23 amino acids are presented with names and abbreviations (Figures 4.2 through 4.8).

Each of the aliphatic amino acids possesses a common structural component, shown within the boxed area of alanine (Figure 4.2). The aliphatic amino acids are glycine, alanine, valine, leucine, and isoleucine. Metabolism of the branched-chain aliphatic amino acids (valine, leucine, and isoleucine) is sometimes prevented, owing to the lack in newborns of an enzyme, a branched-chain α-keto acid dehydrogenase, resulting in an inborn error of metabolism called maple syrup urine disease (MSUD). This disease cannot be corrected but is controllable by limiting these amino acids in the diets of children. Glycine is needed for the synthesis of the porphyrin ring of hemoglobin and myoglobin and is a constituent of a bile acid. Glycine may also function in detoxification. Serine and threonine differ in structure by a methyl group and are the hydroxyl-containing amino acids (Figure 4.3).

Aspartic acid and glutamic acid (Figure 4.4) are acidic amino acids because each possesses two carboxylic acids and only one amino group. These two amino acids differ by only a single methylene, which when added to aspartic acid becomes glutamic acid. The monosodium salt of glutamic acid is commonly used as a flavor enhancer in foods and is known as monosodium glutamate (MSG). Sometimes, protein contains the amide derivatives of aspartic acid, asparagine, and glutamic acid, glutamine. Ammonia (NH₃) from the degradation of protein and amino acids is commonly carried in body fluids as glutamine, the ammonia having been attached to the γ-carboxylic group of glutamic acid. There is some evidence that glutamine

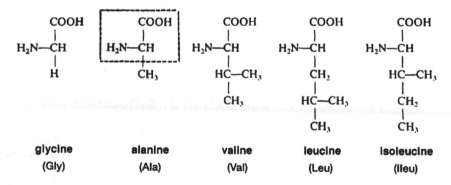

Figure 4.2 Aliphatic amino acids.

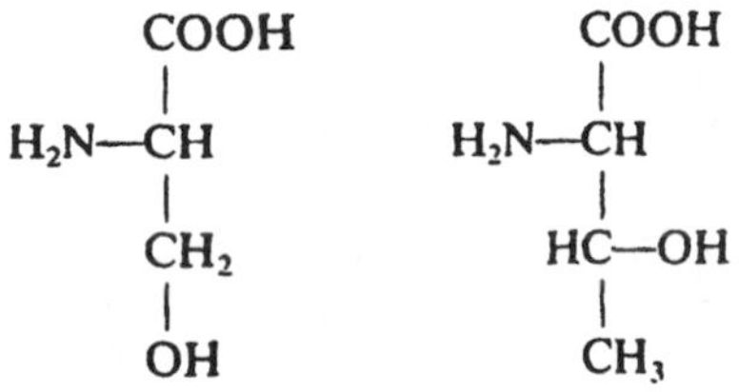

```
        COOH              COOH
         |                 |
   H₂N—CH            H₂N—CH
         |                 |
        CH₂              HC—OH
         |                 |
        OH               CH₃

      serine            threonine
       (Ser)              (Thr)
```

Figure 4.3 Hydroxyl amino acids.

may regulate muscle protein turnover. Glutamic acid is also needed for the synthesis of γ-amino butyric acid (γABA or GABA), a neurotransmitter.

Lysine, arginine, and histidine (Figure 4.5) are the basic amino acids because they each possess at least two amino groups or amine equivalents and only one carboxylic acid. Lysine is nutritionally one of the most important amino acids, as it is often the limiting dietary essential amino acid of plant protein. Arginine is needed for the synthesis of urea. Arginine also appears to be of importance in the immune system perhaps due to its conversion to nitric oxide, a secondary messenger. Nitric oxide helps to regulate blood pressure and perhaps peristalsis. Histamine, a dilator of the capillaries and stimulator of gastric secretion, is synthesized from histidine.

The aromatic amino acids phenylalanine, tyrosine, and tryptophan (Figure 4.6) contribute to the ultraviolet-absorbing property that most proteins possess. Phenylalanine is a tyrosine precursor. Phenylalanine or tyrosine is needed for the synthesis of epinephrine, norepinephrine, and thyroxine. Melanin, a pigment found in skin and hair, is also derived from tyrosine. The methyl ester of phenylalanine and the acidic amino acid aspartic acid are combined as a dipeptide forming the sweetener aspartame, one trade name for which is NutraSweet®. Children born without the enzyme phenylalanine hydroxylase, which converts phenylalanine to tyrosine, have

Proteins

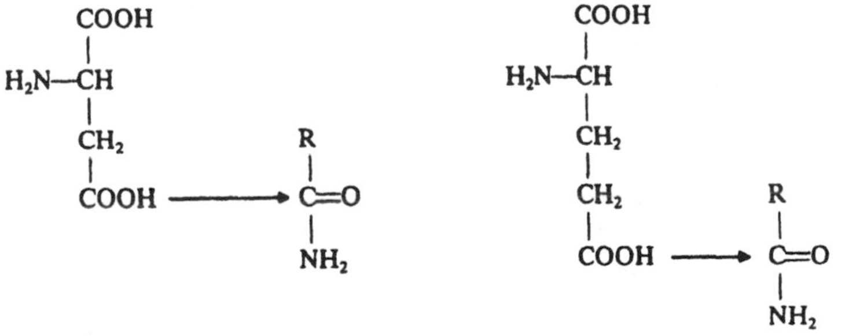

```
        COOH                                COOH
         |                                   |
   H₂N—CH                            H₂N—CH
         |                                   |
        CH₂        R                       CH₂
         |          |                        |
        COOH ——→  C=O                     CH₂         R
                    |                        |          |
                   NH₂                     COOH ——→  C=O
                                                        |
                                                       NH₂

  aspartic acid   asparagine          glutamic acid   glutamine
     (Asp)          (Asn)                 (Glu)          (Gln)
```

Figure 4.4 Acidic amino acids.

```
        COOH              COOH              COOH
         |                 |                 |
  H₂N—CH            H₂N—CH            H₂N—CH
         |                 |                 |
       CH₂               CH₂               CH₂
         |                 |
       CH₂               CH₂
         |                 |           N       NH
       CH₂               CH₂
         |                 |
       CH₂               HN
         |                 |
       NH₂               C=NH
                           |
                          NH₂

     lysine            arginine          histidine
     (Lys)              (Arg)              (His)
```

Figure 4.5 Basic amino acids.

the inborn metabolic disease phenylketonuria (PKU). This disease is managed by controlling the quantity of phenylalanine in the diet. Persons with this disease are cautioned to not use products with NutraSweet because of its phenylalanine content. Tryptophan can be converted by cells in the body to the vitamin niacin. Tryptophan is also a precursor of serotonin, a neurotransmitter.

The sulfur amino acids methionine and cysteine (Figure 4.7) are two predominant sulfur-containing compounds in many cells. Only methionine need be included in the diet, as cysteine is derived from S-adenylsylmethionine, the principal methylating agent of cells. When incorporated into protein, cysteine can undergo oxidation and combine with another oxidized cysteine residue, forming cystine. Cystine, a disulfide, functions as both an interchain and intrachain cross-linking amino acid in protein structure (see also Figure 4.9). Methionine also functions as a methyl group donor. Cysteine is a component of another important thiol compound, glutathione, the tripeptide γ-glutamylcysteinylglycine. This abundant intracellular thiol common

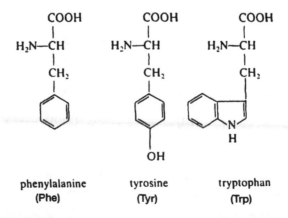

```
        COOH              COOH              COOH
         |                 |                 |
  H₂N—CH            H₂N—CH            H₂N—CH
         |                 |                 |
       CH₂               CH₂               CH₂
```

     phenylalanine   tyrosine   tryptophan
       (Phe)   (Tyr)   (Trp)

Figure 4.6 Aromatic amino acids.

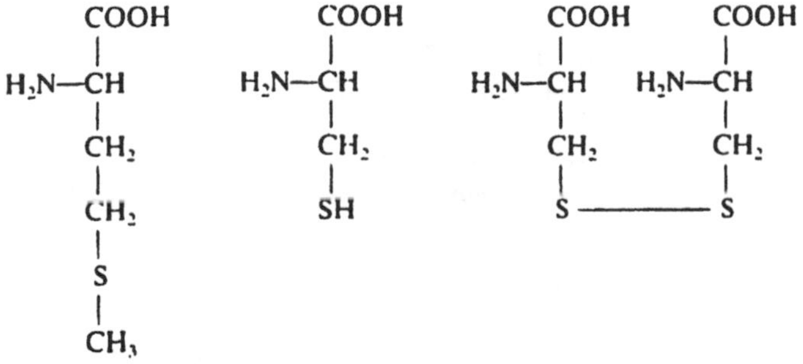

methionine (Met) | cysteine (CySH) | cystine (Cys)

Figure 4.7 Sulfur amino acids.

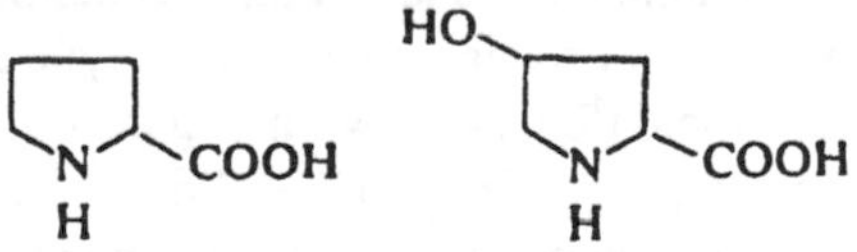

proline (Pro) | hydroxyproline (Hyp)

Figure 4.8 Secondary amino acids.

to all cells functions to prevent harmful oxidation reactions in cells (see Chapter 15). Glutathione also detoxifies carcinogens and xenobiotics by forming glutathione derivatives with these compounds, which are then excreted. Taurine, which is derived from cysteine, appears to be an effective scavenger of peroxidation products and may also function as a neuromodulator. Creatine phosphate, a high-energy compound, is derived from glycine, arginine, and methionine.

Another commonly found amino acid in blood proteins and enzymes is selenocysteine. Selenocysteine is identical to cysteine except that selenium replaces the sulfur in cysteine. Selenocysteine is not a dietary essential amino acid as this amino acid is formed *de novo* from the dietary essential trace element selenium (see Chapter 6).

Proline and hydroxyproline are not primary amino acids but are the only two secondary amino (imino) acids (Figure 4.8). Proline interrupts α-helical formations in protein. Hydroxyproline is extensively found in collagen, a protein of connective tissue. Vitamin C, ascorbic acid, is required for the hydroxylation of proline to make hydroxyproline.

PROTEIN STRUCTURE

All amino acids needed for synthesis of a protein must be in the same cell at the same time. Proteins are assembled from their constituent amino acids, one by

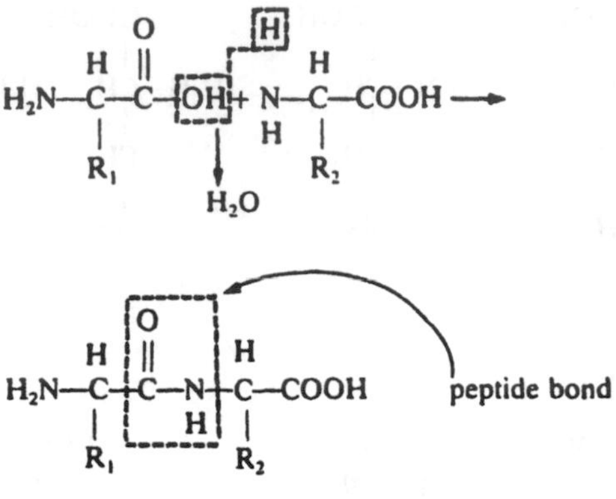

Figure 4.9 Formation of a dipeptide.

one and one at a time. Two amino acids are initially combined, forming a dipeptide by the exclusion of a molecule of water from the carboxylic acid (R_1) and the amino group of the second amino acid (R_2), as shown in Figure 4.9. The result is formation of a dipeptide with its amide, "peptide bond." Addition of a third amino acid to the dipeptide results in the formation of a second peptide bond and a tripeptide (Figure 4.10). To the tripeptide is added, in similar fashion, another amino acid, forming a tetrapeptide, and so, one by one, polypeptides are assembled from amino acids. When polypeptides begin approaching 50 amino acids in length they are called proteins. Hormones of the pituitary gland, thyroid-stimulating hormone (TSH) (MW 30,000) and follicle-stimulating hormone (FSH) (MW 26,000), are moderately large proteins. Other hormones of the pituitary gland, vasopressin, oxytocin (nine amino acid residues), and human β-melanocyte-stimulating hormone with 22 amino acid residues, are polypeptides. Insulin (Figure 4.11), a pancreatic hormone with its 51 amino acids, is a small protein. Proteins vary extensively in size and function and are physically described by their amino composition (primary structure), which determines their molecular weight. Proteins are further described by their α-helical content stabilized by hydrogen-bonding between amino acid residues (secondary

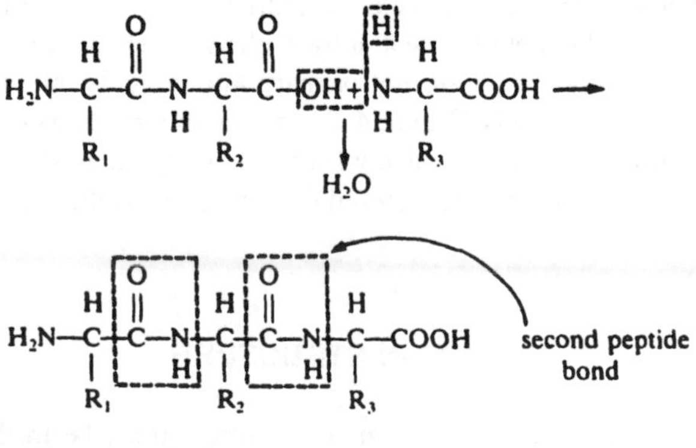

Figure 4.10 Formation of a tripeptide.

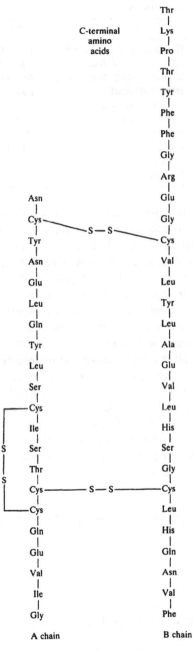

Figure 4.11   Insulin.

Table 4.1 Complex Proteins

Complex	Example	Nonpeptide Moiety
Glycoproteins	Blood antigens A, B, AB, O	Carbohydrates
Lipoproteins	HDLs, LDLs, VLDLs	Triglycerides, cholesterol
Nucleoproteins	Chromosomes, ribosomes	Nucleic acids
Metalloproteins	Metallothionein	Zinc
	Dehydrogenases	Zinc
	Cytochromes	Iron
Chromoproteins	Hemoglobin	Heme iron
	Myoglobin	Heme iron
	Cytochromes	Heme iron
	Ferritin	Non-heme iron

structure), and the spatial arrangement of secondary structure contributed by —S—S— (single bonds) bonding (tertiary structure). Some proteins will assemble themselves by the association of individual subunits (quaternary structure). They are the principal components of muscle, connective tissues, hair, nails, serum, antibodies, and enzymes. It is the catalytic function of proteins that makes all life processes possible. All proteins are three-dimensional configurations of coiled or folded polypeptide chains which form structures that are essentially either fibrous (most structural proteins) or globular (enzymes and antibodies). Proteins are believed to have been the first molecules, for it is their catalytic activity that permits the assembly of the nucleic acids and all the other bioorganic molecules. Proteins do not always exist singularly but are often associated with other compounds. Such complex proteins in association with nucleic acids, lipids, carbohydrates, and minerals are often classified according to the molecule with which the protein associates. These protein complexes, often called conjugated proteins, perform specific functions which neither constituent could properly perform alone. Such protein complexes are named in Table 4.1. Derived proteins come from protein metabolism and include peptides, peptones, and proteoses.

CLASSIFICATION OF AMINO ACIDS BY FUNCTION

W. C. Rose, during the 1930s, demonstrated that some of the amino acids found in proteins were essential or indispensable, while others were *nonessential* or dispensable. The essential amino acids cannot be synthesized *in vivo* from nonprotein sources in sufficient quantity to meet the body's needs, and so must be supplied to humans from either plant or animal proteins. There are nine essential amino acids required in the diet of humans. A decade or so ago, eight amino acids were considered to be essential for the human adult, and nine for infants. J. D. Kopple and M. E. Swendseid have suggested that histidine, the amino acid essential for infants but not thought to be for adults, may also be essential for adults. These essential amino acids are given in Table 4.2. Arginine is not synthesized in amounts sufficient to meet the needs of the young of most mammalian species. It appears that arginine is not required by the human infant, but the need by the premature infant is unknown.

Table 4.2 Essential (Indispensable) Amino Acids

Amino Acids Required by the Human Infant and Adult		Amino Acids Synthesized *In Vivo* (Nonessential Amino Acids)	
Valine	Leucine	Hydroxyproline	Tyrosine
Threonine	Lysine	Glycine	Alanine
Tryptophan	Phenylalanine	Serine	Glutamine
Isoleucine		Glutamic acid	Asparagine
Methionine		Aspartic acid	Proline
Histidine		Cysteine	
Arginine[a]		Cystine	

[a] May not be required by adults, or perhaps even infants.

The amino acids tyrosine and cysteine (also cystine) are sometimes classified as semi-essential amino acids or conditionally essential amino acids. Tyrosine can be synthesized *in vivo* from only the essential amino acid phenylalanine, while cysteine (cystine) can be synthesized *in vivo* from only the essential amino acid methionine. Frequently, humans consume phenylalanine and methionine in low amounts and these two amino acids may not be available for conversion to tyrosine and cysteine (cystine). There is some evidence that arginine, proline, and glycine are conditionally essential for low-birth-weight infants. The body is able to synthesize the nonessential amino acids by transamination utilizing amino groups from other nonessential amino acids and unneeded essential amino acids. A certain quantity of nonessential amino acids is considered to be a dietary essential.

The body's protein needs are both qualitative and quantitative. The body needs each of the essential amino acids in certain proportions and also needs a sufficient quantity of protein. The 1989 Recommended Dietary Allowance (RDA) for protein is 0.75 g/kg body weight for adults, including the elderly. Younger individuals require more protein per kg body weight than adults. The RDAs for protein by age–sex groups, pregnancy, and lactation are given in Chapter 17.

PROTEIN QUALITY

The essential amino acid content of protein foods determines the quality of the protein. Most protein foods contain many different proteins, so the quality of a protein food reflects a composite of the amino acid content of several different proteins. For example, milk contains the proteins lactalbumin and casein.

Complete proteins contain all the essential amino acids needed by the body in proportions and amounts that are adequate. Generally proteins from animal-derived foods are complete; these include meat, poultry, fish, cheese, eggs, and milk. Gelatin is an animal protein that is incomplete, lacking in many of the essential amino acids.

Incomplete proteins do not contain all the essential amino acids needed by the body in amounts that are nutritionally adequate. Incomplete proteins contain one or more essential amino acid(s) in insufficient quantity(ies) to meet the body's needs. Most plant proteins are incomplete. The essential amino acid that is present in the smallest concentration relative to the amount needed for protein synthesis is called the limiting amino acid. The dietary absence of even one essential amino acid will stop most proteins from being synthesized.

Complementary proteins are two or more incomplete proteins whose essential amino acid contents complement each other in such a way that the essential amino acid(s) missing from one protein (the limiting amino acid) is supplied by the other protein. The following are general statements about limiting amino acids in foods (some exceptions exist): vegetables are low in methionine; legumes are low in methionine and tryptophan; grains are low in lysine; seeds are low in lysine; and nuts are low in threonine and sometimes lysine. Combinations which are complementary include the following: legumes + grains, legumes + seeds, vegetables + grains, vegetables + seeds, vegetables + nuts, and grains + nuts. Individuals can obtain adequate protein quality and quantity by eating foods that contain complementary proteins.

PROTEIN STATUS

In a research setting the protein status of humans is most commonly determined by nitrogen balance studies. Most of the body's total nitrogen is found in protein. Nitrogen balance is equal to the nitrogen intake (diet) minus the nitrogen output (in urine and feces; sometimes sweat is also included). Adults need to maintain a net nitrogen balance, while children should have a positive nitrogen balance (retain more nitrogen than is excreted). The aged and individuals with some diseases have negative nitrogen balance (retain less nitrogen than is being excreted).

Unfortunately no one satisfactory measurement is available for the assessment of protein status. Parameters other than nitrogen balance that are utilized for evaluation of protein status of humans include serum total protein, albumin, prealbumin, or transferrin concentrations; serum amino acid ratios; urinary hydroxyproline indices or 3-methylhistidine levels, and urinary urea:creatinine ratios in the fasting state. Several muscle function tests and immunological measurements may also be used in evaluating protein status. Generally the most often used biochemical method for assessing protein status in a hospital or clinic setting is the determination of serum albumin concentration; however, prealbumin, retinal-binding protein, and/or transferrin concentrations are also used.

Somatotrophin (or growth hormone), insulin, testosterone, and estrogen stimulate protein synthesis. Thyroxine increases the metabolic rate, and thus influences both the anabolism and catabolism of proteins. Both gluconeogenesis and ketogenesis from proteins are increased by glucocorticoids.

FUNCTIONS OF PROTEINS IN THE BODY

Amino acids and their specific order in the primary protein structure provides the chemical specificity that dictates their function. Dietary protein provides the amino acids needed for the synthesis of body proteins. Protein synthesis is an anabolic process which builds and maintains body tissues. These body proteins include those needed for cellular structure, enzymes, transport proteins, nucleoproteins, antibodies, blood clotting factors, visual pigments, glutathione, taurine, some hormones, and some neurotransmitters. Body protein is constantly being synthesized and degraded, which is known as protein turnover. Body proteins also function in the maintenance of acid–base balance (as buffers) and in fluid regulation. Proteins can also be used to provide the body with energy; proteins contain approximately 4 kcal/g. Proteins may also be converted to adipose tissue.

PROTEIN CATABOLISM

Only a small reserve of free amino acids exists in the body. Amino acids which are not needed for protein synthesis are deaminated, primarily in the liver, with the resulting carbon skeleton, an α-keto acid, being used for either energy production or adipose tissue formation. The deaminated amino group is converted to urea in the liver and excreted in the urine. The quantity of urea excreted by an individual varies with the protein intake. The metabolism of protein consumed in excess of the body's requirement is referred to as exogenous protein metabolism. The metabolism of body proteins is referred to as endogenous protein metabolism.

Uric acid is the end product of purine catabolism. Purines are components of nucleic acids. A disorder of the catabolism of purines to uric acid is gout which can cause arthritis-like symptoms and kidney stones.

Creatinine is the end product of creatine catabolism which is found in all muscle tissues. Creatine phosphate is a high-energy phosphate reserve. The quantity of creatinine which is excreted is reflective of the lean body mass of an individual. Individuals excrete a relatively constant quantity of creatinine daily. Hence, it is frequently utilized in ascertaining the completeness of 24-hour urine collections and can quantitatively be used to reflect somatic protein status.

PROTEIN-ENERGY MALNUTRITION

Protein-Energy Malnutrition (PEM), formerly known as Protein-Calorie Malnutrition (PCM), is the most widespread form of malnutrition in the world. Around a quarter of the world's population experiences pain from hunger due to lack of food. PEM is prevalent in underdeveloped countries including those in Africa, Asia, and Central and South America. Some cases have been reported in the United States, and PEM is common in at-risk groups, such as the elderly and those under acute catabolic stress (for example, burns and trauma).

Kwashiorkor, or protein deficiency, is caused by insufficient good-quality protein. Kwashiorkor occurs primarily among 2- to 5-year-old children who are weaned to diets of starch cereal pastes. Individuals with kwashiorkor have edema, diarrhea, scaly skin, red flag (reddish pigmentation of the formerly dark hair) or hair that is easily plucked, fatty liver, decreased immunity, decreased growth, and decreased intelligence. Severe and prolonged kwashiorkor may even lead to death. Secondary infections in individuals with kwashiorkor are generally the cause of death. Acute physiologic stress can also predispose individuals to kwashiorkor.

Marasmus is a condition in which there is insufficient dietary protein and calories. Marasmus is starvation in its purest form. In marasmus there is a deficiency of most essential nutrients. The clinical symptoms of marasmus are different from those of kwashiorkor. Symptoms of marasmus include severe muscle wasting, absence of subcutaneous fat, dermatosis, reduced growth, hepatomegaly, anxiety, and decreased intelligence.

The clinical symptoms of PEM can be reversed in four to six weeks with a diet adequate in food energy, nutrients, and high-quality protein. Unfortunately, the effects of PEM on mental development in children are nonreversible. Frequently individuals with PEM also have intestinal parasites and other infectious disorders which also require medical treatment.

EXCESSIVE PROTEIN INTAKES

Individuals can gain weight, particularly as adipose tissue, by the consumption of diets high in protein. Many foods which are high in protein are also high in fat. Individuals may become dehydrated if they consume too much protein. Some studies indicate that there may also be an increased excretion of calcium in people consuming high levels of dietary protein. Dietary restriction of protein may be necessary for individuals having liver or kidney disorders. The National Research Council's Committee on Diet and Health has recommended that protein intake should not exceed twice the Recommended Dietary Allowance.

PROTEIN CONSUMPTION HABITS

In Western countries, people generally consume more high-quality protein than they require. According to NHANESIII data for 1988–91 the median daily protein intakes of men and women, 20 to 59 years old, in the United States are 94 and 64 g, respectively. These median intakes of protein are equivalent to 14.7 and 14.6% of kcal. Median protein intakes of other age–sex groups over a year of age ranged from 12.9 to 16.3% of kcal. Median protein intakes of all age–sex groups were well above the 1989 RDAs, but less than twice the 1989 RDAs.

Third-world people more often than not consume inadequate amounts of protein, which is often the lower-quality protein provided by vegetables and cereal grains containing limited amounts of the essential amino acids lysine and methionine. With world population continuing to grow at disconcerting rates, future droughts, floods, and political disruptions will probably lead to increasing incidences of PEM in the world as has been observed mostly in Africa and presently in North Korea.

Micronutrients:
The Catalysts

CHAPTER 5

Vitamins

Vitamins are organic substances needed in very small amounts for normal functioning of the body that must be provided in the diet. Throughout history, in certain places at certain times, people have suffered not always from a lack of food but from a dietary lack of certain nutrients. Populations of the ancient world were frequently susceptible to the dietary absences and deficiencies of the organic factors the body needed but was not receiving. We know these organic dietary factors today as the vitamins. The lack of these dietary organic factors, vitamin-deficiency diseases, were known to the ancient Chinese and Greeks; the Crusaders of the Middle Ages; the seafaring explorers of Portugal, Spain, Italy, and England; the Japanese; and even to Americans living in the South in the 20th century. The lack of vitamins in the diet of peoples have at times no doubt altered the course of history. Many cultures developed dietary and remedial practices to prevent vitamin-deficiency diseases. Such practices have been passed through the generations and are referred to today as traditional medicine, folklore, and "old wives' tales." Within the 20th century modern Western cultures have replaced such seemingly primitive practices with fortified foods available year round, and vitamin supplements, frequently multivitamin–multimineral supplements (Table 5.1).

No specific chemical knowledge of any vitamin was known before 1900, with one interesting exception. Nicotinic acid was first prepared from nicotine in 1867 by C. Huber, though it remained on the chemist's shelf for many years. With the advent of the purification of proteins, carbohydrates, and inorganics, the stage was set for the discovery of the trace essential dietary organic factors. The discovery of these organic dietary factors we now call vitamins is by any historical measure a contemporary event (Table 5.2). Dietary growth factors were initially discovered and separated based on their solubility in oils (fat) or water. In 1911, nicotinic acid was isolated from rice polishings by C. Funk and given to patients with beriberi, but it was found to have no therapeutic effect. Unfortunately, it was not used in treating pellagra until the mid-1940s. By 1920, E. V. McCullum had identified a fat-soluble vitamine A and a water-soluble vitamine B. Ascorbic acid was soon discovered and became vitamine C in a growing vitamine alphabet. In 1912, C. Funk coined the

Table 5.1 Composition of a Multivitamin/Multimineral Supplement

Each Tablet[a] Contains	Unite of Measurement	% DV[b]	Each Tablet Contains	Unit of Measurement	% DV
Vitamin A (40% as Beta Carotene)	5000 IU	100%	Iodine	150 µg	100%
			Magnesium	100 mg	25%
Vitamin C	60 mg	100%	Zinc	15 mg	100%
Vitamin D	400 IU	100%	Copper	2 mg	100%
Vitamin E	30 IU	100%	Potassium	80 mg	2%
Thiamin	1.5 mg	100%	Vitamin K	25 µg	*c
Riboflavin	1.7 mg	100%	Selenium	20 µg	*
Niacinamide	20 mg	100%	Manganese	3.5 mg	*
Vitamin B_6	2 mg	100%	Chromium	65 µg	*
Folic Acid	400 µg	100%	Molybdenum	160 µg	*
Vitamin B_{12}	6 µg	100%	Chloride	72 mg	*
Biotin	30 µg	10%	Nickel	5 µg	*
Pantothenic Acid	10 mg	100%	Tin	10 µg	*
Calcium	162 mg	16%	Silicon	2 mg	*
Iron	18 mg	100%	Vanadium	10 µg	*
Phosphorus	109 mg	11%	Boron	150 µg	*

a Serving size = 1 tablet.
b DV = Daily Value.
c DV not established.

Recommended Intake: Adults — One tablet daily.

Ingredients: Calcium Phosphate, Magnesium Oxide, Calcium Carbonate, Potassium Chloride, Ascorbic Acid (Vit. C), Ferrous Fumurate, Microcrystalline Cellulose, dl-alpha Tocopheryl Acetate (Vit. E), Gelatin, Crospovidone, Niacinamide, Zinc Oxide, Hydroxypropyl Methylcellulose, Calcium Panthothenate, Vitamin A Acetate/Vitamin D, Titanium Dioxide, Manganese Sulfate, Magnesium Stearate, Stearic Acid, Silicon Dioxide, Pyridoxine Hydrochloride (Vit. B_6), Cupric Oxide, Riboflavin (Vit. B_2), Triethyl Citrate, Thiamin Mononitrate (Vit. B_1), Polysorbate 80, Beta Carotene, FD&C Yellow #6, Folic Acid, Sodium Selenate, Potassium Iodide, Chromium Chloride, Sodium Metasilicate, Sodium Molybdate, Borates, Phytonadione (Vit. K) Biotin, Sodium Metavanadate, Stannous Chloride, Nickelous Sulfate and Cyanocobalamin (Vit. B_{12}).

This is an example of a multivitamin/multimineral formulation. The product is Advanced Formula Centrum®. *Source: Centrum Labeling Information for Advanced Formula*. Reproduced by permission of Lederle Laboratories Division of American Cyanamid Company, Pearl River, NY 10965. Copyright © American Cyanamid Company and reprinted with permission.

Table 5.2 Chronology of Vitamin Discoveries by Publication Date

Vitamin	Year of Isolation	Year Synthesized	Human Deficiency Disease
Niacin	1911	1865	pellagra
Thiamin	1926	1936	beriberi
Vitamin C	1928	1933	scurvy
Vitamin A	1931	1947	xerophthalmia, night blindness, dermatitis
Vitamin D	1931	1936	rickets, osteomalacia
Riboflavin	1933	1935	ariboflavinosis
Biotin	1935	1942	—
Vitamin K	1935	1939	antihemorrhagic factor
Vitamin E	1936	1937	—
Vitamin B_6	1938	1939	varied symptoms
Pantothenic acid	1938	1940	—
Folic acid	1941	1946	megaloblastic anemia
Vitamin B_{12}	1948	1973	megaloblastic anemia, pernicious anemia

term "vitamine" to describe the newly discovered growth factors because they were thought to be vital to life and quite mistakenly amines. The term "vitamine" stuck, and with the omission of the "e," deleting the reference to any chemical constituent, the reference to these organic dietary factors as vitamins continues today.

Today, we recognize vitamin C and eight members of the B-complex of vitamins as the dietary essential water-soluble vitamins. Thiamin, vitamin B_1, was first isolated in 1926, but its chemical structure was not fully elucidated until 1936. As the water-soluble vitamins were identified as individual dietary factors, each was designated with a subscript numeral — B_1, B_2, and so on — following a convention introduced by the British. Along the way of vitamin discoveries, compounds once believed to be water-soluble vitamins and so designated were later found not to be vitamins at all. Examples include p-aminobenzoic acid, inositol, lipoic acid, vitamins P (for permeability) and M (for monkey), and coenzyme Q (ubiquinone). Even pangamic acid and laetrile have been incorrectly designated as water-soluble vitamins B_{15} and B_{17}, for which no vitamin function is known.

FAT-SOLUBLE AND WATER-SOLUBLE VITAMINS

From early research, beginning with the identification of a fat-soluble growth factor in milk (vitamin A), four fat-soluble factors have now been identified as the vitamins A, D, E, and K. These vitamins possess characteristics which, in addition to their solubility, are much different from those of the water-soluble vitamins. The water-soluble vitamins are vitamin C and B-complex vitamins or B-vitamins. The B-vitamins are thiamin, riboflavin, niacin, vitamin B_6, folacin, vitamin B_{12}, pantothenic acid, and biotin. The water-soluble B vitamins all function as coenzymes in enzyme systems, are required in the diet, do not exhibit appreciable tissue storage, and are relatively nontoxic except at quite high dietary levels. Deficiencies of water-soluble vitamins can develop rather rapidly. The water-soluble vitamins are also more labile than those which are fat-soluble, meaning that there is generally greater loss of water-soluble vitamins during food preparation. In contrast, fat-soluble vitamins, with the possible exception of vitamin K, are not known to function like the classical coenzymes. Most of the fat-soluble vitamins and other antioxidants are absorbed with lipids in the small intestine with bile and pancreatic secretions required for efficient absorption. Provitamin D, 7-dehydrocholesterol, is synthesized in the skin and is converted to vitamin D in the presence of adequate sunshine. Vitamin E functions as an antioxidant; other antioxidants can act synergistically with vitamin E with regard to much of its functioning. Vitamin K is synthesized by the intestinal flora of mammals and absorbed from the human intestinal tract. Biotin, likewise, is synthesized by the intestinal microflora and absorbed by the human intestinal tract. Fat-soluble vitamins are stored in the lipid components of adipose tissue, liver, and cell membranes. When ingested in large amounts, fat-soluble vitamins A and D can be quite toxic, as they will continuously accumulate in lipids of liver and adipose tissues. Deficiencies of fat-soluble vitamins are slow to develop due to this significant storage in tissues.

Some of the vitamins have known pharmacologic functions. Niacin may lower serum total cholesterol and triglycerides and raise HDL cholesterol levels when taken in excess of 1200 mg daily. Pharmacologic doses (25 to 100 mg/day) of vitamin B_6 may be of benefit in the treatment of mental diseases. Some people have overdosed on vitamins, and toxicities were thus noted. For many of the vitamins, optimal, pharmacologic, and toxic intake levels are known to exist.

The concentration of serum homocysteine has been associated with the incidence of coronary heart disease. Folate, vitamin B_6, and vitamin B_{12} function with relation to homocysteine metabolism. Hence, a deficiency of any of these three vitamins could possibly increase the incidence of coronary heart disease. Cysteine by itself seemingly is not able to act as a redox catalyst, but homocysteine appears to do so, generating free radicals.

VITAMINS AS COENZYMES

All B vitamins, many nonvitamin organic factors (e.g., lipoic acid and ubiquinone), and minerals function as coenzymes, cofactors, and prosthetic groups in enzyme systems (also called holoenzymes). Unlike enzymes, which do not participate directly in biological reactions but affect the rates of reactions, coenzymes participate in the reactions directly and are required for catalysis to occur. Most enzymes are of moderate to large molecular weight, but in comparison, coenzymes are of very small molecular weight. Most coenzymes are found loosely bound to enzymes, with others being covalently bound to enzymes. All enzymes act catalytically on substrates to produce products. In Figure 5.1, an enzyme (E) combines

$$\text{E} + \text{S} \xrightarrow{\text{association}} [\text{E} - \text{S}] \xrightarrow{\text{dissociation}} \text{E} + \text{P}$$

Figure 5.1 Enzyme catalysis without coenzyme.

Enzyme–coenzyme (vitamin) catalysis.

$$E + Co\text{-}E \xrightarrow{\text{association 1}} [E\text{-}Co\text{-}E] + S \xrightarrow{\text{association 2}} [E\text{-}Co\text{-}E\text{-}S] \xrightarrow{\text{dissociation 1}}$$
$$P + [E\text{-}Co\text{-}E] \xrightarrow{\text{dissociation 2}} E + Co\text{-}E$$

Figure 5.2 Enzyme reaction requiring coenzyme.

with its substrate (S) at the active site to form a transient enzyme–substrate (E–S) association complex. Catalysis occurs within this (E–S) complex, resulting in dissociation of a product(s), renewing the enzyme for further catalysis. In enzyme reactions that require coenzymes (Figure 5.2), the enzyme (E) must first combine with the coenzyme (Co–E), as in association 1, to complete the structural integrity of the active site of the enzyme for the binding of the substrate (association 2).

The enzyme–coenzyme–substrate complex (E–Co–E–S) is functionally analogous to the (E–S) complex of Equation 5.1. A product(s) is (are) produced from this complex (dissociation 1); the (E–Co–E) complex may recycle and combine with another substrate molecule (S) or dissociate as in dissociation 2. In enzymatic reactions requiring coenzymes, the reactions do not take place without participation of the coenzyme in a continuous recycling manner.

Some vitamins function without biochemical modification. Other vitamins, however, have to be converted by the body into their metabolically active form(s), while other vitamins serve as components of even larger coenzymes. The vitamins are presented in Table 5.2 in chronological order of their published discovery, accounting for the lack of a strict alphabetical listing. Each of the vitamins will be discussed, beginning with the fat-soluble vitamins and followed by those which are water soluble.

VITAMIN A

Name: Retinoids
Active form: Retinol, retinal, retinoic acid
Function: Weak antioxidant, visual cofactor, growth, immunity
Activity: 1 RE =1 μg all-trans retinol
        6 μg all-trans β-carotene
        12 μg other provitamin A carotenoids
        3.33 IU vitamin activity from retinol
        10 IU vitamin activity from β-carotene
Precursor: β-carotene and some other carotenoids (mostly β-carotene)

Vitamin A, as one may guess, was the "first" fat-soluble vitamin to be recognized, and it was first separated by E. V. McCollum in 1920. McCollum was later to discover that his vitamin A also contained another lipid-soluble factor, vitamin D.

Forms of the Vitamin

Both retinoids and carotenoids have vitamin A activity. The retinoids are also known as previtamin A. About 50 of the 600 characterized carotenoids, including β-carotene, are known as provitamin A compounds or vitamin A precursors, as they can be converted to vitamin A, if needed, by the body. Some of the retinoids and β-carotene are shown in Figure 5.3. Retinoids are consumed in foods as retinyl esters of fatty acids, usually palmitate (retinyl palmitate), in which the ester stabilizes the molecule from peroxidation. Retinoids are digested and absorbed in association with lipids, with bile and pancreatic secretions and the presence of antioxidants increasing absorption efficiency. Retinol is the major circulating retinoid, and is carried by the retinol-binding protein (RBP) and as transthyretin or thyroxine-binding prealbumin. Retinal (formerly known as retinene) functions in vision. Retinoic acid, the excretory form of retinoids, can function in tissue growth and healing. Retinoids are stored, primarily in the liver, as retinyl esters along with lipids. Carotenoids are converted to retinol, if needed, in the small intestine and liver via a dioxygenase reaction. One molecule of β-carotene is converted *in vivo* to one molecule of retinol. β-carotene is the most potent and prevalent form of provitamin A, with approximately one in six molecules ultimately being converted to retinol as shown in Figure 5.4.

Functions

The best known function for vitamin A is its role as a coenzyme with the protein opsin, found in rods and cones, the photoreceptor cells of the eye (Equation 5.1). The visual protein pigments, rhodopsin (rods), responsible for low light vision, and iodopsin (cones), responsible for color and bright light vision, both contain retinol (as 11-*cis*-retinal). Rhodopsin and iodopsin are the visual pigments of the eye, which in the presence of light are "bleached." Bleaching results in the conversion of vitamin A to the all-trans retinal by light energy, release of opsin, and the interruption of optic nerve electric impulses by Ca^{2+} (dark current), which are amplified and interpreted by the visual center of the brain as light (Figure 5.5). Both niacin and riboflavin have coenzyme redox functions in the vitamin A visual cycle.

Vitamin A is required for normal growth of epithelial tissues (eyes, skin, respiratory tract, digestive tract, urogenital tract) and skeletal tissues, affecting protein synthesis, bone cell differentiation, and enamel formation. Vitamin A also functions in mucopolysaccharide synthesis, including that of mucus which lubricates the linings of all body openings. Vitamin A plays an important role in reproduction and immune functioning (see Chapter 15).

Vitamin A is a weak fat-soluble antioxidant. High plasma levels of retinoids are associated with a decreased incidence of chronic diseases, particularly coronary heart disease and epithelial cancers. A high correlation exists between high blood levels of both nutritionally active and inactive carotenoids and decreased incidence of chronic disease. Most of these associations have been observed in epidemiological studies. It may be that the carotenoids and retinoids have protective effects in reducing oxidative effects, and thus decreasing the risk of chronic disease.

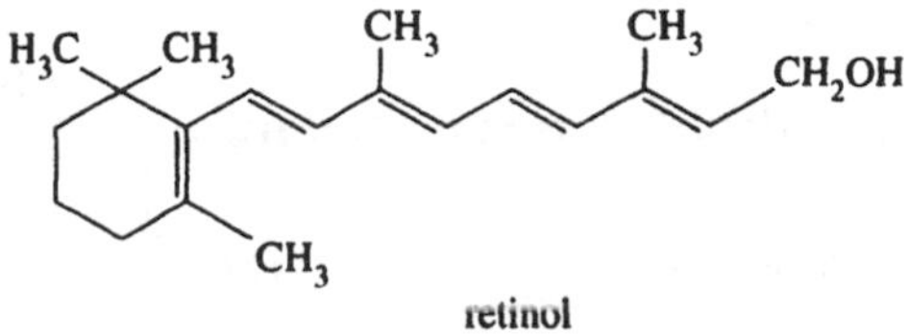

retinol

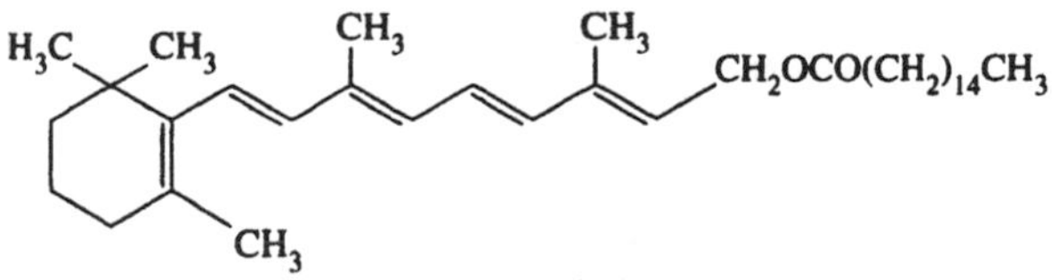

retinyl palmitate

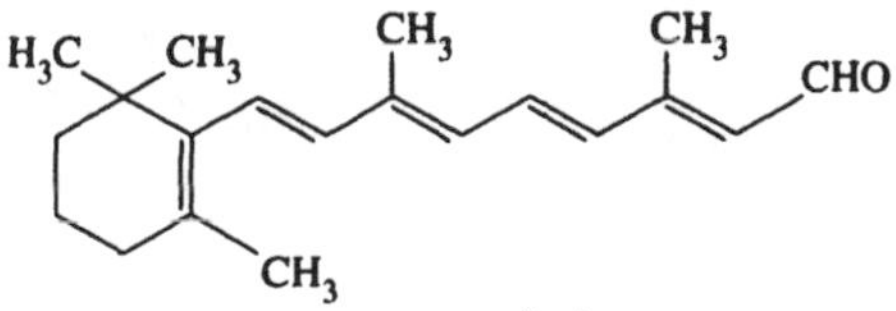

retinal

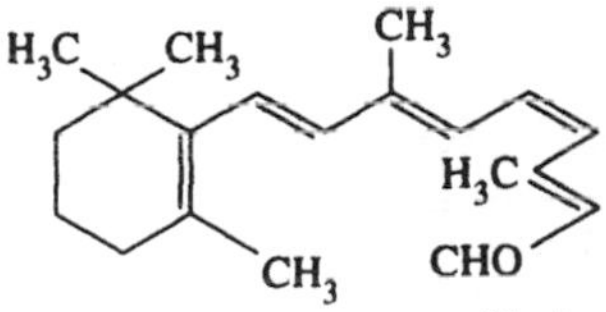

11-*cis*-retinal

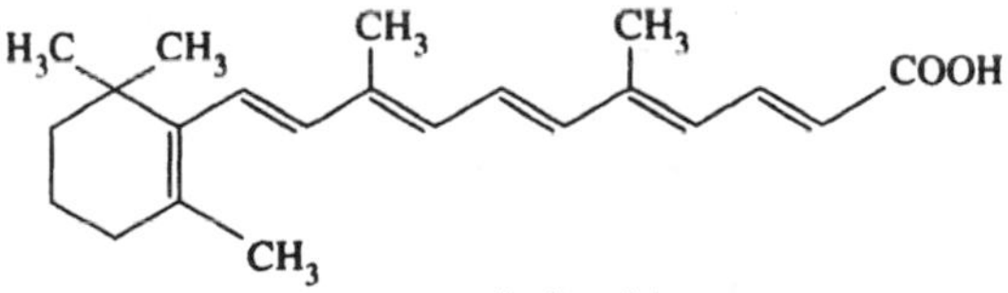

retinoic acid

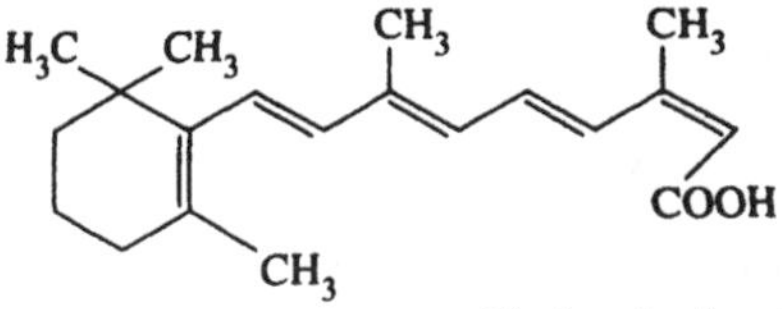

13-*cis*-retinoic acid

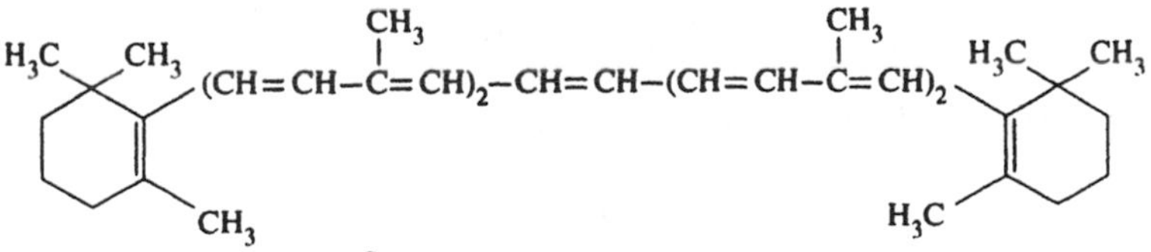

β-carotene

Figure 5.3 Vitamin A (retinol), retinoids, and β-carotene.

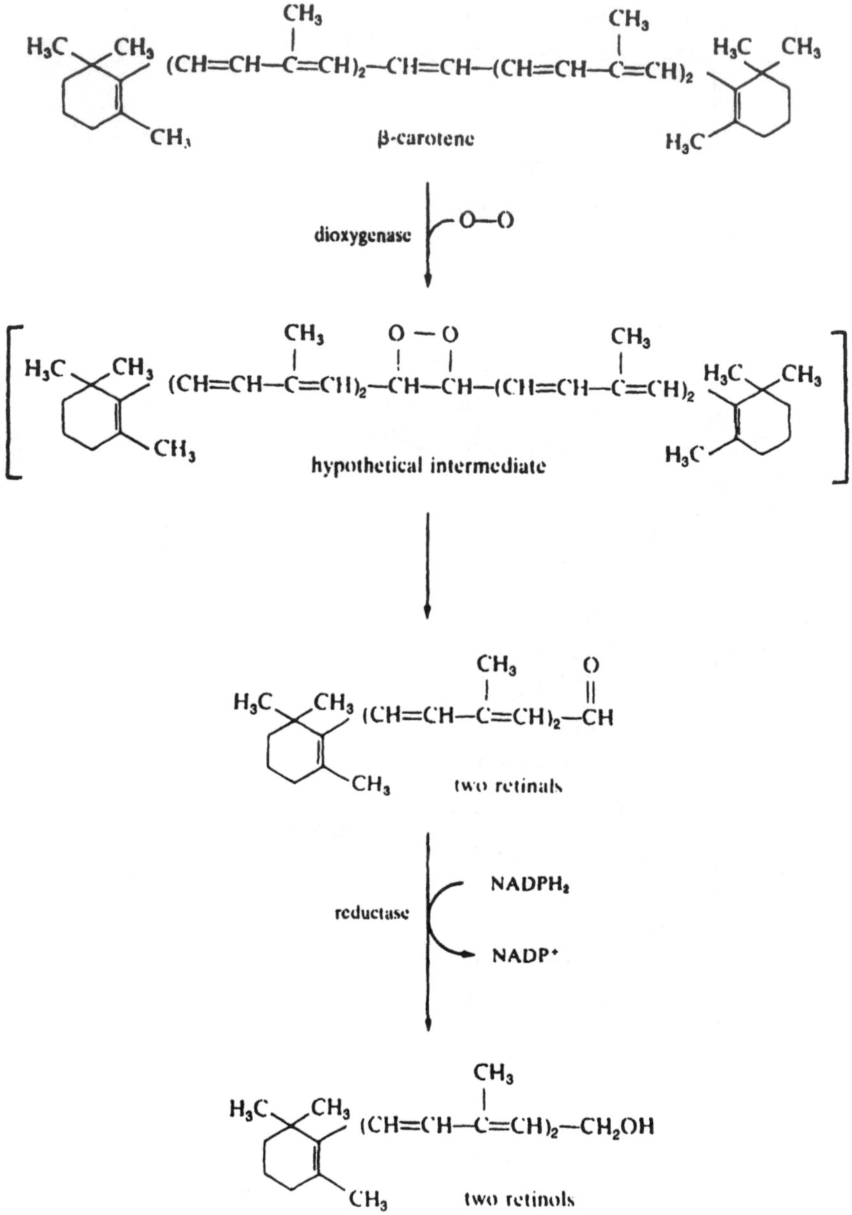

Figure 5.4 Scission of β-carotene by dioxygenase.

$$\text{11-}cis\text{-retinal}-\overset{\overset{\textstyle O}{\|}}{C}-\underset{\underset{\textstyle H}{|}}{N}-(CH_2)_4\text{-opsin.}$$

Equation 5.1 Vitamin A as it functions in vision.

Food Sources

Preformed vitamin A is found only in animal foods, particularly organ meats, egg yolks, and fortified food products. Non-fat and low-fat dairy products are frequently fortified with retinoids. Carotenoids are found in dark green, leafy vegetables and yellowish-orange fruits and vegetables. Individuals living in the United States generally get about a quarter of their vitamin A from carotenoids; however, individuals in developing countries get most of their vitamin A from the conversion of carotenoids into retinol. Retinoids and carotenoids are relatively stable in common food preparation procedures, but somewhat sensitive to oxidation.

Dietary Recommendations

The recommendations of the National Research Council for vitamin A intakes are given in retinol equivalents (RE) as µg. The 1989 RDA for men and women is 1000 and 800 RE, respectively. The different forms of the retinoids and carotenoids have different vitamin A activities, with retinoids having higher potencies than carotenoids. Commercial vitamin A supplements are used fairly extensively by the American public. According to NHANESIII, the median vitamin A intakes of men and women, 20 to 59 years, in the United States are 739 and 581 RE, respectively. These intakes are below 1989 RDA levels, but the incidence of this population having low serum vitamin A levels was low.

Deficiency

Symptoms characteristic of early vitamin A deficiency include reduced appetite, weight loss, skin disorders, decreased mucus production, and follicular hyperkeratosis, a hardening of the skin around the hair follicle. Night blindness, a vitamin A deficiency disease, was recognized and treated by the ancient Chinese, the early Egyptians, and even Hippocrates himself. A more severe vitamin A deficiency can lead to xerophthalmia (dry eye) and if untreated, permanent blindness. Xerophthalmia among children of Southeast Asia remains an almost permanent contemporary problem. Vitamin A deficient individuals characteristically have Bitot's spots, foamy spots on the eyes. Depressed growth and decreased immune function are observed in vitamin A deficient individuals. Vitamin A is transported in the blood by proteins; thus, vitamin A status is influenced by protein deficiency. Vitamin A deficiency is usually associated with PEM, low fat intake and malabsorption, gastrointestinal distress, and respiratory disease. Although rare in the United States, vitamin A deficiency is the most prevalent nutrient deficiency worldwide, and resulting blindness and death are relatively common. Vitamin A status is usually evaluated by measuring plasma levels of the vitamin, which sometimes includes β-carotene.

Pharmacologic Doses

Large oral doses (~60 mg 1 to 3 times yearly) of retinoids have been used prophylactically in infants and children in developing countries where vitamin A

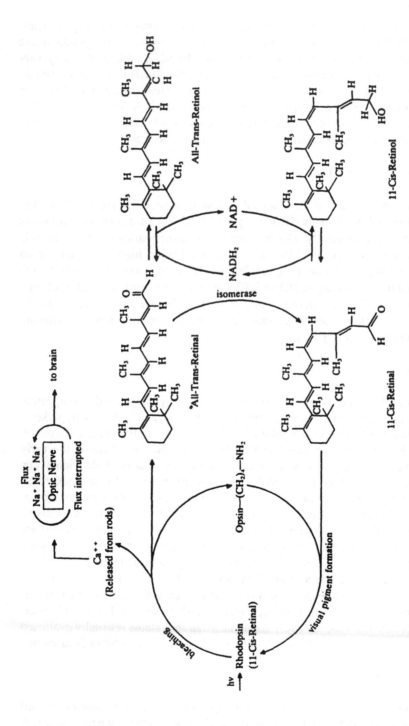

Figure 5.5   Vitamin A in the visual cycle. Release of all-*trans*-retinal from rhodopsin causes Ca^{2+} to be released from rods interrupting a continuous flux of Na$^+$ within the optic nerve. The interruption of Na$^+$ flux is interpreted by the brain as vision by the pattern of rods and/or cones so affected by light (*hν*). Rhodopsin is regenerated from retinal, retinol, or hydrolysis of retinyl esters.

deficiency is prevalent. Many retinoids have been used with some efficacy in treating severe acne and other skin disorders and some types of cancer. RetinA® may be of benefit in the treatment of some skin disorders. In that high doses of retinoids are generally required for maximal effectiveness, toxic effects are frequent.

Toxicity

Vitamin A toxicity symptoms are variable but may include headache, insomnia, dry skin, loss of hair, dryness and fissuring of lips, menstrual irregularities, weight loss, bone abnormalities, spontaneous abortions, birth defects, and hepatomegaly. Hypervitaminosis A may also adversely affect the rods and cones in the eyes. Toxicity occurs with sustained daily intakes, from foods and supplements, exceeding about 6,000 RE daily in infants and young children and 15,000 RE daily in adults. Hypervitaminosis A is reversible in its early stages.

Carotenoids are relatively nontoxic when consumed in large quantities, partially because of their reduced absorption efficiency. However, carotenoids are absorbed well enough to produce orangish-yellow adipose tissues, including subcutaneous tissues. Hypercarotenosis results in yellowish skin, palms of hands, and soles of feet. The yellowish color disappears when high intake is discontinued.

VITAMIN D

Name: Calciferol
Active form: 1,25-$(OH)_2$ D and 24,25-$(OH)_2$ D
Function: Facilitates utilization of calcium and phosphorus, insulin secretion, cell differentiation, immunity, skin cell development
Activity: 1 µg D_2 or D_3 = 40 IU
Precursor: 7-dehydrocholesterol

Vitamin D is known as the antirachitic vitamin. Vitamin D deficiency is the cause of rickets, a crippling disease of children. In adults, vitamin D deficiency is expressed as osteomalacia. These diseases have been a scourge on humankind throughout history. Especially plagued with the disease have been those people living in the northernmost latitudes of Europe, Asia, and North America. The Industrial Revolution and its extensive use of coal added to the number of cases of rickets in both Europe and the United States. Vitamin D is not a vitamin at all in the classic sense of dietary need and coenzyme function. Vitamin D is a vitamin–hormone produced in the skin of people in amounts adequate to prevent rickets and osteomalacia when exposed directly to the ultraviolet light of the sun. Those factors necessary to produce rickets and osteomalacia were all present for people living in northern latitudes in cities of the Industrial Revolution. Long winters, indoor confinement, overcast skies, heavy clothing, and polluted cities all contributed to reduced ultraviolet light exposure and vitamin D synthesis. Such environmental circumstances were compounded by the lack of significant vitamin D in the diet. Vitamin D is a vitamin in the classic sense as a result of environmental life-style.

In the early part of this century, E. Mellanby produced and then cured rickets with cod-liver oil in dogs. E. V. McCollum in 1922 found the antirachitic factor in cod-liver oil not to be vitamin A, and named the fat-soluble substance vitamin D. The ultraviolet light conversion of fat-soluble factors into vitamin D came into practice and was made possible by H. Steenbock and A. Black in 1924. Their discovery followed the 1919 observations of K. Huldskinsky, who was curing rachitic children with ultraviolet light. A U.S. patent (1,680,818) covering the irradiation of ergosterol for the synthesis of vitamin D was issued in 1928 to the University of Wisconsin.

Forms of the Vitamin

The precursors of vitamin D are ergosterol in plants and 7-dehydrocholesterol in the skin of animals and humans, these compounds having chemical structures nearly identical to cholesterol. In the presence of ultraviolet light, ergosterol is converted into vitamin D_2 in plants and 7-dehydrocholesterol into vitamin D_3 in animals (Figure 5.6). As shown in Figure 5.6, ultraviolet light results in the scission of the β-sterol ring. The chemical structures of vitamins D_2 and D_3 differ only with respect to unsaturation occurring between C_{22} and C_{23} in ergosterol. Vitamins D_2 and D_3 have equivalent vitamin D potency, and both forms are used in supplements. The absorption of dietary vitamin D is enhanced by the presence of dietary lipids and the secretion of bile. Vitamin D from the skin or intestine is carried in the blood by a vitamin D–binding protein. Vitamin D is stored in the liver, skin, muscles, and adipose tissues.

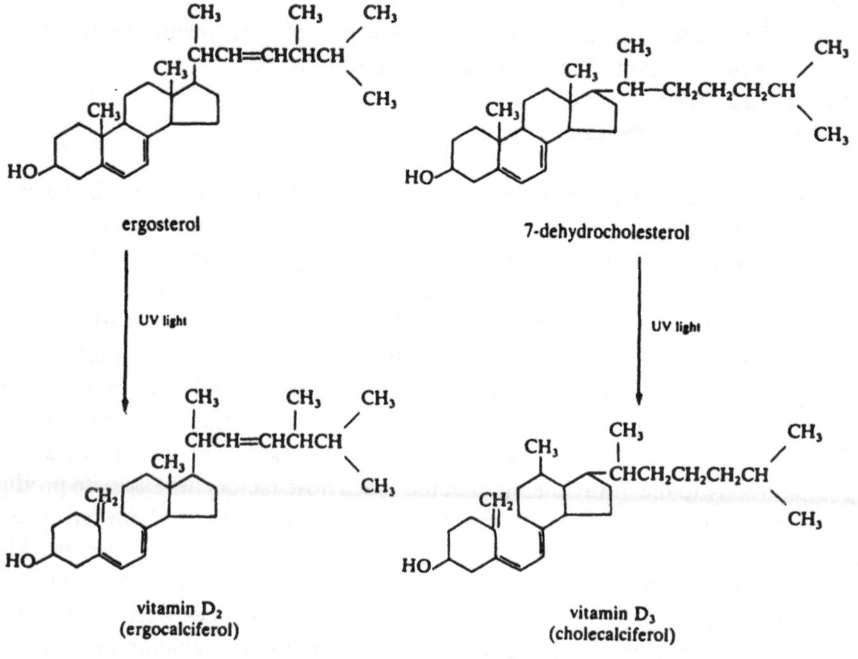

Figure 5.6 Ultraviolet conversion of provitamins D_2 and D_3.

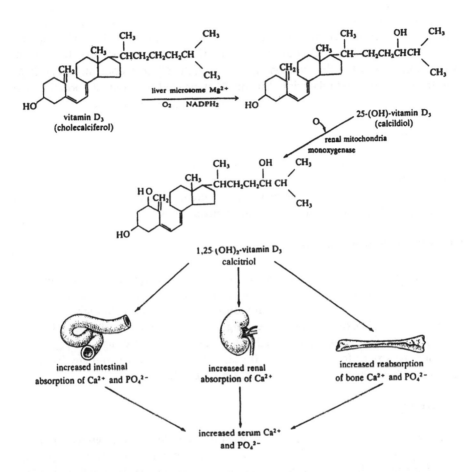

Figure 5.7 Metabolism of vitamin D₃.

Vitamins D₂ and D₃ are prohormones to the active vitamin derivative which is a hormone. In a series of brilliant experiments by J. Lund and H. F. Deluca, beginning in 1966, the metabolism of vitamin D began to unfold. Following dietary absorption of vitamin D₂ or D₃ or synthesis of vitamin D₃ in the skin, vitamins D₂ and D₃ in mammals are hydroxylated in the liver by enzymes requiring molecular oxygen, Mg^{2+}, and niacin (as NADPH₂), producing 25-(OH)-vitamin D, often referred to as 25(OH)D. The 25(OH)D, transported by the α-globulin from the liver to the kidney, undergoes a second renal hydroxylation by a mixed-function oxygenase to yield 1,25(OH)₂D, calcitriol, and 24,25(OH)₂D (Figure 5.7). 1,25(OH)₂D is the most active form of vitamin D, but 24,25(OH)₂D does have some vitamin D activity.

Function

Vitamin D, as 1,25(OH)₂D, along with the parathyroid hormone (PTH) functions in the regulation of mineral homeostasis, particularly that of calcium and phosphorus, by its influence on the intestines, kidneys, bones, and parathyroid glands. $24,25(OH)_2D$ is known to increase absorption of calcium, phosphorus, and perhaps other bone minerals. Serum levels of calcium and phosphorus effectively regulate $1,25(OH)_2D$ and $24,25(OH)_2D$ synthesis. $1,25(OH)_2D$ is also essential for normal insulin secretion, cell differentiation, immunity, skin cell development, and perhaps muscle contraction and relaxation. Vitamin D is needed to maintain normal serum calcium levels by increasing calcium absorption from the duodenum.

Food Sources

With the exception of fatty fish and fish liver oils, the amount of vitamin D present in unfortified foods is small and variable. Most dairy products and margarines are fortified with vitamin D as are many of the cereals and chocolate mixes. Vitamin D is quite stable to various food preparation procedures.

Dietary Recommendations

An individual whose skin is exposed to sufficient sunlight is able to synthesize sufficient vitamin D to meet needs. In that many individuals in the United States are not exposed to much light, especially during certain seasons of the year, dietary need for vitamin D exists for those spending inadequate amounts of time in the sun. The 1997 Adequate Intake (AI) for individuals up to 50 years of age is 5 μg, or 200 IU, daily. AI values for adults 51 to 70 years of age for the vitamin are 10 μg per day, while those for adults over 70 years are 15 μg daily.

Deficiency

Rickets is the vitamin D deficiency disease in children, and osteomalacia is the deficiency disease in adults. Without vitamin D, calcium, phosphorus and perhaps other bone minerals are not deposited in the collagenous matrix of bones. Rachitic bones are unable to support the body and withstand weight. Bowlegs, knock-knees, enlarged joints, curvature of the spine, pigeon breast, and frontal bossing of the skull result. There is also inadequate mineralization of tooth dentin and enamel. Deformities of the chest, pelvis, spine, and limbs and even bone fractures are seen in osteomalacia, where there is an inability of reabsorbed bone to recalcify. Vitamin D deficiency is rare in the United States today, primarily due to the fortification of dairy products with the vitamin. However, rickets and osteomalacia are still observed worldwide.

Vitamin D status may be evaluated by quantitating the various forms of the vitamin in plasma or indirectly and more frequently evaluated by measuring serum calcium concentrations. Vitamin D status may also be evaluated by quantitating plasma alkaline phosphatase activity.

Pharmacologic Doses

In that toxicities of vitamin D have been observed at relative low doses (~40 μg daily), vitamins D_2 and D_3 are not utilized therapeutically. Individuals with bone diseases due to bone, kidney, or parathyroid malfunctioning have been successfully treated with 25(OH)D and 1,25(OH)$_2$D. These individuals are unable to synthesize 25(OH)D or 1,25(OH)$_2$D. The 1997 Tolerable Upper Intake Level for vitamin D for adults is 50 μg or 2,000 IU daily.

Toxicity

Vitamin D toxicity is a serious consequence of excessive vitamin intake. Early symptoms include nausea, vomiting, excessive thirst and urination, muscular weakness, and joint pain. Consequences of severe hypervitaminosis D include hypercalcemia and hypercalciuria, with death possible from irreversible calcification of the heart, lungs, major arteries, and kidneys. It is not possible to get hypervitaminosis D by overexposure to sunlight.

VITAMIN E

Name: Tocopherols and tocotrienols
Active form: α-, β-, γ-, and δ-tocopherols and tocotrienols
Function: Lipid-soluble antioxidant
Activity: 1 RE =1 mg d-α-tocopherol
2 mg β-tocopherol
10 mg γ-tocopherol
3.34 mg α-tocotrienol
1.49 IU

Vitamin E was recognized and named by H. Evans in 1925 as the fertility factor that prevented reproductive failure in female rats fed a rancid diet and whole wheat. Present in the oil of the wheat germ was vitamin E. Isolated as a pale yellow oil, and identified structurally in 1938 by E. J. Fernholz, vitamin E was found to be a derivative of tocol and was named α-tocopherol, meaning childbirth (*tokos*, Greek) and to carry or bear (*pherin*), in that it was required for pregnant rats to bear young. It is also required for reproduction in male rats.

Forms of the Vitamin

Eight compounds have been isolated that have vitamin E activity; these are α-, β-, γ- and δ-tocopherols and tocotrienols (Figure 5.8). The most active form of vitamin E is d-α-tocopherol. In plants and seeds (oils) α-tocopherol may constitute only 10 to 15% of the total tocopherols, but in animals and fish, α-tocopherol normally accounts for >90% of all tocopherols. The various forms of the vitamin have different amounts of vitamin E activity. Commercial tocopherols are stabilized and supplied as either the acetate or succinate esters. Absorption of dietary tocopherols is about 20 to 40%, and is facilitated by lipids, bile, and pancreatic secretions. Absorbed into the lymph and subsequently the blood, vitamin E circulates with all the lipoproteins and membranes of erythrocytes. In general, vitamin E penetrates

Structure	Common name	Biological activity in international units per milligram
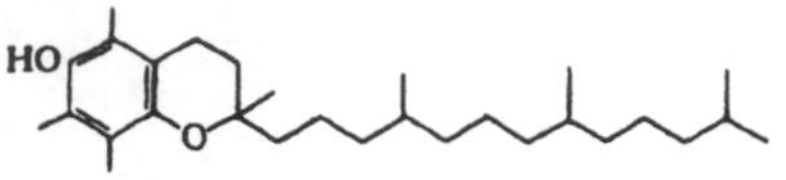	d-α-tocopherol (5,7,8 trimethyltocol)	1.49
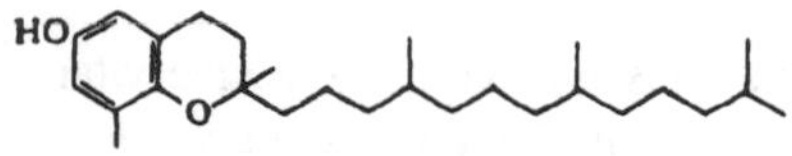	d-β-tocopherol	0.75
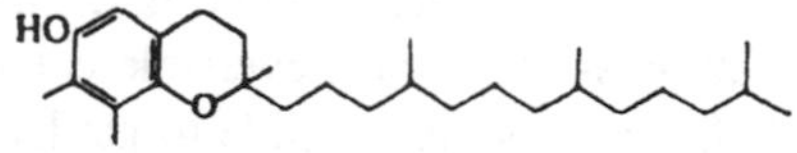	d-γ-tocopherol	0.15
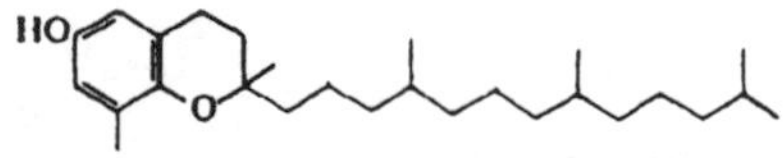	d-δ-tocopherol	0.05
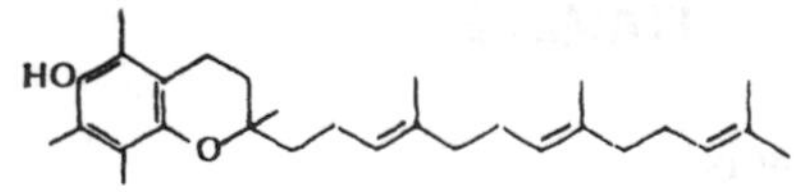	d-α-tocotrienol	0.45
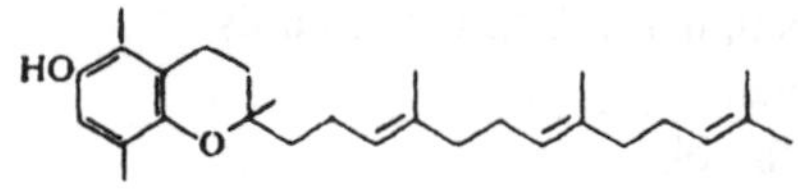	d-β-tocotrienol	Not determined
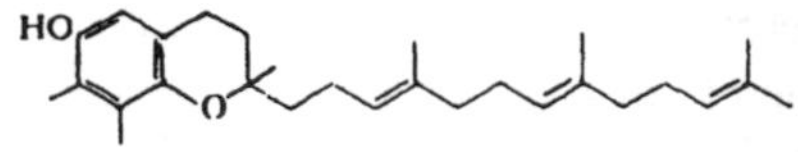	d-γ-tocotrienol	Not determined
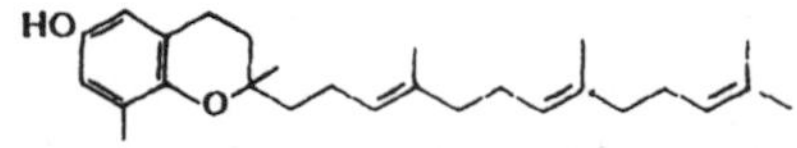	d-δ-tocotrienol	Not determined
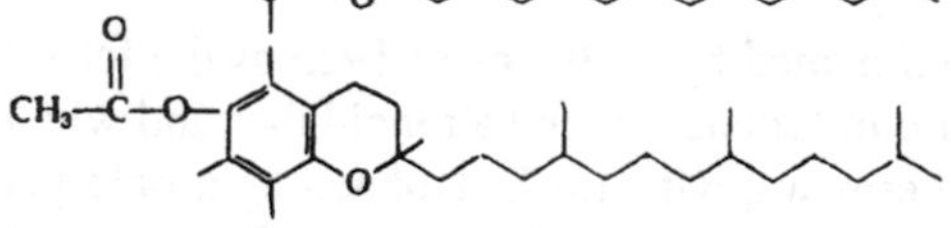	d-α-tocopherol acetate	1.36
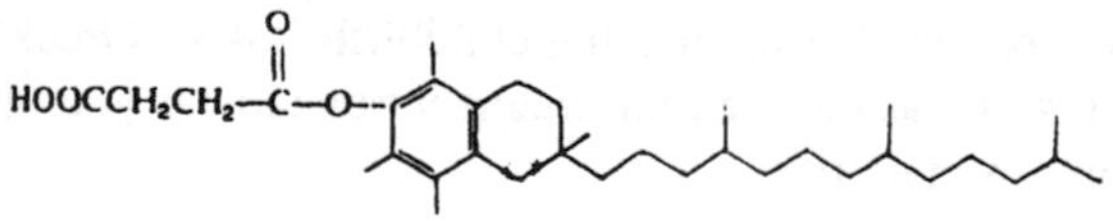	d-α-tocopherol succinate	1.21

Figure 5.8 Natural and synthetic occurring forms of vitamin E.

and is found associated with the lipid fraction of cells and membranes. Its concentration is particularly high in association with adipose tissue, adrenals, liver, and muscle tissues.

Function

The only function attributed to vitamin E is its role as an antioxidant (see Chapter 15). Vitamin E protects unsaturated lipid components of cells from free-radical attack by itself becoming oxidized. Vitamin E is found in cellular membranes and subcellular membranes associated with polyunsaturated fatty acids. Vitamin E is probably the body's major defense against potentially harmful oxidations. Vitamin C, β-carotene, and selenium frequently function with vitamin E as antioxidants. Vitamin E also protects the skeletal muscles, nervous system, and ocular retina from oxidation via its functioning as an antioxidant. Vitamin E, a potent fat-soluble antioxidant, protects circulating LDL and lipoprotein membranes in the various kinds of tissues from oxidation. Male and female rats need vitamin E for reproduction. There is no evidence to relate malfunction of the reproductive process in humans with an increased need for vitamin E.

Vitamin E is essential for normal immune function. High plasma levels of vitamin E, particularly α-tocopherol, have been associated with decreased incidence of coronary heart disease and certain cancers. Most of these associations were observed in epidemiological studies, though some were from clinical studies.

Vitamin E may reduce the toxicity of metals, particular iron and lead, likely owing to its antioxidant properties. Vitamin E may also protect against environmental pollutants such as ozone, and effects of tobacco usage. Vitamin E is also protective against the hepatotoxicity of alcohol and certain drugs. Toxic minerals, air pollution, smoke, alcohol, and some drugs all produce free radicals (see Chapter 15).

Vitamin E affects arachidonic and prostaglandin metabolism. Several, but not all, studies indicate that vitamin E inhibits platelet aggregation. The suggestion has been made that vitamin E may serve as a repressor for the synthesis of some enzymes and may serve as an electron acceptor in the electron transport chain. Vitamin E may be performing these functions as an antioxidant, or perhaps the vitamin has other functions yet to be discovered.

Food Sources

The richest food sources of vitamin E are vegetable oils and food products containing vegetable oils. Nuts, wheat germ, and seeds also are rich sources of vitamin E. Frequently as much as half of the vitamin E in a food is lost during food processing and cooking as it is particularly susceptible to destruction by oxygen, light, and extended use of oils in deep-frying.

Dietary Recommendation

The requirement for vitamin E is dependent on the quantity of polyunsaturated fatty acids consumed, with the ratio of 0.4 mg d-α-tocopherol to each gram of polyunsaturated lipids being recommended as adequate. The 1989 RDA for vitamin E for men and women is 10 and 8 mg α-TE (α-tocopherol equivalents), respectively. The various tocopherols and tocotrienols have different vitamin E potencies. Median intakes for adult men and women, 20 to 59 years, reported in NHANESIII were 8.63 and 6.26 mg α-TE, respectively. Median intakes of vitamin E were below 1989 RDA values for people 1 year of age and older. Many individuals, particularly older adults, in the United States take supplements containing vitamin E.

Deficiency

Rats made dietarily deficient of both vitamin E and the trace element selenium are subject to liver necrosis and death from oxidative stress and lipid peroxidation. In other animal species, conditions attributed to vitamin E deficiency included muscular myopathies, accumulation of tissue lipofusin pigments, anemia, hemolysis, cataracts, and retinal degeneration. Vitamin E deficiency in humans occurs in PEM and in individuals with lipid malabsorption problems and abetalipoproteinemia. Vitamin E status is clinically evaluated indirectly by measuring erythrocyte hemolysis. Vitamin E status is generally assessed by quantitating the amount of the individual or combined forms of the vitamin in plasma or serum. Research laboratories frequently quantitate plasma levels of the individual forms of the vitamin. Accepted criteria for their interpretation have not been agreed upon. Newborn infants have low reserves of vitamin E as the vitamin does not cross the placenta during pregnancy. Symptoms of vitamin E deficiency observed in these infants include a hemolytic anemia, thrombocytosis, retinopathy, and occasional edema. Vitamin E deficiency occurs in about half the children with chronic cholestasis, and may also be found in children with neuromuscular disorders. Vitamin E deficiency symptoms reported in adults include abnormalities of the nervous system eventually affecting the muscles and the retina. Recently, low-normal vitamin E status has been associated with an increased risk of atherosclerosis, cancer, cataract formation, and other diseases associated with aging.

Pharmacologic Doses

Several diseases have been reported to be responsive to the administration of large doses of vitamin E. Much of the evidence is anecdotal or from poorly controlled and short-term studies. Large supplements of vitamin E (200 to 800 IU/day) appear to be beneficial with regard to intermittent claudication and various infectious and chronic diseases in humans. The evidence from epidemiological studies and a limited number of clinical studies in older people, suggests that large doses of vitamin E may be beneficial in decreasing the risk of coronary heart disease, certain cancers, and cataracts, as well as perhaps being useful in reducing exercise-induced oxidative stress in muscle tissues.

Toxicity

Vitamin E taken orally is relatively nontoxic. Large intakes of vitamin E may exacerbate the coagulation defect of vitamin K deficiency, adversely affect individuals taking anticoagulant therapy, decrease the absorption of vitamin A, and increase the quantity of iron needed for a hematologic response in anemic individuals.

VITAMIN K

Name: Phylloquinone, menaquinone, menadione
Active form: Unknown

Function: Cofactor in carboxylations of blood coagulation factors II, VII, IX, and X
Note: Form of vitamin synthesized by intestinal microflora

Vitamin K was the first of a series of fat-soluble compounds derived from 2-methyl-1,4-naphthoquinone to be isolated and identified by E. A. Doisy in 1939. The vitamin had earlier been observed as an unidentifiable lipid-soluble factor that produced hemorrhaging in chicks fed a fat-free diet. This lipid-soluble factor present in plants was recognized in 1935 by H. Dam and named vitamin K after the Dutch word *koagulation*. In 1939, Dam isolated vitamin K from alfalfa.

Forms of the Vitamin

Formulas for the three forms of vitamin K are given in Figure 5.9. Phylloquinone (vitamin K_1) is the form of the vitamin found in green plants. Menaquinone (vitamin K_2) is the form of the vitamin synthesized by bacteria in the intestinal microflora. This bacterially synthesized form of vitamin K is absorbed by humans and other monogastric animals excluding chicks. Humans get about half of their vitamin K, ranging from 5 to 95% (large individual differences) via synthesis by the intestinal microflora. Foods from animal sources contain both phylloquinone and menaquinones. Dietary vitamin K is absorbed more efficiently in the presence of lipids, bile, and pancreatic secretions.

Menadione (vitamin K_3) is a synthetic form of the vitamin. Menadione is utilized clinically as a coagulant. Menadione is the most potent form of vitamin K, having about twice the vitamin activity of vitamin K_1. Vitamin K_2 has about 75% of the vitamin activity of vitamin K_1. Phylloquinone is the form of the vitamin generally utilized in supplements.

Coumarins and their derivatives (such as dicumarol), which are used clinically as anticoagulants and warfarin, a rodenticide, are vitamin K antagonists (Figure 5.10). The same is true of certain indandiones and their derivatives. Any drugs that

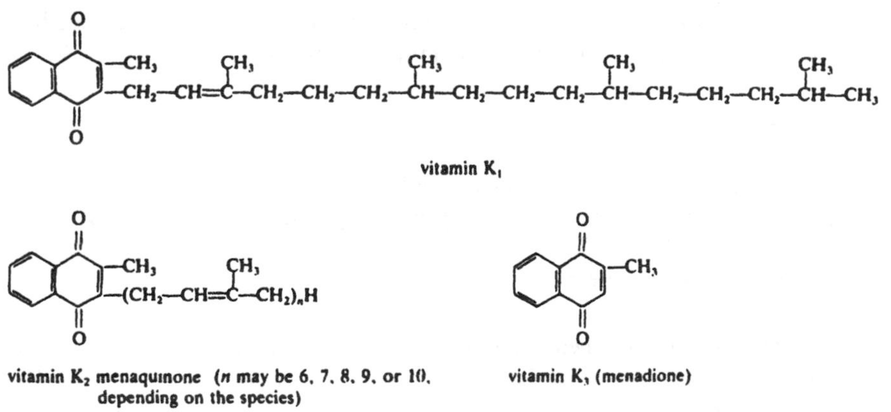

vitamin K_1

vitamin K_2 menaquinone (*n* may be 6, 7, 8, 9, or 10, depending on the species)

vitamin K_3 (menadione)

Figure 5.9 Phylloquinone (vitamin K_1) and analogs.

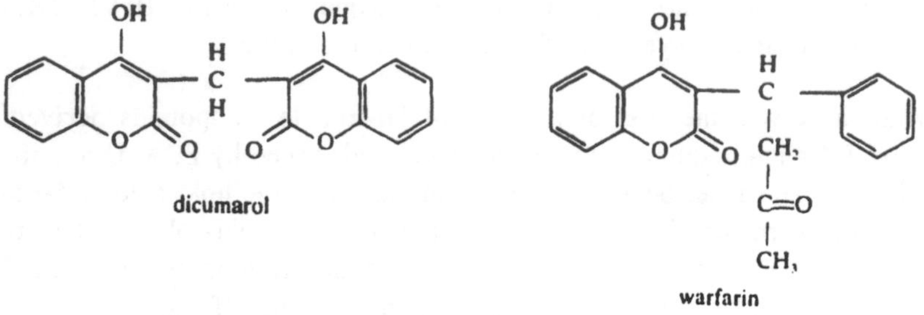

Figure 5.10 Anticoagulants: dicumarol and warfarin.

function in decreasing the intestinal microflora also decrease its ability to synthesize vitamin K_2.

Function

The process of blood coagulation (clotting) involves a highly complex and not fully understood process involving cells: thrombocytes, platelets, erythrocytes, numerous protein factors, and the Ca^{2+} ion. The net result of this complex process is the conversion of a highly soluble protein, fibrinogen, into a highly insoluble protein matrix, insoluble fibrin. Vitamin K is known to be needed for the synthesis of four coagulation factors and two protein factors which also function in coagulation. In 1974, prothrombin was found to contain many residues of carboxylated γ-glutamate. In the following two years it was demonstrated using *in vitro* systems that vitamin K was a necessary cofactor in a γ-carboxylase enzyme system which functions in converting precursor proteins to coagulation factors (Figure 5.11). Vitamin K functions in the synthesis of prothrombin (factor II), proconvertin (factor VII), the Christmas factor (factor IX), and the Stuart–Prower factor (factor X), as well as that of proteins C and S (Table 5.3).

Vitamin K also is required for the synthesis of some of the proteins in bone, kidney, liver, and plasma. Vitamin K metabolism in these tissues may not be as sensitive to the coumarins, which are vitamin K antagonists.

Food Sources

Green leafy vegetables and liver are rich sources of vitamin K. Limited data indicate that vitamin K is stable to food processing and cooking procedures.

Dietary Recommendations

Humans get much of their vitamin K (~50% on the average) from bacterial synthesis in the intestines which is absorbed primarily in the ileum. The 1989 RDA for men and women, 25+ years of age, for vitamin K is 80 and 65 μg, respectively.

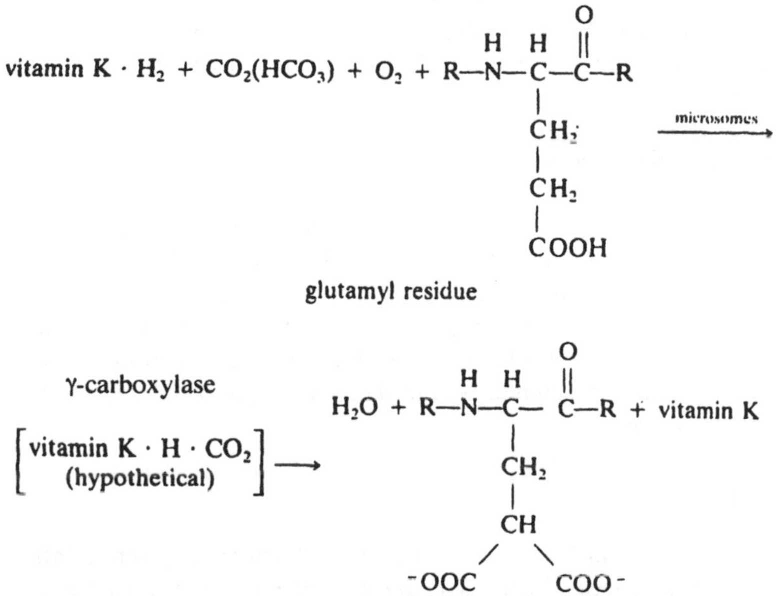

$$\text{vitamin K} \cdot H_2 + CO_2(HCO_3) + O_2 + R-N-\overset{H}{\underset{|}{C}}-\overset{O}{\overset{\|}{C}}-R$$

$$\begin{array}{c} H \quad H \\ | \quad | \\ CH_2 \\ | \\ CH_2 \\ | \\ COOH \end{array}$$

$\xrightarrow{\text{microsomes}}$

glutamyl residue

γ-carboxylase

$$\left[\begin{array}{c} \text{vitamin K} \cdot H \cdot CO_2 \\ \text{(hypothetical)} \end{array} \right] \longrightarrow \quad H_2O + R-N-\overset{H}{\underset{|}{C}}-\overset{O}{\overset{\|}{C}}-R + \text{vitamin K}$$

$$\begin{array}{c} CH_2 \\ | \\ CH \\ / \quad \backslash \\ {}^-OOC \qquad COO^- \end{array}$$

Figure 5.11 Scheme for the γ-carboxylation of glutamate residues by vitamin K.

Table 5.3 Clotting Factors in Blood Coagulation

	Factor	Name
	I	Fibrinogen
	II	Prothrombin
	III	Thromboplastin (tissue)
Vitamin K dependent	IV	Ca^{2+}
	V	Labile factor
	VI	No name assigned
	VII	Proconvertin
	VIII	Antihemophilic factor (AHF)
	IX	Christmas factor
	X	Stuart–Prower factor
	XI	Plasma thromboplastin antecedent
	XII	Hageman factor
	XIII	Fibrinase

Deficiency

Hemorrhaging is observed in vitamin K deficiency as there is decreased synthesis of prothrombin and other vitamin K-dependent coagulation factors. Vitamin K deficiency is relatively rare in individuals over the age of about 1 year and when observed, is associated with lipid malabsorption or decreased intestinal microflora generally caused by prolonged use of antibiotics. Due to poor placental transfer of vitamin K and a lack of vitamin K_2-producing intestinal microflora, newborns, particularly those who are pre-term, frequently have inadequate vitamin K status and are hemorrhagic. Vitamin K deficiency is also frequently seen in infants. Vitamin K status is most often evaluated by determining plasma or blood prothrombin concentration.

Pharmacologic Doses

Menadione or phylloquinone is frequently administered clinically to individuals having problems getting the blood to clot. All commercial infant formulas contain added phylloquinone. Phylloquinone is given to individuals who have accidentally ingested large quantities of anticoagulants. Phylloquinone or menadione is also given to individuals who have had long-term treatment with broad-spectrum antibiotics or long-term hyperalimentation as well as those with lipid malabsorption and chronic biliary obstruction.

Toxicity

Excessive vitamin K, as menadione not phylloquinone, given to infants results in increased incidence of hemolytic anemia, hyperbilirubinemia, kernicterus, and liver damage, especially in premature infants who have erythroblastosis. A problem with vitamin K overdosing in adults is reduced effectiveness of anticoagulants.

VITAMIN C

Name: Ascorbic acid or hydroascorbic acid
Active form: Reduced ascorbic acid
Function: Aqueous antioxidant, hydroxylations

A human ascorbic acid, vitamin C inadequacy produces scurvy, a nutritional deficiency disease described by ancient authors, including Hippocrates, the Greek physician of the fifth century. Scurvy ravaged the 13th-century French (crusaders) in Palestine, and it became perilous for sailors of the 16th and 17th centuries to be at sea for more than four or five months. A voyage of six months or more meant almost certain death. One hundred Portuguese sailors led by Vasco da Gama died of scurvy. The French explorer J. Cartier described the disease in 1535 while waiting out the long North American winter on the St. Lawrence River, near Quebec City, Canada.

> "The unknown sickness began to spread itself amongst us accompanied by the most marvelous and extraordinary symptoms ... in as much as some did lose all their strength and could not stand on their feet. Their legs became swollen, the sinews contracted and turned black as coal... . Others had their skin spotted with spots of blood of a purple color; then did it creep up to their hips, thighs, shoulders, arms, and neck. Their mouths became stinking, their gums so rotten that all the flesh did fall off, even to the root of the teeth... . The disease spread out ... so widely that,

by February, out of our group of 110, there were not 10 left in good health... . We had already 8 men dead and there remained over 50 whom we had given up for lost."

Many other observations of scurvy were later to be made and recorded. Admiral Richard Hawkins of the British Royal Navy wrote in 1662 "that sour oranges and lemons" were effective against the disease, but scurvy continued to be the primary cause of death of sailors at sea. It was the great sea plague. Not until Royal Navy Surgeon J. Lind did his human experiments with scorbutic sailors using oranges, lemons, cider, and seawater aboard the *Salisbury* at sea (May 20, 1747) was the value of citrus fruits appreciated. Published in 1753, Lind's *Treatise on the Scurvy* and other publications led the British admiralty in 1795 to order rations of lemons to sailors at sea. Lemons, often referred to as limes by the British, resulted in future sailors of the Royal Navy being called limeys.

The principal factor contributing to scurvy was the lack of dietary ascorbic acid. This anti-scorbutic factor was isolated in 1932 by C. G. King and W. A. Waugh, and independently by J. L. Surbely and A. Szent-Györgyi, who received the Nobel Prize for this discovery in 1937. Ascorbic acid's molecular composition was determined and its synthesis accomplished in 1933.

Forms of the Vitamin

Vitamin C, ascorbic acid, is similar in structure but functionally different from D-glucose or D-galactose (Figure 5.12). Vitamin C is dietarily required by humans, other primates, and several other animals such as the guinea pig. The guinea pig is

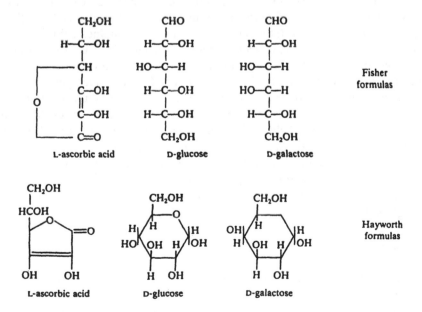

Figure 5.12 Hexoses: ascorbic acid, glucose, and galactose.

most often employed in vitamin C research as an animal model. Most animals possess the enzyme L-gulono-γ-lactone oxidase, which is needed for the synthesis of vitamin C from glucose or galactose (Figure 5.13).

Ascorbic acid is a strong reducing agent and upon oxidation, dehydroascorbic acid is formed. Dehydroascorbic acid is the most active form of the vitamin. Further oxidation produces diketoglutamic acid which has no vitamin activity. The water-soluble vitamin C is absorbed in the small intestine and goes via the circulatory system to the body tissues. Vitamin C is found in the liver, adrenals, kidneys, and spleen, where it apparently is in equilibrium with serum levels. Large amounts are excreted primarily as ascorbic acid, oxalic acid, and other metabolites.

Function

One of the major functions of ascorbic acid is that of an antioxidant, protecting cells and cellular components from free-radical attack (see Chapter 15). As a strong reducing agent, vitamin C may facilitate the absorption of ferric iron (Fe^{3+}) by its reduction to ferrous iron (Fe^{2+}), and of cupric copper (Cu^{2+}) by its reduction to cuprous copper (Cu^+). Vitamin C functions in the cytochrome series in conjunction with iron. Vitamin C also plays a role in transferring iron from its blood carrier transferrin to the storage form ferritin. In hydroxylation reactions in which either iron or copper must remain in a reduced state for the function of an enzyme, vitamin C is needed. Vitamin C also functions in oxidation–reduction reactions sparing vitamin E and glutathione.

As a coenzyme, vitamin C functions in the hydroxylation of the amino acids proline and lysine in the formation of collagen, of cholesterol to bile acids, of tyrosine in the formation of norepinephrine, of tryptophan in the formation of 5-hydroxytryptophan, of histidine in the formation of histamine, and in the detoxification of certain toxic compounds (Figure 5.14). Vitamin C is also involved in the conversion of the folic acid found in foods to its active form, in corticosteroid synthesis, in carnitine synthesis, in enzymatic amidation of neuropeptides, in the immune response, and possibly in wound healing and allergic reactions. In some manner, the vitamin functions in bone and tooth formation. Recent evidence indicates that vitamin C may help in the regulation of protein translation. Vitamin C may reduce the formation of nitrosamines, which are weak carcinogens formed from nitrates. Epidemiological studies and some clinical studies indicate that the incidence of coronary heart disease, some cancers, and cataracts may be lower in individuals having high plasma vitamin C levels, with some studies contradicting these generalizations.

Food Sources

The richest food sources of vitamin C are citrus fruits and juices as well as vegetables and organ meats. Vitamin C is the most labile nutrient, with considerable quantities of the vitamin being destroyed during common food preparation procedures. When possible, vitamin C-rich foods should be eaten raw. Vegetables retain more vitamin C if microwaved or steamed as opposed to boiled.

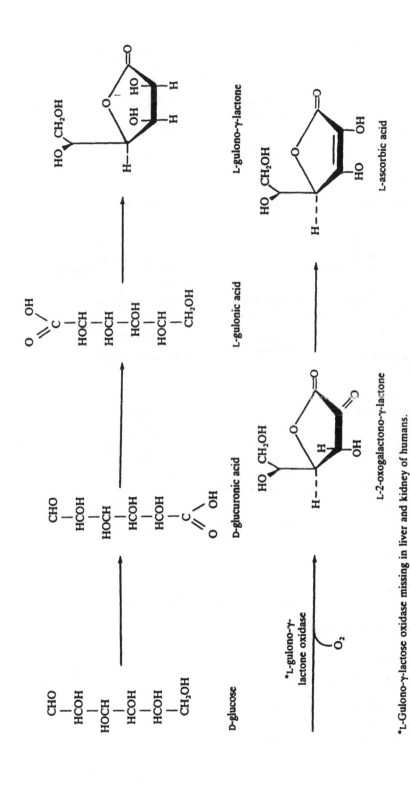

Figure 5.13 Synthesis of ascorbic acid by animals from glucose.

*L-Gulono-γ-lactose oxidase missing in liver and kidney of humans.

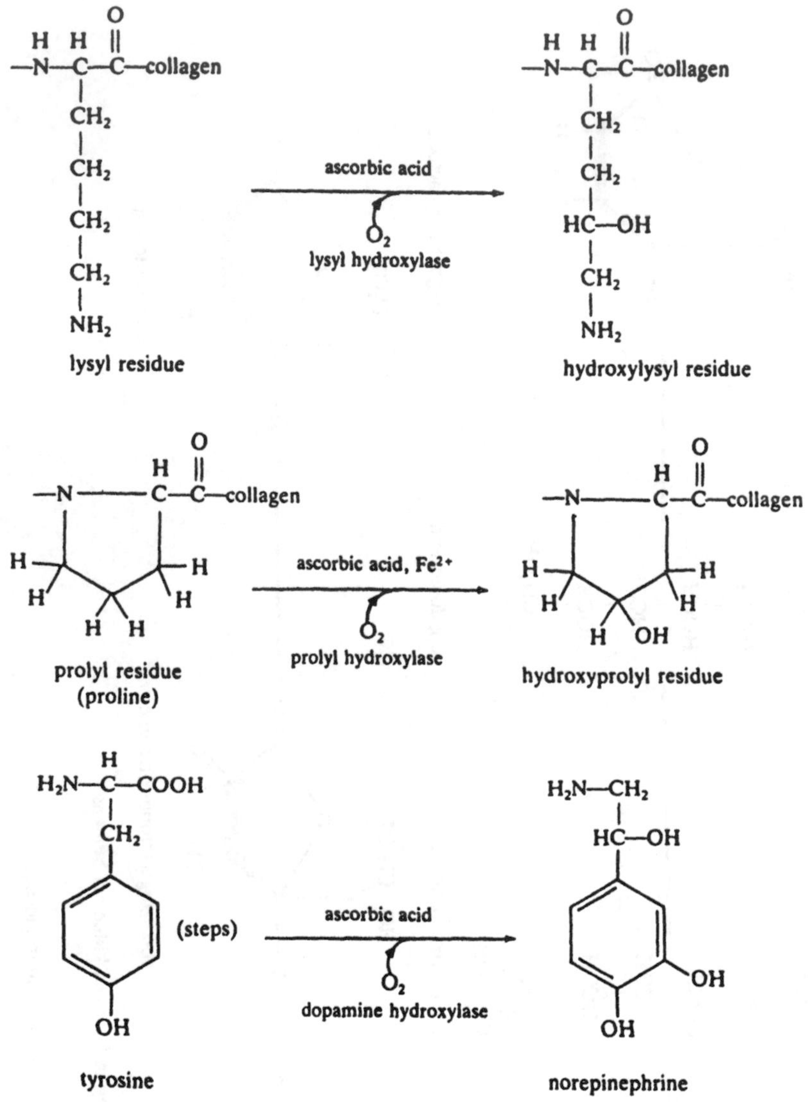

Figure 5.14 Some hydroxylation reactions with ascorbic acid (abbreviated). (See also bile acid synthesis and xenobiotic metabolism hydroxylation reactions in Figure 16.4.)

Dietary Recommendations

The 1989 RDA for adults is 60 mg daily, and cigarette smokers should ingest at least 100 mg vitamin C daily. Research indicates that a daily intake of about 200 mg of vitamin C daily seems to provide for maximal body retention of the nutrient and perhaps optimal immune function. The median vitamin C intakes of men and women, 20 to 59 years, in NHANESIII were 85 and 67 mg, respectively. Many individuals in the United States report taking vitamin C supplements.

Deficiency

The disease from ascorbic acid deficiency is scurvy. Symptoms include fatigue, perifollicular hyperkeratosis, swollen or bleeding gums, joint pain, ocular hemorrhaging, lethargy, followed by death. In the United States scurvy appears primarily in alcoholics and elderly men living alone. Scurvy is still found worldwide and is often associated with poverty. Vitamin C status is most often evaluated by measuring plasma vitamin C concentrations.

Pharmacologic Doses

Higher-than-adequate intakes of vitamin C have been suggested to accelerate wound healing, increase immunoresistance, prevent or reduce the severity of the common cold, and reduce the risks of cardiovascular disease and cancer. The true effective value of higher-than-recommended dietary intake of vitamin C remains to be elucidated more fully.

Toxicity

Many people take gram levels of ascorbic acid without apparent toxicity. However, reports exist indicating adverse effects when consuming over 4 g daily on a habitual basis. Reported adverse effects include nausea, diarrhea, development of kidney stones, mobilization of bone minerals, iron overabsorption, increase in serum cholesterol concentrations in atherosclerotic patients, systematic conditioning to higher intakes, and abortion. These effects have not been found in all studies and the risk of sustained ingestion of these quantities of vitamin C is unknown.

THIAMIN

Name: Thiamin, vitamin B_1
Active form: Thiamin pyrophosphate
Function: Oxidative decarboxylations, transketolations

Dietary deficiency of thiamin leads to a neurological condition known as beriberi. The disease sometimes involves atrophy of cardiac muscles and paralysis of involuntary muscles. The Dutch physician C. Eijkman is credited with the 1897 discovery that rice polishings prevented nutritional polyneuritis in chickens fed polished rice and that the disease in chickens was similar to beriberi in humans. The antineuritic factor in rice bran and yeasts was indirectly investigated until its isolation and identification as thiamin by B. C. P. Jansen and W. F. Donath in 1926. Its organic synthesis was completed in 1936 by R. R. Williams and J. K. Cline.

Forms

Thiamin is comprised of pyrimidine and thiazole rings connected by a methylene ($—CH_2—$) bridge. The active form of thiamin as a coenzyme is thiamin pyrophos-

thiamin pyrophosphate (TPP)

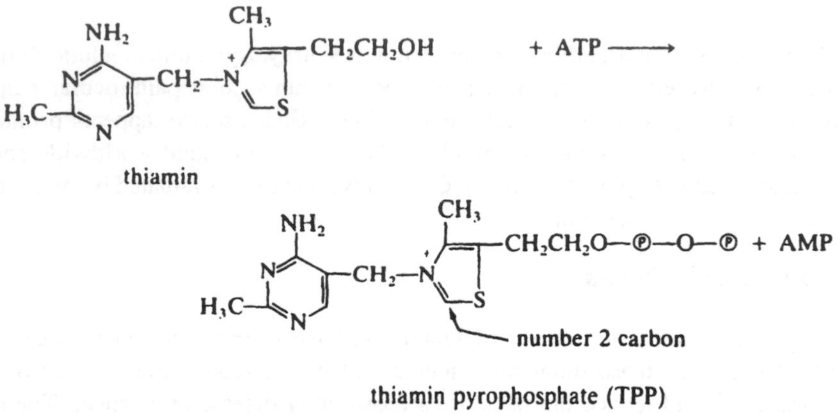

Figure 5.15 Phosphorylation of thiamin.

phate (TPP), which is formed by phosphorylation of thiamin with ATP *in vivo*; Mg^{2+} is required for this phosphorylation, which usually takes place in the intestinal mucosa during thiamin absorption (Figure 5.15). Thiamin is transported in erythrocytes and plasma and is stored primarily in the liver, heart, kidneys, skeletal muscles, and brain. The vitamin is excreted in the urine. Thiamin was formerly known as vitamin B_1.

Functions

The best known coenzyme functions for TPP are the oxidative decarboxylation (Figure 5.16) of α-keto acids and the transfer of ketones (—C=O) from α-keto acids in transketolase reactions (Figure 5.17). The oxidative decarboxylase and transketolase reactions usually require a divalent cation, either Mg^{2+} or Mn^{2+}. The oxidative decarboxylation of pyruvic acid and α-ketoglutaric acid, which is part of the TCA (tricarboxylic acid or Krebs) cycle, are examples of α-keto acid oxidative decarboxylations (Figure 5.18). These reactions are part of the aerobic metabolism of oxidizable substrate for the generation of ATP. Valine, leucine, isoleucine, methionine, and threonine can also undergo oxidative decarboxylations. The transketolase reaction involves the hexose monophosphate shunt or pathway (also referred to as the

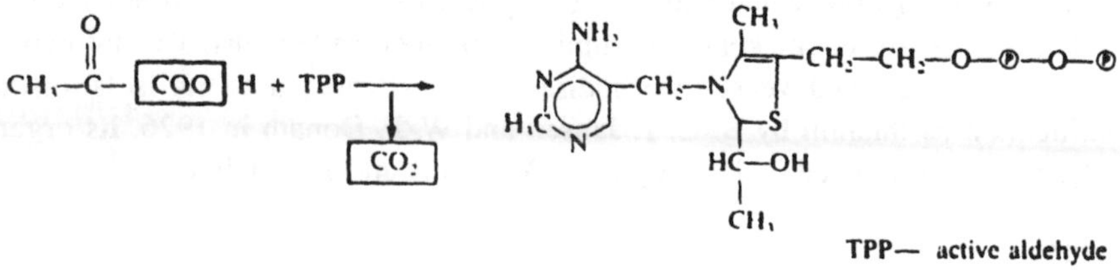

TPP— active aldehyde

Figure 5.16 Oxidative decarboxylation of pyruvate by TPP.

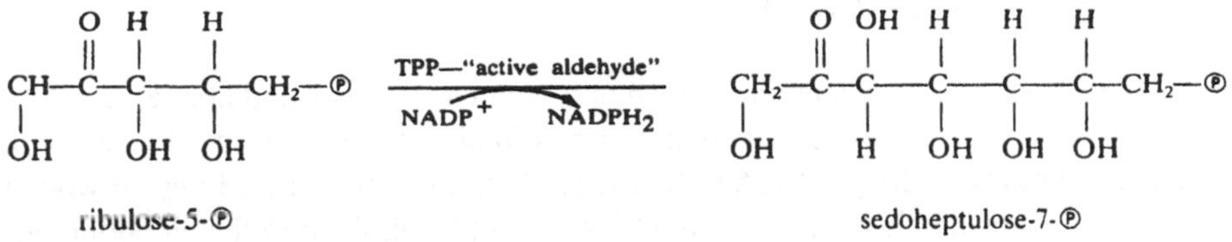

Figure 5.17 Transketolase reaction by TPP.

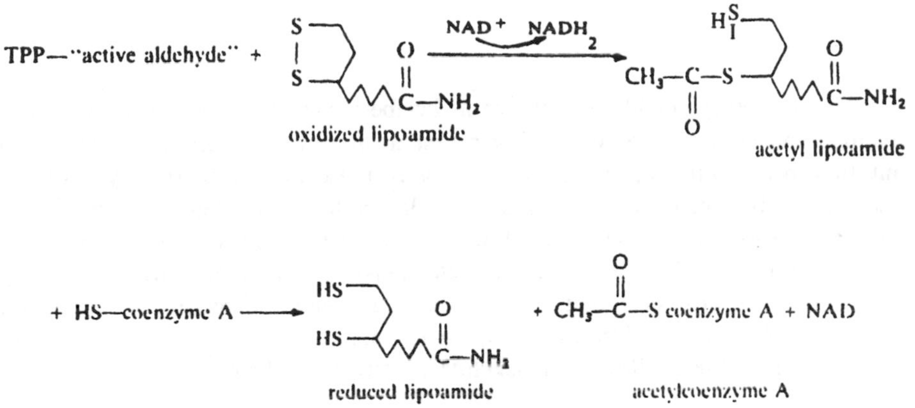

Figure 5.18 Formation of acetylcoenzyme A from TPP and acetyllipoamide.

pentose phosphate shunt or pathway and as the direct oxidative shunt) which uses TPP to transfer a ketol to an aldose (aldehyde carbohydrate), thereby adding two new carbons to the carbohydrate. In this manner, three-, four-, five-, six-, and seven-carbon sugars are interconvertible. The hexose monophosphate shunt is an alternate pathway for the oxidation of glucose, and is a major source of pentoses for synthesis of nucleic acids and NADPH (contains niacin) for the synthesis of fatty acids. TPP is also concentrated in the nerve tissues, affecting the chloride permeability and functioning in these cells.

Food Sources

Rich sources of thiamin include baker's and brewer's yeasts, pork, wheat germ, organ meats, cereal germs, whole grains, nuts, and dried legumes. Thiamin is the second most labile nutrient and is frequently used as an "index nutrient" in research studies on nutrient retention. Much of the thiamin present in foods is destroyed during the cooking process. Much of the thiamin is lost in the production of polished rice and white flour; rice, flour, and many baked products are frequently enriched with thiamin.

Dietary Recommendations

The 1998 RDA for thiamin for men and women, 19 years and above, is 1.2 and 1.1 mg/day, respectively. The median thiamin intake of adults 20 to 59 years in the United States according to NHANESIII is 1.77 mg for men and 1.23 mg for women. Thiamin deficiency in developed countries is mainly confined to the alcoholic population. Many individuals in the United States report taking multivitamin preparations containing thiamin hydrochloride. The deficiency is still seen in developing countries in populations consuming unenriched polished rice as their dietary staple.

Deficiency

The deficiency condition is known as beriberi. Symptoms observed in beriberi include anorexia, degenerative changes first in the lower extremities followed by multiple peripheral neuritis, mental confusion, muscular weakness (dry beriberi), edema (wet beriberi), ataxia, tachycardia, enlarged heart, and death. Dry beriberi is associated with both energy deprivation and physical inactivity; whereas, wet beriberi is associated with a high carbohydrate intake and strenuous physical activity. Thiaminase, an enzyme found in raw fish, is a thiamin antagonist, but is only a problem if about 10%+ of the diet is raw fish. Thiamin status is most often evaluated by determining the erythrocyte transketolase activity coefficient.

Pharmacologic Doses

Thiamin is sometimes used in the treatment of alcoholism. Because some individuals are hypersensitive to the vitamin, parenteral administration of the vitamin is used only in specific cases. No Tolerable Upper Intake Level has been set for thiamin.

Toxicity

No toxic effects other than gastric upset have been reported with high doses (up to 1 g daily) of thiamin other than in some individuals who are hypersensitive to the vitamin. Parenteral administration of thiamin has lead to conditions resembling anaphylactic shock in these individuals.

RIBOFLAVIN

Name: Riboflavin, vitamin B_2
Active form: Flavin mononucleotide (FMN), flavin adenine dinucleotide (FAD)
Function: Hydrogen carrier (oxidases, dehydrogenases)

Riboflavin was recognized early as a separate entity often found in the presence of thiamin. As a separate growth factor for animals, it was named vitamin B_2, following the convention established for naming the vitamins by the British, and as

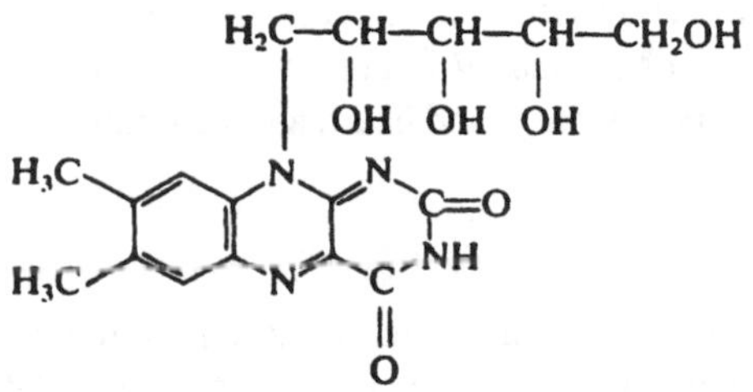

Figure 5.19 Structure of riboflavin.

vitamin G in the United States. Riboflavin was first isolated in 1934 from egg whites by P. György, and was synthesized by R. K. Khun and P. Karrer in 1935.

Riboflavin is a bright orange-yellow colored compound. Its color gives the slight yellow color to egg "whites," where it is found as ovoflavin. One of only two highly colored vitamins, it is strongly fluorescent in solution, and its ability to absorb ultraviolet light causes it to be chemically unstable. Former names of riboflavin include vitamin B_2, vitamin G, lactoflavin, and ovoflavin.

Forms

Riboflavin consists of a conjugated isoalloxazine ring (flavin) and a five-carbon carbohydrate, ribitol (Figure 5.19). Riboflavin forms part of and is the functional moiety of two larger coenzymes, flavin mononucleotide (FMN) and flavin adenine dinucleotide (FAD); these two coenzymes are called flavoproteins. Riboflavin is absorbed in the small intestine, phosphorylated (Figure 5.20) in the intestinal mucosa

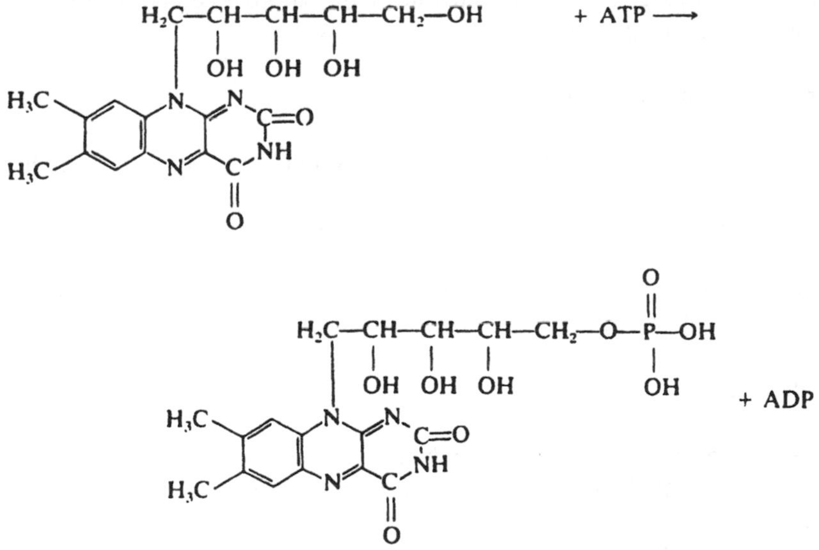

Figure 5.20 Phosphorylation of riboflavin.

to FMN, and sometimes converted in the liver to FAD. Both of these phosphorylation reactions require Mg^{2+}. FMN and FAD are easily interconvertible. The vitamin is found primarily in the liver, kidney, and heart, and generally is excreted as riboflavin.

Functions

Riboflavin as FMN or FAD functions in oxidation–reduction reactions (particularly as a hydrogen carrier) as a component of oxidases and dehydrogenases (Figure 5.21). FMN and FAD designate the oxidized forms of the respective riboflavin coenzymes, while $FMNH_2$ and $FADH_2$ designate the reduced forms of the coenzymes. The flavoproteins function in conjunction with amino acid oxidases (catabolism of amino acids), xanthine oxidase (production of uric acid; enzyme also contains iron and molybdenum), cytochrome reductase (part of electron transport chain), succinic dehydrogenase (part of TCA cycle), acyl-coenzyme A dehydrogenase (needed for catabolism of fatty acids), in fatty acid synthesis, α-glycerophosphate dehydrogenase (part of glycolysis), lactic acid dehydrogenase (needed for conversion of lactic acid), kynurenine 3-hydroxylase (needed for conversion of tryptophan to niacin), and aldehyde oxidases such as that which functions in the interconversion of two forms of vitamin B_6. Free riboflavin exists in the retina, but how it functions there is unknown.

Food Sources

Rich food sources of riboflavin include baker's and brewer's yeasts, meats, dairy products, and enriched cereals and breads. Asparagus, broccoli, collard and turnip greens, and spinach are rich sources of the vitamin. The vitamin is relatively stable to various food processing and cooking methods, but losses do occur if the food is exposed to ultraviolet light.

Dietary Recommendations

A riboflavin intake of 0.6 mg/1000 kcal should meet the needs of healthy individuals, with a minimum intake of 1.2 mg daily for adults. The 1989 RDA for men and women, 19 to 50 years, is 1.7 and 1.3 mg daily, respectively. The median daily intakes of the vitamin for men and women, 20 to 59 years, living in the United States according to NHANESIII is 2.11 and 1.49 mg, respectively. Many individuals ingest riboflavin as part of a multivitamin preparation.

Deficiency

Riboflavin deficiency symptoms include seborrheic dermatitis, lacrimation, burning and itching of the eyes, cheilosis, angular stomatitis, purple swollen tongue (geographic tongue), normocytic anemia, photophobia, and presenile cataracts. In that riboflavin is needed for the functioning of vitamin B_6 and niacin, some of the symptoms of the deficiency are actually due to functional insufficiencies of the other

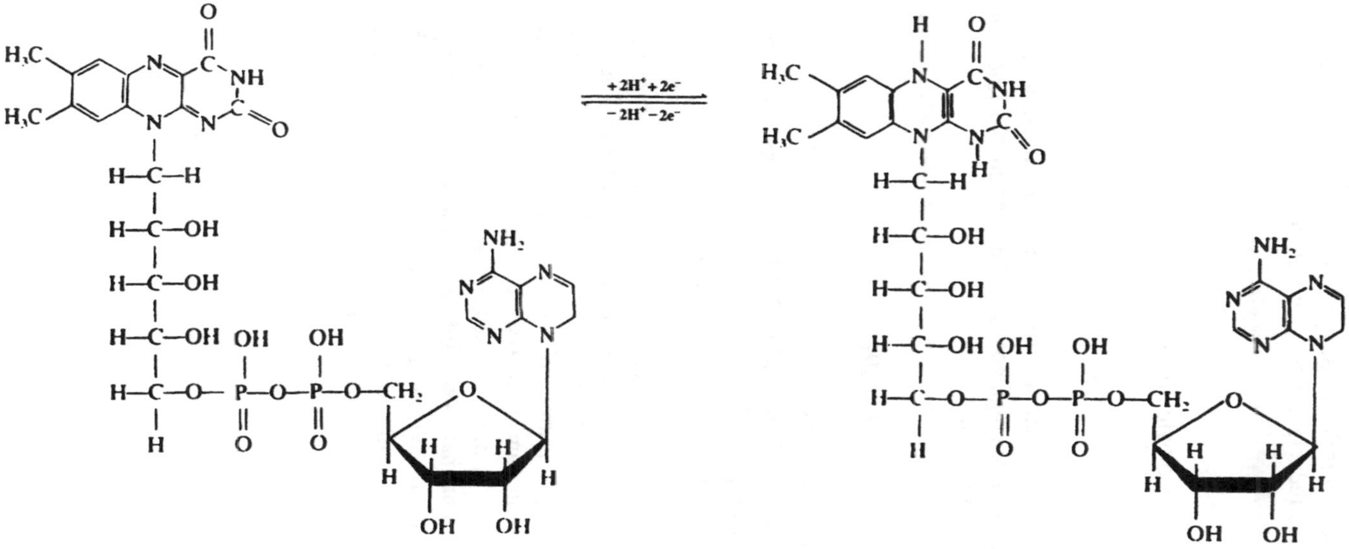

Figure 5.21 Oxidation–reduction of a riboflavin coenzyme.

two B-vitamins. Clinical signs of riboflavin deficiency are rarely seen in developed countries, except in chronic alcoholics. Riboflavin deficiency is seen in conjunction with PEM. The accepted method for evaluating riboflavin status is a determination of the erythrocyte glutathione reductase activity coefficient.

Pharmacologic Doses

There are no known pharmacologic effects of riboflavin.

Toxicity

Riboflavin toxicity has not been reported in humans. Riboflavin will precipitate in the kidneys and hearts of rats given high doses of the vitamin. No Tolerable Upper Intake Level has been set for riboflavin.

NIACIN

Name: Nicotinic acid and nicotinamide
Active form: Nicotinamide adenine dinucleotide (NAD), nicotinamide adenine dinu-
cleotide phosphate (NADP)
Function: Hydrogen carrier (dehydrogenases, reductases)

Niacin is the generic term for nicotinic acid and nicotinamide (Figure 5.22). The discovery of nicotinamide as a vitamin was tied to the search for the cause of human pellagra (meaning "rough skin") in the southern United States by J. Goldberger of the U.S. Public Health Service just prior to World War I. Believing that pellagra was an infectious disease, Goldberger and four assistants failed at attempts to transfer pellagra to healthy individuals. In dogs, a disease comparable to human pellagra, black tongue, developed when animals were fed human diets that knowingly caused the disease. At the University of Wisconsin in the 1930s, C. A. Elvehjem and associates were feeding nicotinic acid and nicotinamide to dogs with black tongue. Nicotinic acid, then packaged in bottles with a skull and crossbones, and liver-isolated nicotinamide both cured black tongue in dogs and were later found to prevent human pellagra.

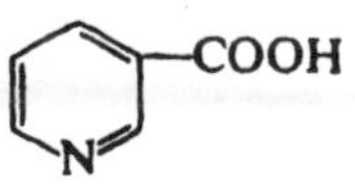

nicotinic acid

(provitamin)

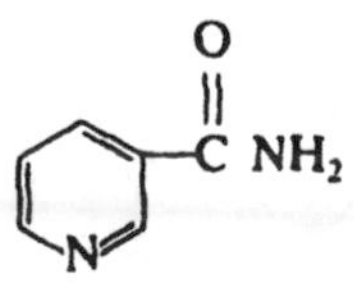

nicotinamide

(vitamin)

Figure 5.22 Structure of nicotinic acid and nicotinamide.

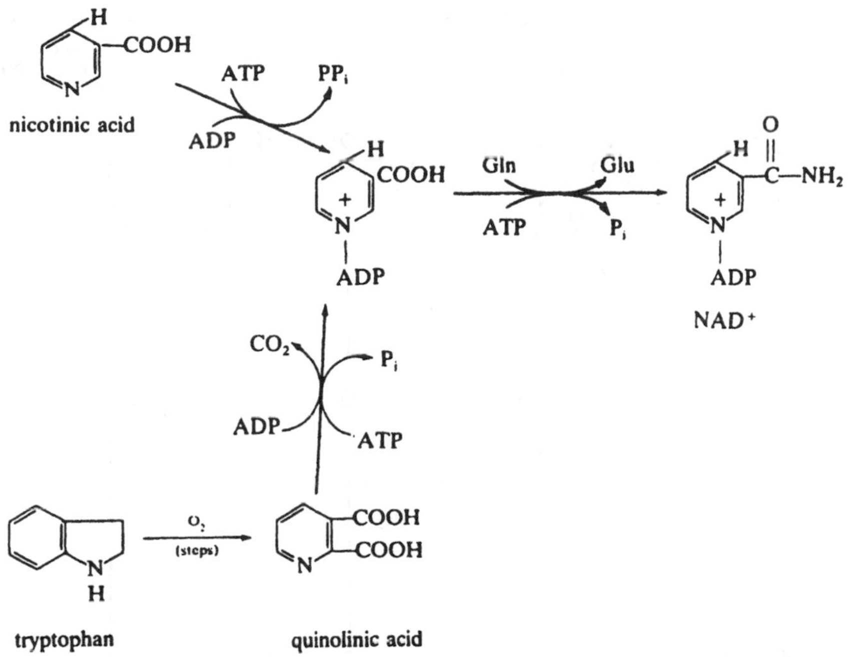

Figure 5.23 Conversion of nicotinic acid and tryptophan into nicotinamide of NAD⁺.

Forms

Nicotinic acid is known to be converted to nicotinamide (also known as nia-cinamide) by the liver in a series of reactions involving ATP, ADP, and glutamine, which provides the amine in the conversion of nicotinic acid to nicotinamide. Tryptophan, an essential amino acid, in a series of biochemical transformations, is also capable of being transformed by the liver into nicotinamide, as first demon-strated in rats; however, vitamin B_6, copper, riboflavin, iron, magnesium, and niacin itself are required for this conversion (Figure 5.23).

Niacin, or more specifically, nicotinamide, like riboflavin forms a portion of two larger redox coenzymes nicotinamide adenine dinucleotide (NAD⁺) and nicotina-mide adenine dinucleotide phosphate (NADP⁺). These two coenzyme molecules, both shown in their reduced form, differ only by the addition of the phosphate ester supplied by ATP to the 2'-hydroxyl of ribose (Figure 5.24).

Niacin and its precursor tryptophan are absorbed in the small intestine. Tissue stores of the vitamin are small. Niacin is excreted as N'-methyl-nicotinamide and its pyridones.

Functions

NAD and NADP are present and function in all cells in oxidation–reduction reactions primarily as hydrogen carriers (Figure 5.25). NAD⁺ is utilized in most catabolic (oxidation) reactions, while $NADPH_2$ is the coenzyme for most anabolic

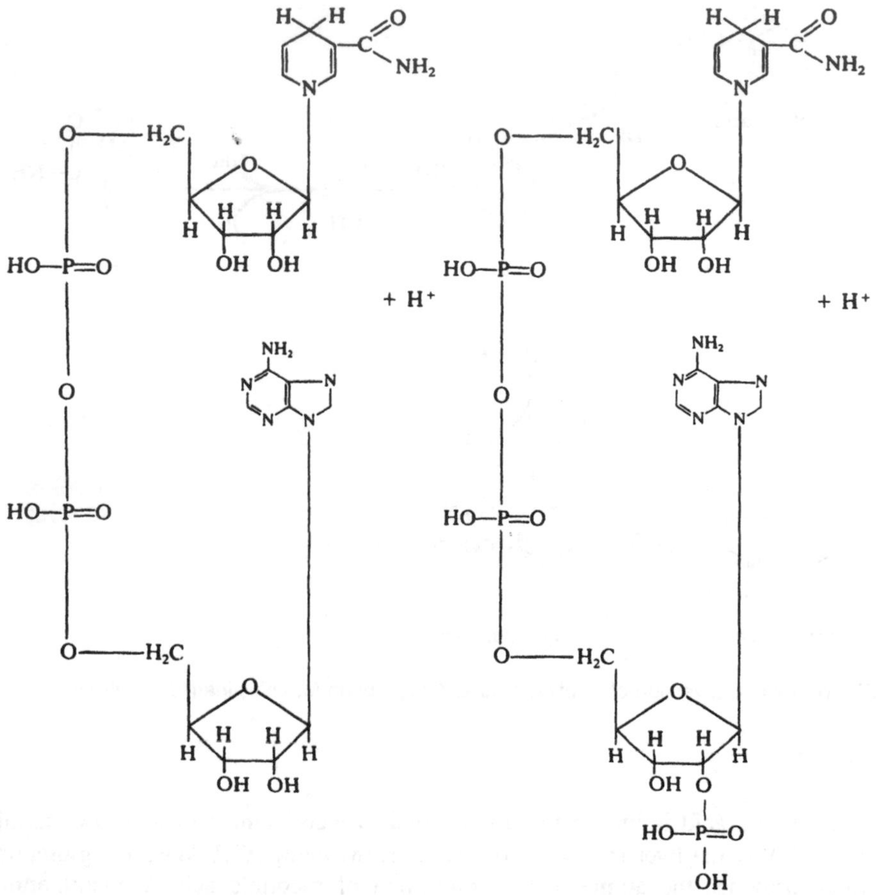

Figure 5.24 Coenzymes of niacinamide.

(reduction) reactions. These coenzymes are noncovalently bound components of dehydrogenases and reductases. NAD is a component of the electron transport chain and functions in the TCA cycle and glycolysis. NADP functions in fatty acid and steroid synthesis. Niacin functions in the vitamin A visual cycle and in the inter-conversion of choline and betaine.

Food Sources

Rich sources of niacin include baker's and brewer's yeasts, organ meats, lean meats, poultry, fish, nuts, and enriched products such as cereals and grains. The amino acid tryptophan can be converted to niacin with rich dietary sources of

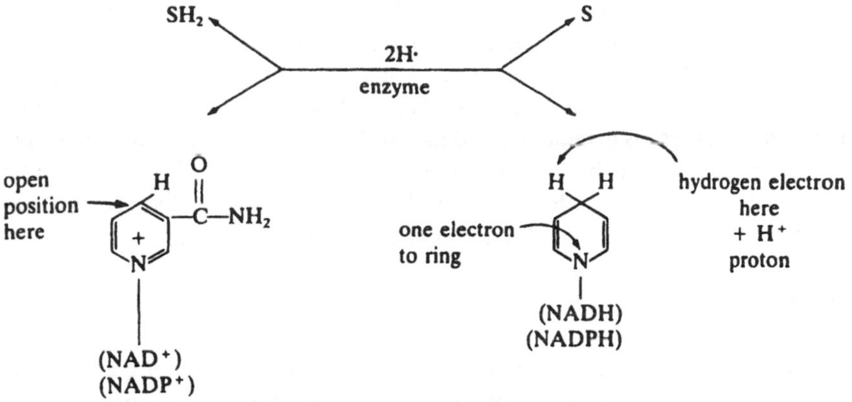

Figure 5.25 Oxidation–reduction reactions of nicotinamide coenzymes.

tryptophan including lean meats, fish, poultry, and nuts. Little niacin or tryptophan is lost during the cooking of foods.

Dietary Recommendations

In that tryptophan can be converted to niacin, recommendations are given as niacin equivalents (NE). Approximately 60 mg tryptophan may be converted to 1 mg niacin. The 1998 RDA for men and women 19 years and over is 16 and 14 mg NE (frequently referred to as simply NE), respectively. The median niacin intakes for men and women 20 to 59 years in the United States according to NHANESIII are 26.2 and 17.5 mg daily not counting the tryptophan. Many people ingest the vitamin as part of a multivitamin preparation.

Deficiency

The niacin deficiency disease is known as pellagra or the 3 or 4 D's (diarrhea, symmetric dermatitis, dementia, and death). Early symptoms include insomnia, anorexia, anemia, weight loss, muscle loss, numbness, and nervousness. The nervous system becomes malfunctional in the advanced stages. Pellagra is a wasting disease slow in its development. The deficiency is rare in developed countries, being seen only in malnourished alcoholics and in individuals having disorders of tryptophan metabolism. Pellagra is still seen in individuals in the Near East and Africa. Niacin status most often is evaluated by determining the urinary excretion of N'-methyl-nicotinamide (and sometimes also its pyridones) following a tryptophan test dose.

Pharmacologic Doses

Pharmacologically nicotinic acid and nicotinamide are dissimilar. Large doses (1200+ mg/day) of nicotinic acid can reduce serum cholesterol, free fatty acids, and total lipid levels and elevate LDL levels. Large doses of nicotinic acid may improve vascular tone and decrease fatty acid mobilization from adipose tissue during exercise. Side effects of these large doses include acute flushing of the skin with a concomitant itching and feeling of heat, elevation of blood glucose levels, and possible liver damage. If choline or another methyl group donor is given along with nicotinic acid, there is decreased incidence of fatty liver. Nicotinic acid was thought for years to be useful in the treatment of mental disorders, but evidence now indicates that this is not true. A Tolerable Upper Intake Level of 35 mg NE has been established for adults; this level was based upon the adverse effect of flushing.

Toxicity

Both nicotinic acid and nicotinamide can be toxic when 3 to 9 g are consumed. Hypertension, gastrointestinal problems, and hepatic toxicity are among the problems associated with nicotinic acid toxicity, while individuals chronically taking excessive quantities of nicotinamide are unable to focus their eyes.

VITAMIN B$_6$

Name: Pyridoxal, pyridoxol, pyridoxamine, pyridoxal phosphate, pyridoxol phosphate, pyridoxamine phosphate
Active form: Pyridoxal phosphate
Function: Transaminations, nonoxidative deaminations, desulfhydrations, decarboxylations, dehydrations

Vitamin B$_6$ was initially recognized as an antidermatitis factor in rats by J. Goldberger and R. Lillie in 1926, and was again recognized as the same antidermatitis factor by P. György, who in 1934 proposed the vitamin's name. Independently isolated by three research teams in 1938, vitamin B$_6$ was then synthesized in the following year (1939).

Forms

Since 1945 it has been known that vitamin B$_6$ could be isolated in three different forms (isomers): two in animal tissues, pyridoxal and pyridoxamine, and one from plants, pyridoxol (also known as pyridoxine). Pyridoxine is not another name for vitamin B$_6$, but is the name of one of the forms of the vitamin. These three forms are shown in Figure 5.26. The three forms also exist as 5'-phosphorylated vitamers: pyridoxal phosphate, pyridoxol phosphate, and pyridoxamine phosphate. ATP is required for the formation of the phosphorylated forms of the vitamin. Riboflavin as FMN functions in the conversion of pyridoxal phosphate to pyridoxol phosphate and pyridoxamine phosphate. The vitamin is absorbed in the small intestine and may be phosphorylated in the intestinal mucosa. The liver and muscle are where most of the reserve is located, with very little vitamin B$_6$ being stored in the body. The major excretion product of the vitamin is urinary 4-pyridoxic acid.

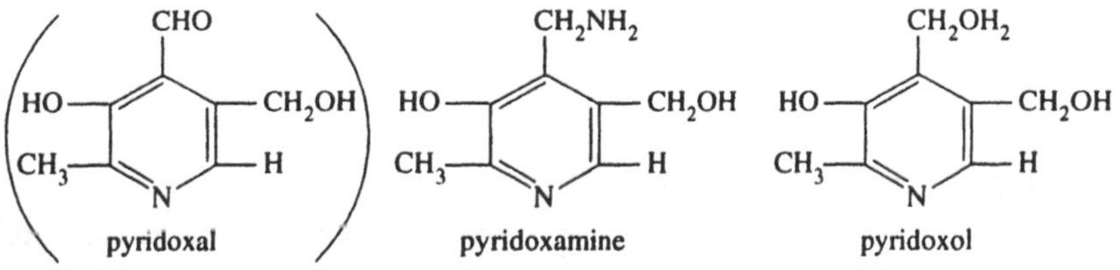

Figure 5.26 Isomers of vitamin B$_6$.

Function

   Vitamin B$_6$, like all other B vitamins, participates in enzymatic reactions as a coenzyme. Its coenzyme functions in the metabolism of predominantly amino acids. Pyridoxal phosphate (Figure 5.27) participates as a coenzyme in several enzymatic reactions in the metabolism of the essential and nonessential amino acids. The enzymatic reactions in which pyridoxal phosphate participates are transamination reactions, in which α-amino acids are converted to α-keto acids with the concurrent transfer of the amino moiety to a different α-keto acid, forming a second and usually different amino acid (Figure 5.28). Such transamination reactions are responsible for the synthesis of the nonessential amino acids from α-keto acids. These α-keto acid substrates exist as metabolic intermediates of carbohydrate and lipid catabolism. Other vitamin B$_6$-requiring reactions add hydrocarbons or cleave the side chain (R) of amino acids, providing for the racemization, deamination, or desulfhydration of amino acids. Vitamin B$_6$ is needed in hemoglobin formation. The vitamin also functions in the conversion of glycogen to glucose (actually glucose-1-phosphate), the synthesis of the fatty acid arachidonic acid from linoleic acid, the formation of sphingolipids for the myelin sheath, the synthesis of niacin from tryptophan, the synthesis of norepinephrine and epinephrine, and the synthesis of nucleic acids. The vitamin is required for the synthesis of the neurotransmitter γ-amino-butyric acid (γABA or GABA), dopamine, serotonin, taurine, and histamine. The vitamin is also needed for the functioning of the immune system.

Food Sources

   Rich sources of vitamin B$_6$ include baker's and brewer's yeasts, organ meats, bananas, most legumes, seeds, rice polishings, and egg yolks. Beef, pork, poultry,

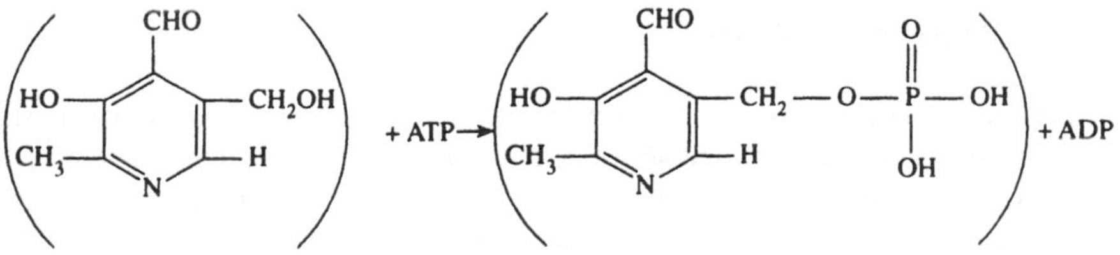

Figure 5.27 Formation of the active coenzyme pyridoxal phosphate (PLP).

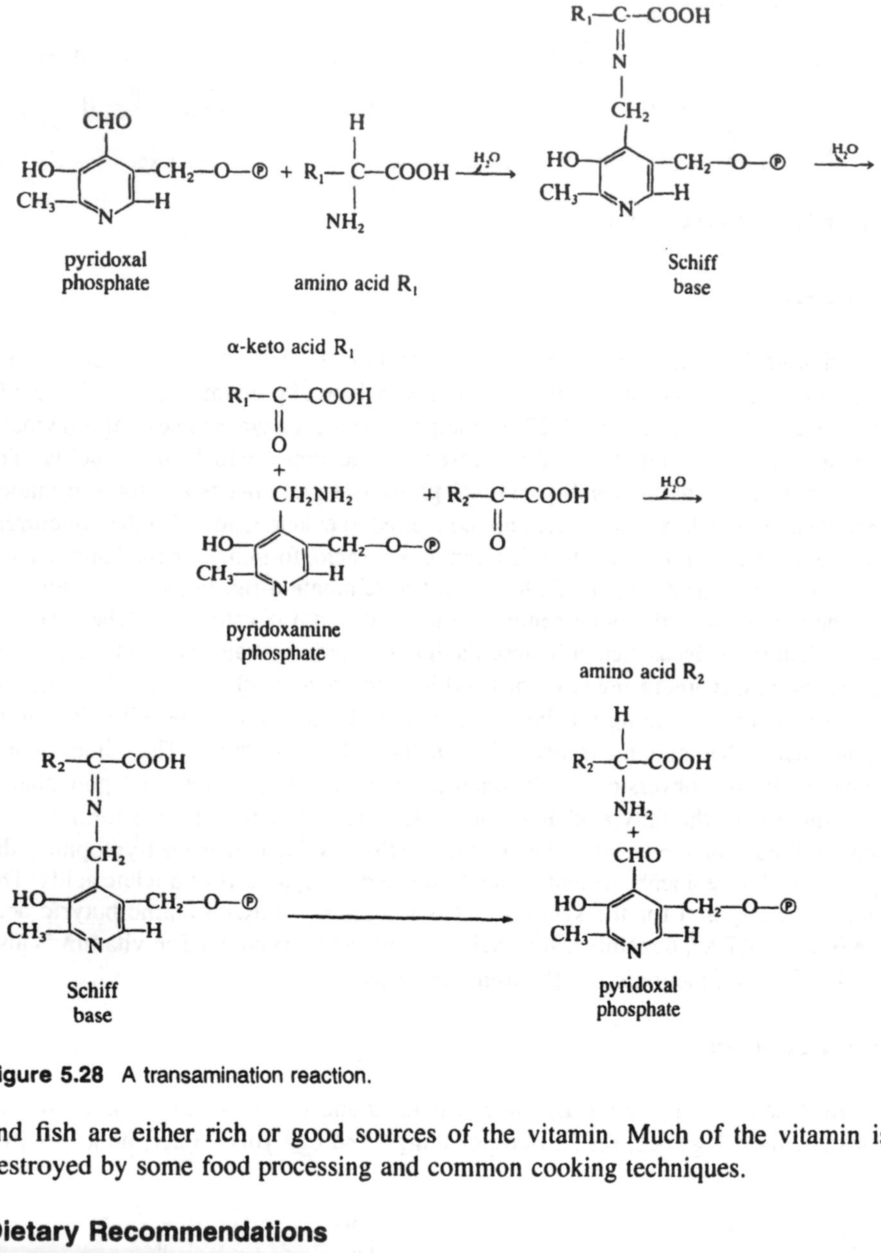

Figure 5.28 A transamination reaction.

and fish are either rich or good sources of the vitamin. Much of the vitamin is destroyed by some food processing and common cooking techniques.

Dietary Recommendations

The 1998 RDA for both men and women 19 to 50 years is 1.3 mg, while that for men and women 51 years and above is 1.7 and 1.5 mg, respectively. The median intake of men and women 20 to 59 years in the United States according to NHANES-III is 1.97 and 1.31 mg, respectively. Elderly individuals in the United States frequently consume less vitamin B_6 than is recommended. Many individuals in the United States ingest pyridoxine hydrochloride as part of a multivitamin preparation.

Deficiency

Vitamin B_6 deficiency due to inadequate intake of the vitamin is relatively rare; however, many drugs and medications are known to interfere with the functioning of the vitamin. Deficiency symptoms include dermatitis, dental caries, microcytic anemia, stomatitis, abdominal distress, irritability, depression, decreased immune function, epileptiform seizures, and convulsions. Infants fed a milk formula which had been subjected to moist heat developed irritability followed by epileptiform seizures. The infants recovered when pyridoxine hydrochloride was administered. Abnormal electroencephalograms have been reported in infants and adults who are deficient in vitamin B_6. Most individuals who are deficient in vitamin B_6 are also deficient in other nutrients, and frequently are also alcoholics.

Many methods exist for evaluation of vitamin B_6 status, yet no one method is the best. Vitamin B_6 status most commonly is evaluated by determining the plasma pyridoxal phosphate content using a C^{14}-radioenzymatic method.

Pharmacologic Doses

Vitamin B_6 metabolism is altered in several diseases and disorders. Pyridoxine hydrochloride has been utilized pharmacologically (25 to 50 or 100 mg doses daily) in treating several of these diseases and disorders including Down's syndrome, premenstrual syndrome, gestational diabetes, morning sickness, carpal tunnel syndrome, hyperoxaluria, autism, radiation sickness, diabetic neuropathy, various kidney disorders, depression, coronary heart disease, and alcoholism. Researchers have reported variable success in treating individuals with these diseases and disorders with the vitamin. Patients taking isoniazid, cycloserine, and penicillamine are often given vitamin B_6 as these drugs interfere with metabolism of the vitamin.

Toxicity

Neuropathies and ataxias have been reported in individuals who have self-dosed with pyridoxine hydrochloride at intakes of 400 mg and perhaps even as low as 200 mg daily for over eight months. Vitamin B_6-dependency has also been reported in normal adults who took 200 mg of pyridoxine hydrochloride daily for 33 days. The Tolerable Upper Intake Level of vitamin B_6 for adults is 100 mg daily.

FOLIC ACID

Name: Folacin
Active form: Tetrahydrofolic acid
Function: One-carbon metabolism

Folic acid or folate, also known as folacin, is chemically named pteroylmonoglutamic acid. It is composed of pteridine, p-aminobenzoic acid, and glutamic acid (Figure 5.29). A. Biermer, in 1872, called an anemia observed in a group of pregnant

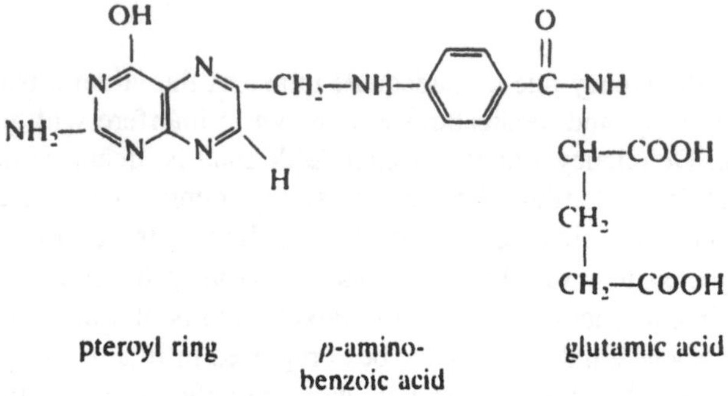

Figure 5.29 Structure of folic acid.

women a "progressive pernicious anemia." L. Wills and co-workers during the early 1930s observed that pregnant females having a severe type of megaloblastic anemia, improved when given yeast extracts (Wills factor). Monkeys fed diets similar to that consumed by the women developed macrocytic anemia, which was cured by yeast or wheat germ extract (vitamin M). This substance was also shown to be a growth factor for chicks (vitamin B_c) as well as for the lactic acid bacteria *Lactobacillus casei* (*L. casei* or lactic acid factor). The name folic acid was coined in 1941 by H. K. Mitchell and co-workers. By the late 1940s it was found that all the above-mentioned factors and vitamins were the same compound. Found in plants, folic acid was both identified as an animal and bacterial nutrient factor and was synthesized in 1946.

Forms

Most of the folic acid found in foods is in the form of pteroylpolyglutamates, which contain a pteridine, *p*-aminobenzoic acid, and three to seven or even eleven glutamic acid molecules. Vitamin B_{12} functions as part of a deconjugase in converting the pteroylpolyglutamates to pteroylmonoglutamates, the active form. Vitamin C and niacin (as NADPH) functions in reducing folate. During or following absorption primarily in the jejunum, pteroylmonoglutamate in its reduced form is converted to methyl-tetrahydrofolic acid. Small stores of folic acid exist primarily in the liver, cerebrospinal fluid, bone marrow, spleen, and kidneys. Folic acid acquires 1-carbon units at the N^5 or N^{10} or between these two positions. The 1-carbon units can be formyl, methyl, hydroxymethyl, methenyl, and formimino moieties, and form various intraconvertible tetrahydrofolic acid compounds (Figure 5.30). The different forms of the vitamin vary in nutritional effectiveness and stability. Bile contains folate due to enterohepatic circulation of the vitamin. Most folate is excreted in the urine.

Function

Folic acid functions as a 1-carbon donor/recipient. The vitamin is needed for the synthesis of the purines adenine and guanine and the pyrimidine thymine, and thus

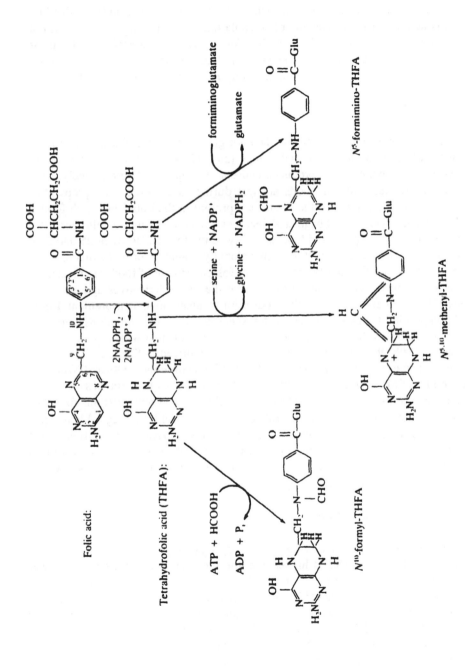

Figure 5.30 Reduction and coenzyme forms of folic acid.

functions in DNA and RNA synthesis and cell growth in general. Folic acid functions in amino acid metabolism in the interconversion of serine and glycine (vitamin B_6 also needed), the oxidation of glycine, and the synthesis of methionine from homocysteine (vitamins B_6 and B_{12} also needed) and of glutamic acid from histidine. Folate is needed for the conversion of ethanolamine to choline and of nicotinamide to N'-methyl-nicotinamide. Folate also functions as a nonspecific 1-carbon donor/recipient in reactions in which no specific 1-carbon donor/recipient is required. Folate is needed for the synthesis and maturation of both red and white blood cells.

Food Sources

Rich sources of folic acid include the dark green leafy vegetables, organ meats, legumes, wheat germ and bran, and orange juice. Good sources include bananas, egg yolks, nuts, whole grain products, and enriched grains. Approximately 20 to 75% of the folates found in foods are lost during food storage and preparation (including cooking). Some of the folates are present in the liquid in which food is cooked. Foods such as cabbage and legumes contain conjugase inhibitors that decrease dietary absorption and bioavailability of the folates. Between 25 and 50% of the dietary folates are thought to be nutritionally available for metabolism. Older tables and portions of currently used tables of folacin content of foods are inaccurate in that precautions were not taken to preserve the folate derivatives and all of the folic acid was not extracted from the foods prior to quantitative measurement. Better food composition tables are needed with respect to folic acid estimations. Enriched grains in the United States have been required to be fortified with folic acid since January 1, 1998; this fortification has also been authorized in Canada.

According to the recent (1998) report of the Panel on Folate, Other B Vitamins, and Choline of the Food and Nutrition Board, folic acid from food sources has nearly 50% lower bioavailability than synthetic folic acid. The recommendations for folate intake are now expressed as dietary folate equivalents (DFEs); 1 µg DFE is equal to 1 µg food folate. Folic acid taken with food is 85% bioavailable and food folate is about 50% bioavailable; hence, folic acid taken with food is 1.7 (85/50) times more bioavailable. Differences also exist as to whether folate acid is taken on an empty stomach or with meals.

Dietary Recommendations

The 1998 RDA for folate is 400 µg dietary folate equivalents (DFE) daily for both men and women. This is higher than the previous RDA of 1989 which was 200 µg for men and 180 µg for women. Many nutrition researchers believed that the recommended intakes should be raised to 300 to 400 µg daily in order to provide a more adequate safety allowance for populations at risk, particularly premenopausal women. Women of childbearing age should consume 400 µg of folate according to 1992 recommendations of the United States Public Health Service. The Panel on Folate, Other B Vitamins, and Choline, Food and Nutrition Board, in 1998 stated that "to reduce the risk of neural tube defects for women capable of becoming pregnant, the recommendation is to take 400 µg of synthetic folic acid daily, from fortified foods and/or supplements, in addition to consuming food folate from a varied diet." The median daily intakes of men and women 20 to 59 years in the United States according to NHANESIII are 280 and 189 μg, respectively. Many individuals, particularly premenopausal and pregnant women in the United States and Western Europe, have low plasma or erythrocyte folic acid levels. Many individuals in the United States ingest folate as part of a multivitamin preparation.

Deficiency

Folate deficiency is probably the most common vitamin deficiency in humans. Deficiency symptoms include apathy, irritability, poor growth, megaloblastic macrocytic anemia, leukopenia, thrombocytopenia, glossitis, and gastrointestinal disturbances. Women who consume inadequate quantities of folic acid prior to conception are more likely to have infants with neural tube defects than those consuming adequate amounts. The folic acid nutriture of the woman for about two months prior to and about one month following conception is critical in reducing the incidence of neural tube defects in their newborns. Folate status is most often evaluated by determining plasma or erythrocyte folic acid levels radiometrically. Plasma homocysteine and folic acid levels are also utilized in evaluating folate status.

Folic acid deficiency is commonly caused by malabsorption of folate or of vitamin B_{12}. Alcoholics are frequently folate deficient in that alcohol impairs folate absorption and also appears to block methyl-tetrahydrofolate release from the liver. Individuals taking anticonvulsants, oral contraceptives, and folate antagonists (aminopterin, amethopterin) frequently are folate deficient due to absorption and metabolic impairments. Protein malnutrition may impair folate utilization.

Pharmacologic Doses

Supplements exceeding 400 μg daily are considered to be pharmacologic. Folate may partially reverse the antiepileptic effects of phenobarbital and other anticonvulsants. Folate acid antagonists are generally used in treating malignancies, with these drugs being used in massive amounts, and then "rescue therapy" is undertaken, giving folates. Folate supplements are also being given to decrease the risk of cardiovascular disease as they may lower plasma homocysteine levels.

Since January 1, 1998, specified amounts of folic acid must be added to every 100 g of enriched flour, bread, pasta, and other grain products according to Food and Drug Administration regulations. This mandate was in recognition of the importance of adequate intakes of folic acid with regard to protection against neural tube defects in infants at birth and atherosclerosis later in life. The upper limit of daily folic acid intake should be 1 mg according to a 1992 recommendation of the United States Public Health Service. The Tolerable Upper Intake Level for folic acid for adults is 1000 μg daily of folic acid, exclusive of folate from foods.

Toxicity

Large doses of folates may obscure diagnosis of vitamin B_{12} deficiency in that it relieves the megaloblastic anemia caused by vitamin B_{12} deficiency, but the irreversible damage to the central nervous system continues. Doses of 5 mg/day can prevent the hematologic relapse in individuals with pernicious anemia. Otherwise, daily doses up to 15 mg of folate to adults seem to be without toxic effects. Rats given massive doses (~500 mg/kg body weight) of folate develop renal toxicity because of folate precipitation, and convulsions have been observed in rats given 45 to 125 mg folate intravenously.

VITAMIN B₁₂

Name: Cobalamin
Active form: Methylcobalamin, adenosylcobalamin (including 5′-deoxyadenosylco-
        balamin), hydroxocobalamin
Function: One-carbon metabolism

Vitamin B_{12} is a group of cobalamins (Figure 5.31) or cobalt-containing corrinoids which have the biological activity of cyanocobalamin. The vitamin is also known as the anti-pernicious anemia factor, the extrinsic factor of W. B. Castle, and the animal protein factor. Vitamin B_{12} is very different from all other water-soluble vitamins in that it possesses a mineral, cobalt, coordinate covalently bonded within a corrin ring (which is four reduced pyrrole rings linked together). Vitamin B_{12} has the largest molecular weight of all the vitamins.

As early as the 1820s J. S. Combe described a fatal anemia due to "some disorder of the digestive and assimilative organs." This anemia was fatal for at least another century, and therefore was known as pernicious anemia. G. R. Minot and W. P. Murphy received the Nobel Prize for finding in the 1920s that the disease could be treated by eating liver. W. B. Castle, in 1929, found that the liver extrinsic factor required an intrinsic factor secreted by the stomach for absorption. The active component present in liver was later found to be vitamin B_{12}. Vitamin B_{12} was the last of the vitamins to be isolated in crystalline form. It was first isolated in 1947 by K. Folkers and E. Rickers of Merck & Co. from a fermentation process using *Lactobacillus lactis*. From a blood-red solution formed dark-red crystals of the long-sought anti-pernicious anemia factor named vitamin B_{12} by K. Folkers. The synthesis of vitamin B_{12} was completed in 1973 by R. B. Woodward and a team of scientists. In 1975 the Nobel Prize in Chemistry was awarded for the synthesis of the vitamin.

Forms

The vitamin B_{12} found in foods usually is attached to polypeptides, which are hydrolyzed in the stomach and duodenum. The intrinsic factor, a glycoprotein produced by the parietal cells of the gastric mucosa, binds vitamin B_{12} as a dimer (IF–B_{12}–IF). The intrinsic factor delivers the vitamin to receptor sites in the ileum, where calcium is needed for attachment of the intrinsic factor–vitamin B_{12} complex to the receptor sites. Approximately half of the vitamin B_{12} found in foods is

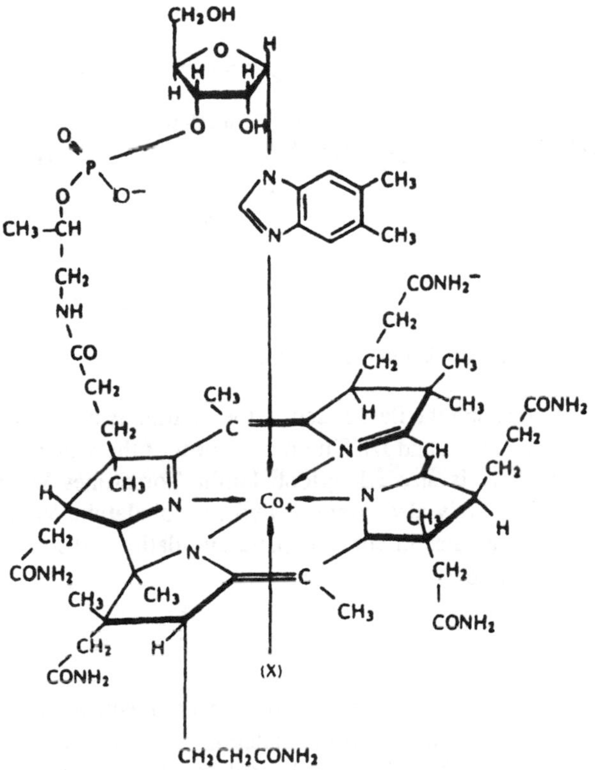

vitamin B$_{12}$

(X) = —NO$_2$ nitrocobalamin
   = —H$_2$O aquacobalamin
   = —CN in cyanocobalamin
   = —OH in hydroxocobalamin
   = —CH$_3$ in methylcobalamin   (coenzyme B$_{12}$)

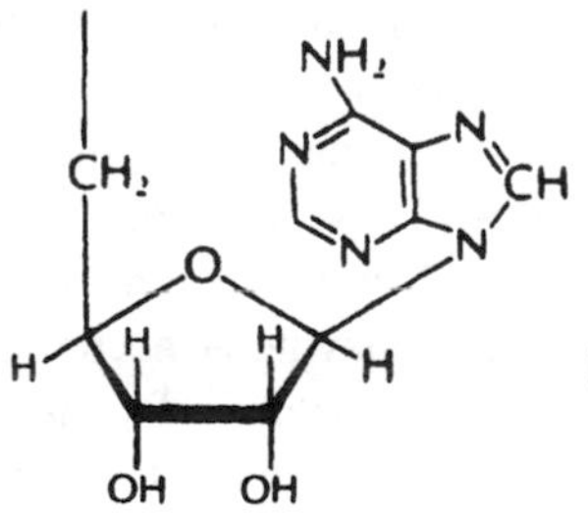

in 5'-deoxyadenosylcobalamin   (coenzyme B$_{12}$)

Figure 5.31 Structure of vitamin B$_{12}$ and coordinate substitutes.

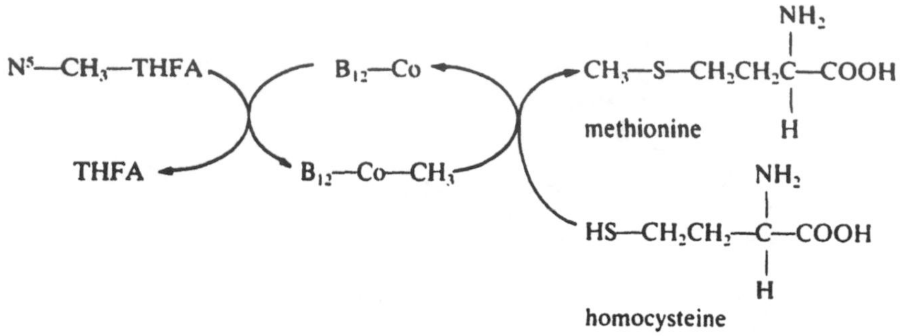

$$N^5—CH_3—THFA \qquad B_{12}—Co \qquad CH_3—S—CH_2CH_2\overset{\overset{\displaystyle NH_2}{|}}{C}—COOH$$

$$THFA \qquad B_{12}—Co—CH_3 \qquad methionine \qquad H$$

$$HS—CH_2CH_2—\overset{\overset{\displaystyle NH_2}{|}}{C}—COOH$$

$$H$$

homocysteine

Figure 5.32 Conversion of homocysteine to methionine.

absorbed. Once absorbed through the ileal mucosa, the vitamin is bound to transport proteins, the transcobalamins I, II, and III. The major form of the vitamin in plasma is methylcobalamin, but there is also adenylcobalamin (sometimes known as 5′-deoxyadenylcobalamin). The body also contains hydroxocobalamin. Vitamin B_{12} is secreted in the bile and participates in enterohepatic circulation. Absorbed vitamin B_{12} is also excreted in the urine.

Function

There are only two reactions in humans that have been unequivocally shown to require vitamin B_{12} as a coenzyme. Methylcobalamin is an intermediate in the transfer of a methyl group from N^5-methyl-tetrahydrofolate to homocysteine to form methionine (Figure 5.32); if vitamin B_{12} is not available, N^5-methyl-tetrahydrofolate is trapped (called the folate or methyl trap) and cannot be converted to tetrahydrofolate, and then to other folates. Vitamin B_{12} enables the tetrahydrofolates to perform their functions. These folates function in DNA and RNA synthesis (see Chapter 14). Hence, both folic acid and vitamin B_{12} are needed for the synthesis of nucleic acids, cell division, and growth in general. A decrease in DNA synthesis results in megaloblastosis. Methylcobalamin is also needed for the conversion of homocysteine to methionine along with folic acid and vitamin B_6. Adenosylcobalamin (actually 5′-deoxyadenosylcobalamin) is needed for the interconversion of methyl-malonyl-coenzyme A and succinyl-coenzyme A. These reactions are involved in the energy metabolism of both carbohydrate and fat metabolites. These reactions are also involved in the catabolism of odd-chain fatty acids and certain amino acids. If adequate vitamin B_{12} is not available, methyl-malonyl-coenzyme A accumulation may inhibit myelin sheath formation and cause neuropathy. Vitamin B_{12} may also function in reactions in which no specific 1-carbon donor/recipient is required.

Food Sources

Vitamin B_{12} is present only in foods containing animal proteins. Rich sources of the vitamin include organ meats, beef, pork, lamb, seafood, eggs, some sea vegetables, and fermented foods. A variety of fermented products are available which contain varying quantities of the vitamin. Vitamin B_{12} is relatively stable to dry heat, but is lost when foods are cooked at an alkaline pH or by prolonged exposure to high temperature.

Dietary Recommendations

The 1998 RDA for vitamin B_{12} was estimated as follows. The minimum quantity of vitamin B_{12} required for maintenance of individuals with pernicious anemia is 1.5 µg daily as judged by maintenance of adequate hematologic and serum vitamin B_{12} values, while the estimate of loss due to lack of reabsorption of biliary vitamin B_{12} is 0.5 µg daily; so, 1.5 µg minus 0.5 µg is 1.0 µg daily. Vitamin B_{12} in foods is approximately 50% bioavailable, so the requirement of normal individuals for vitamin B_{12} from food is 2.0 µg, and the 1998 RDA is 2.4 mg daily for adults. The median vitamin B_{12} intakes of adults 20 to 59 years according to NHANESIII are 4.83 and 3.03 µg daily. Many people ingest the vitamin in the form of cyanocobalamin as part of a multivitamin supplement. Many middle-aged and even more elderly individuals are unable to absorb sufficient vitamin B_{12} from foods or oral supplements due to the lack of IF secretion, and are given the vitamin by intramuscular injections. According to the 1998 report of the Panel on Folate, Other B Vitamins, and Choline, Food and Nutrition Board, individuals over 50 years of age should meet their RDA by consuming foods fortified with vitamin B_{12} or taking supplements containing vitamin B_{12} in that 10 to 30% of older people may be unable to normally absorb the naturally occurring vitamin.

Deficiency

The most common cause of vitamin B_{12} deficiency is an inadequacy of intrinsic factor secretion rather than an inadequate dietary intake of the vitamin. Individuals cannot absorb vitamin B_{12} if sufficient intrinsic factor is not available. Most of the symptoms of vitamin B_{12} deficiency are similar to those of folate deficiency. These include weakness, tiredness, dyspnea, poor growth, glossitis, megaloblastic macrocytic anemia, leukopenia, thrombocytopenia, and gastrointestinal abnormalities. These symptoms are primarily caused by a secondary deficiency of reduced folate. There is also irreversible degeneration of the central nervous system in vitamin B_{12} deficiency, with early symptoms including paresthesia, numbness and tingling sensations of hands and feet, moodiness, confusion, and depression. The neuropathy is due to a generalized demyelinization of nervous tissue.

Clinical signs of pernicious anemia are not evident until 5 to 7 years after cessation of intrinsic factor secretion primarily because of the enterohepatic circulation of the vitamin. The ability to synthesize and secrete intrinsic factor is inherited as an autosomal dominant trait mainly affecting individuals past middle-age, though pernicious anemia has been observed in children. Vitamin B_{12} deficiencies due to low dietary intakes have been reported in vegans who do not consume fermented products, as well as in infants of lactating vegan mothers. Also, impairment of gastrointestinal function for an extended period is of concern with regard to malabsorption of vitamin B_{12} and resulting deficiency of the vitamin.

Nutritional status with regard to vitamin B_{12} is most often evaluated by determining plasma or erythrocyte vitamin B_{12} concentration by radioimmunoassay. All radiodilution kits used in assessment of vitamin B_{12} in the United States must contain purified intrinsic factor as the cobalamin-binding protein. Typical hematologic status parameters are also utilized in the evaluation of vitamin B_{12} status.

Pharmacologic Doses

Individuals with pernicious anemia typically are treated with vitamin B_{12} injections given intramuscularly, thus bypassing the defective absorption, with daily injections of 1 µg being adequate. Frequently 15 to 100 µg of the vitamin are injected following diagnosis of the deficiency. Following recovery about 1 µg is injected intramuscularly daily or more often, 30 to 100 µg (or even 1 mg) at monthly intervals. Individuals with gastric atrophy are treated with 25 µg to 1 mg of the vitamin. No success has been reported in treating neural disorders not caused by the deficiency with large doses of the vitamin. No Tolerable Upper Intake Level has been set for vitamin B_{12}.

Toxicity

Rare allergic reactions probably due to impurities in the vitamin B_{12} preparation have been reported. There is some evidence that large doses of vitamin B_{12} may obscure diagnosis of folic acid deficiency in that it relieves the megaloblastic macrocytic anemia caused by folic acid deficiency. No toxicity symptoms have been observed in animals given several times their requirement of the vitamin.

BIOTIN

Name: Biotin
Active form: Biocytin
Function: Carboxylations
Note: Synthesized by intestinal microflora

Biotin is one of only two vitamins to contain sulfur. It also contains a ureido ring and a valeric acid side chain (Figure 5.33). Around 1900 F. Wildiers found that some yeasts required a factor found in yeast and wort for their growth, and the factor was called "bios." Bios later was found to contain what is now known as biotin, pantothenic acid, and myo-inositol. M. Boas in 1927 noted that "egg white injury" was cured by "protective factor X," which is now known as biotin. P. György in 1931 also discovered this factor and named it vitamin H (*Haut* is German for *skin*). This vitamin was first isolated from egg yolks by F. Kögl and B. Tönnis in 1936.

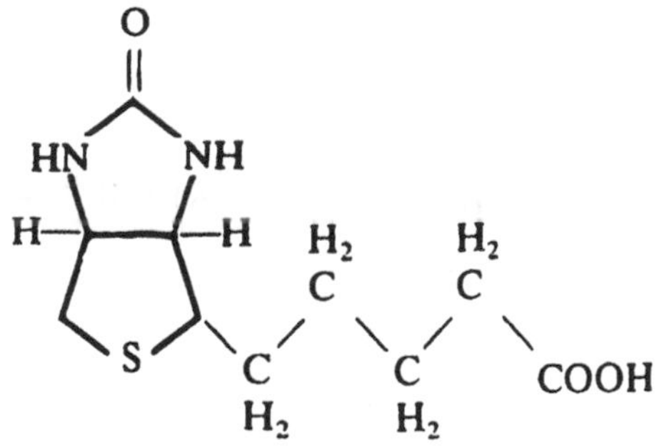

Figure 5.33 Structure of D-biotin.

The chemical synthesis of biotin was first accomplished by S. A. Harris and co-workers in 1945.

Form

Biotin has been isolated or chemically synthesized in eight isomeric forms. Only D-biotin is biologically active as a coenzyme. In tissues, D-biotin is covalently attached to enzymes by an amide bond linking the vitamin to a lysine residue of the enzyme. This conjugation is facilitated by ATP and Mg^{2+}, and the vitamin–enzyme conjugate is known as biocytin. D-biotin and biocytin are absorbed in the proximal small intestine, and likely transported by a biotin-binding protein. Biotin-producing microorganisms and fungi exist in the intestinal tract; some of the biotin produced by this microflora is absorbed and utilized by humans, but not enough is obtained to meet dietary requirements for the vitamin. Careful balance studies in man have shown that urinary excretion of biotin normally exceeds intake.

Function

Biotin as biocytin (Figure 5.34) functions in carboxylation reactions (Figure 3.35). Major carboxylation reactions involving biocytin permit the conversion of odd-numbered hydrocarbons into even-numbered hydrocarbons, which are then metabolized in the major metabolic pathways (Figure 5.36). Both odd-numbered amino acids and fatty acids are converted to even-numbered hydrocarbons by carboxybiocytin. Major carboxylase reactions include the conversion of pyruvate into oxaloacetate, acetyl-coenzyme A into malonyl-coenzyme A, and propionyl-coenzyme A into methyl-malonyl-coenzyme A (Figure 5.37). The biotin containing 3-methyl-crotonyl-coenzyme A carboxylase is needed in the catabolism of branched-chain amino acids. Biocytin is additionally important in the synthesis of carbamyl-phosphate, used in the synthesis of the pyrimidines and in the formation of urea. Thus, biotin is needed for the synthesis and degradation of fatty acids and gluconeogenesis.

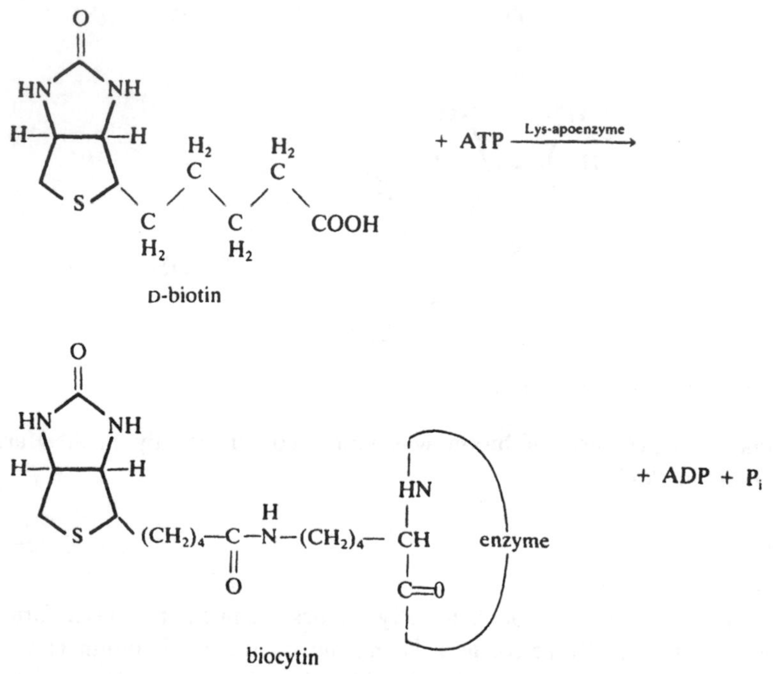

Figure 5.34 Conversion of biotin to biocytin.

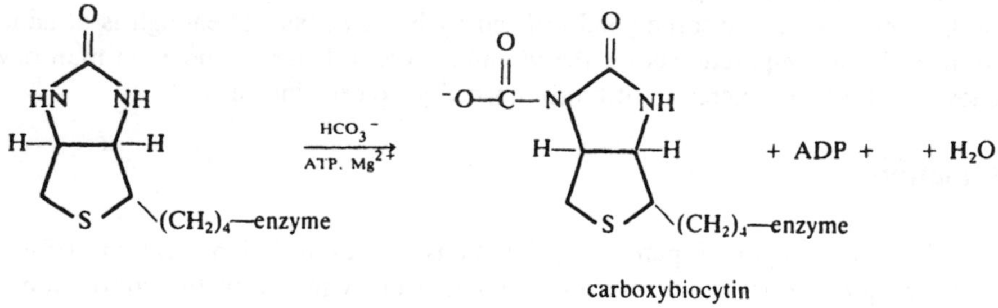

Figure 5.35 Formation of carboxybiocytin.

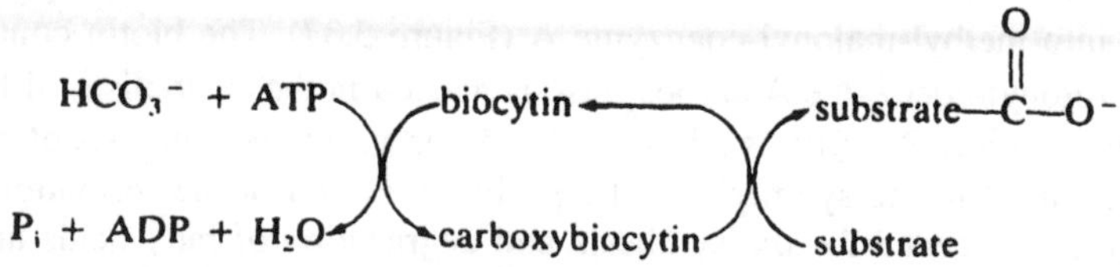

Figure 5.36 Formation of carboxybiocytin and carboxylase reaction.

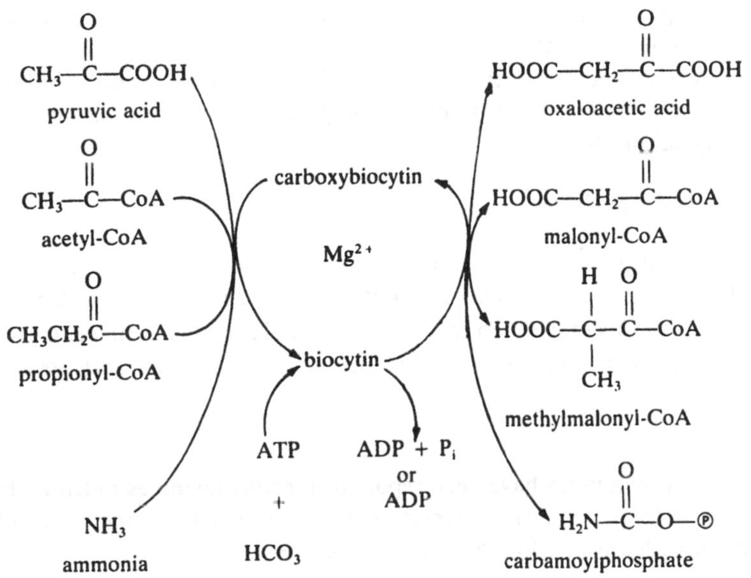

Figure 5.37 Carboxylation reactions showing substrate and product resulting from carboxy-biocytin and carboxylase activity.

Food Sources

Rich sources of biotin include organ meats, egg yolks, soybeans, and baker's and brewer's yeasts. A relatively small percentage of biotin is lost during normal cooking procedures. Not all of the biotin present in foods is bioavailable. Many individuals in the United States ingest biotin as part of a multivitamin preparation.

Dietary Recommendations

The body gets considerable amounts of the vitamin from the absorption of the biotin synthesized by the intestinal microflora which varies greatly from individual to individual. The 1998 Adequate Intake for adults of all ages is 30 μg daily. Most individuals consume adequate quantities of the vitamin.

Deficiency

In humans biotin deficiency may be induced by the consumption of large amounts of raw egg whites (about 10% of diet). Egg white contains the glycoprotein avidin, which can bind biotin and prevent its absorption, but which is denatured when the egg white is cooked. Biotin deficiency symptoms include anorexia, nausea, pallor, scaly dermatitis, atrophy of lingual papillae, graying of mucous membranes, lassitude, depression, muscle pains, hypercholesterolemia, and electrocardiographic abnormalities. Seborrheic dermatitis of infants less than 6 months of age may be due to biotin deficiency as the condition reverses promptly when infants are given biotin (~5 mg) intramuscularly or intravenously. Erythematous rash has been observed in adults on total parenteral nutrition (TPN). Biotin deficiency in humans is rare; however, some inborn errors of metabolism exist with regard to biotin. Biotin status is most often evaluated by determining plasma levels of the vitamin using microbiological methods.

Pharmacological Doses

Biotin (~5 mg) given orally, intramuscularly, or intravenously has been shown to heal skin lesions in the vast majority of infants with seborrheic dermatitis. Patients with biotin-responsive inborn errors of metabolism have improved when given large doses (~10 mg) of biotin. No Tolerable Upper Intake Level has been set for biotin.

Toxicity

No toxicity symptoms have been reported in adults taking as much as 10 mg of the vitamin daily. Controversial reports exist as to whether large doses of biotin affect the reproductive performance of female rats.

PANTOTHENIC ACID

Name: Pantothenic acid
Active form: Forms portion of coenzyme A
Function: Two-carbon metabolism

Pantothenic acid, discovered by R. J. Williams in 1933, is one of the B-complex vitamins. The Greek word "pantos" means everywhere, and it was and is found in a variety of biological materials. T. H. Jukes, in 1939, identified the factor as the "antidermatitis factor" in chicks. Pantothenic acid (Figure 5.38) is composed of pantoic acid and β-alanine.

Form

Unlike the other B vitamins, pantothenic acid does not function independently as a coenzyme; rather it forms a portion of a much larger and very important coenzyme, coenzyme A (Figure 5.39), often abbreviated CoA or CoASH. The remaining components comprising coenzyme A are β-mercaptoethylamine and adenosine diphosphate (ADP).

Function

Pantothenic acid as a component of coenzyme A functions in the synthesis of fatty acids, sterols, membrane phospholipids, choline, and acetylcholine as well as the oxidative degradation of fatty acids and amino acids. Coenzyme A also functions in the tricarboxylic acid (TCA) cycle, and thus functions in energy metabolism. Coenzyme A is needed for the synthesis of the porphyrin ring found in hemoglobin

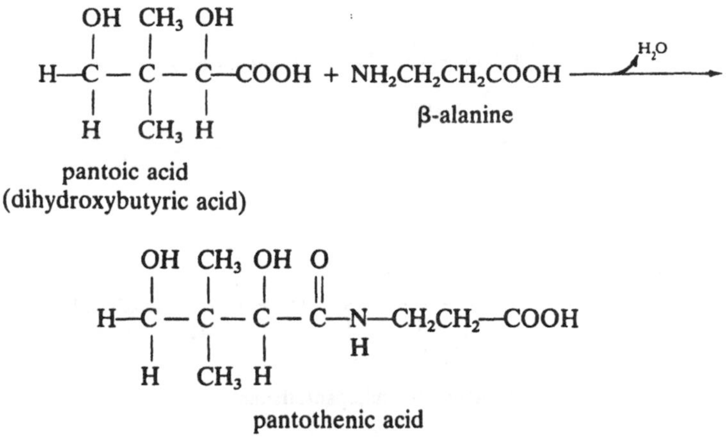

Figure 5.38 Synthesis of pantothenic acid by plants.

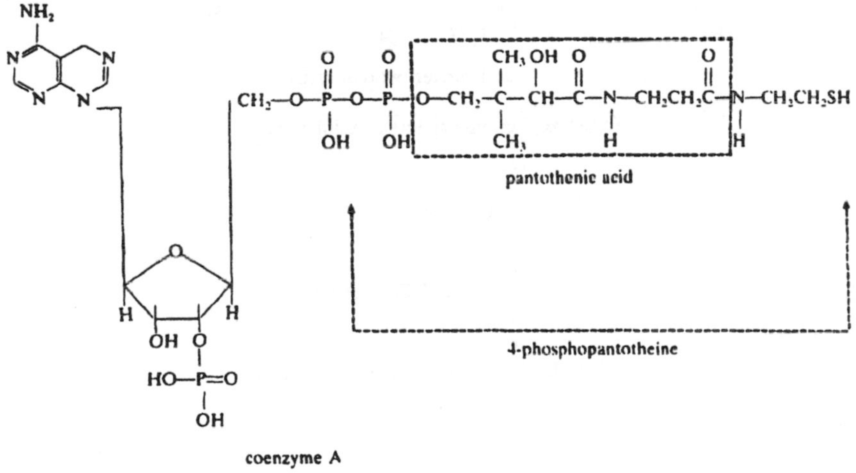

Figure 5.39 Coenzyme A containing pantothenic acid.

and myoglobin, as well as for acylation reactions in general and can function as a nonspecific acetate (2-carbon) donor/recipient. Pantothenic acid, when attached to a carrier protein (ACP) serves as the point of attachment of fatty acids synthesized *de novo* (Figure 5.40).

Food Sources

Pantothenic acid is widely distributed in foods. Rich sources include all meats, egg yolks, whole grains, and molasses. About a third of the pantothenic acid present in foods is lost during ordinary cooking.

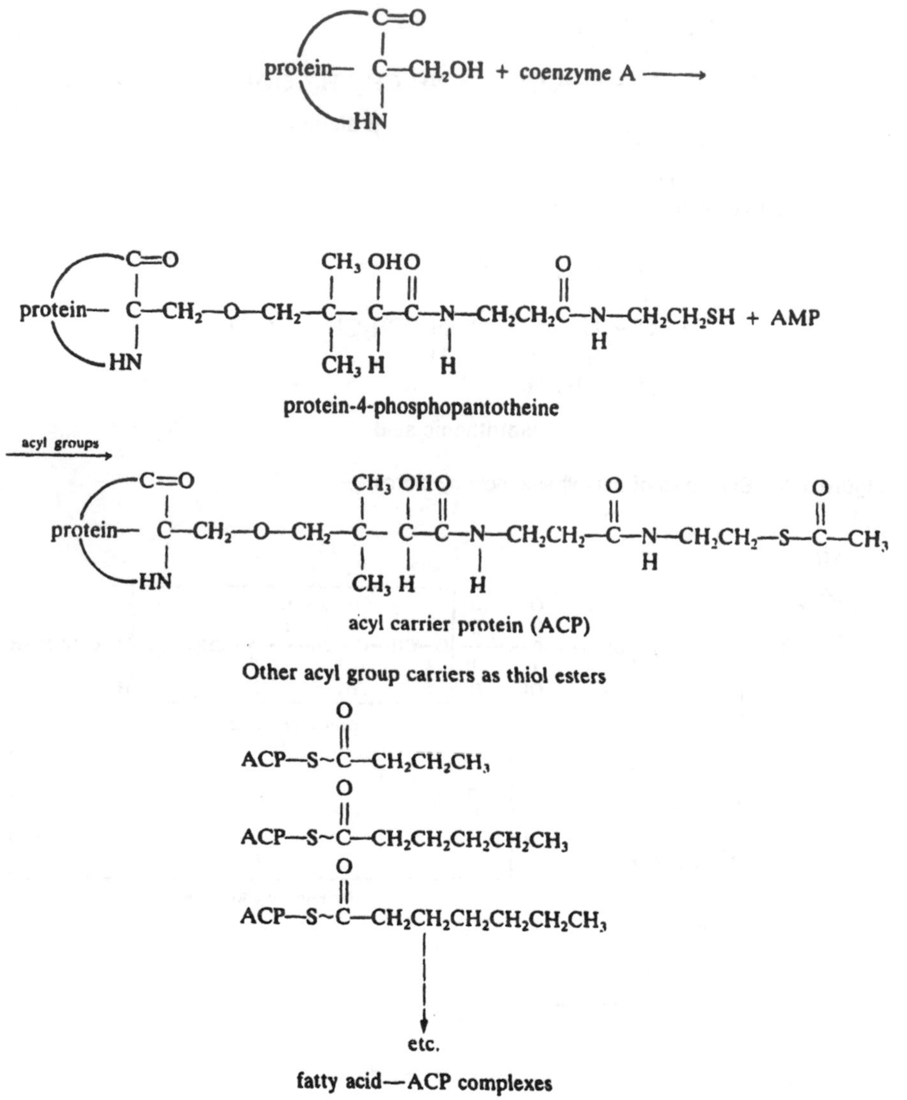

$$
\text{protein—}\ \overset{\displaystyle \overset{\textstyle C=O}{|}}{\underset{\displaystyle \underset{\textstyle HN}{|}}{C}}\text{—}CH_2OH\ +\ \text{coenzyme A} \longrightarrow
$$

$$
\text{protein—}\ \overset{\overset{C=O}{|}}{\underset{\underset{HN}{|}}{C}}\text{—}CH_2\text{—}O\text{—}CH_2\text{—}\overset{\overset{CH_3}{|}}{\underset{\underset{CH_3}{|}}{C}}\text{—}\overset{\overset{OH}{|}}{\underset{\underset{H}{|}}{C}}\text{—}\overset{O}{\overset{||}{C}}\text{—}\underset{H}{N}\text{—}CH_2CH_2\overset{O}{\overset{||}{C}}\text{—}\underset{H}{N}\text{—}CH_2CH_2SH\ +\ AMP
$$

protein-4-phosphopantotheine

acyl groups
⟶

$$
\text{protein—}\ \overset{\overset{C=O}{|}}{\underset{\underset{HN}{|}}{C}}\text{—}CH_2\text{—}O\text{—}CH_2\text{—}\overset{\overset{CH_3}{|}}{\underset{\underset{CH_3}{|}}{C}}\text{—}\overset{\overset{OH}{|}}{\underset{\underset{H}{|}}{C}}\text{—}\overset{O}{\overset{||}{C}}\text{—}\underset{H}{N}\text{—}CH_2CH_2\text{—}\overset{O}{\overset{||}{C}}\text{—}\underset{H}{N}\text{—}CH_2CH_2\text{—}S\text{—}\overset{O}{\overset{||}{C}}\text{—}CH_3
$$

acyl carrier protein (ACP)

Other acyl group carriers as thiol esters

$$
ACP\text{—}S\text{~}\overset{O}{\overset{||}{C}}\text{—}CH_2CH_2CH_3
$$

$$
ACP\text{—}S\text{~}\overset{O}{\overset{||}{C}}\text{—}CH_2CH_2CH_2CH_2CH_3
$$

$$
ACP\text{—}S\text{~}\overset{O}{\overset{||}{C}}\text{—}CH_2CH_2CH_2CH_2CH_2CH_3
$$

etc.

fatty acid—ACP complexes

Figure 5.40 Formation of acyl carrier protein (ACP) and fatty acids *de novo.*

Dietary Recommendations

Usual pantothenic acid intakes of adults in the United States are 5 to 10 mg daily. The 1998 Adequate Intake for pantothenic acid for adults is 5 mg daily. Many individuals ingest pantothenic acid as a component of multivitamin preparations.

Deficiency

Pantothenic acid deficiency has not been observed in humans, except in those who are chronically malnourished. Pantothenic acid deficiency has been reported to cause the "tingling foot syndrome" or "burning foot syndrome" during World War II among prisoners fed little but watery potato soup, as well as in malnourished individuals in the Far East. Deficiency symptoms include numbness and tingling of the extremities, gastric distress and nausea, insomnia, irritability and emotional instability, and muscular weakness. Administration of large doses of the vitamin reportedly reversed these symptoms. Pantothenic acid utilization may be impaired in alcoholics. Pantothenic acid status is most often evaluated by determining plasma or urinary levels of the vitamin using microbiological techniques.

Pharmacologic Doses

Pantothenic acid administration appears to have no pharmacologic effects in humans. A study with rats indicates that pantothenic acid may have a protective effect against radiation sickness. A Tolerable Upper Intake Level has not been set for pantothenic acid.

Toxicity

No toxic effects were reported when 10 g calcium pantothenate were given to young men for 6 weeks. Occasional diarrhea and water retention has been observed in several studies when humans took 10 to 20 mg of the vitamin daily.

SELECTED OTHER SUBSTANCES IN FOODS HAVING SOME CHARACTERISTICS OF VITAMINS

Several other substances in foods have some of the characteristics of vitamins. Generally, knowledge is inadequate as to whether the substance performs a function in humans or whether humans can synthesize sufficient amounts of the nutrients to meet needs. Some of these substances are known to be vitamins for other animals, but not known to be essential for humans. Taurine, carnitine, and myo-inositol are vitamins for some other animals but not humans; data are inconclusive as to whether choline belongs in this category.

CHOLINE

Name: Choline
Active form: Acetylcholine, phosphatidylcholine
Function: Neurotransmission

Choline (Figure 5.41), a water-soluble substance, was discovered in 1862 by A. Strecker. The pathway for synthesis of choline was described in 1942 by V. duVigneaud et al. Choline can be synthesized in humans from ethanolamine and a methyl group donor such as methionine, folate, or vitamin B_{12} (Figure 5.42). The ability of humans to synthesize choline is variable. Limited data exist as to whether

$$HO–CH_2–CH_2–\overset{+}{N}(CH_3)_3$$

Figure 5.41 Structure of choline.

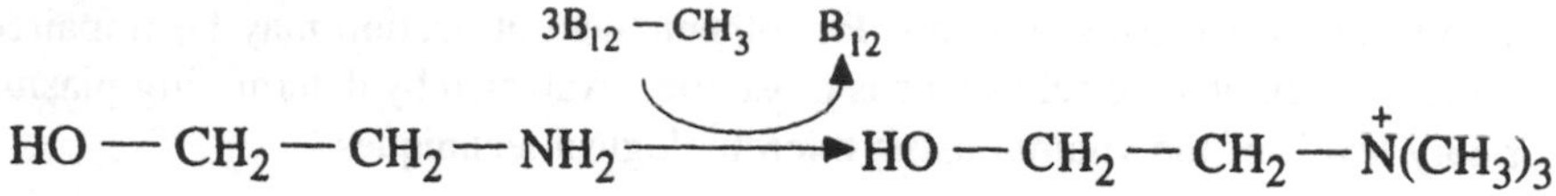

$$HO—CH_2—CH_2—NH_2 \xrightarrow{\quad 3B_{12}—CH_3 \qquad B_{12}\quad} HO—CH_2—CH_2—\overset{+}{N}(CH_3)_3$$

Figure 5.42 Synthesis of choline from methylcobalamin.

choline is a dietary essential during all stages of the life cycle. Perhaps the choline requirement can be met by synthesis within the body during some of the life stages. Human culture cells do require choline.

Form

Choline in foods is primarily in the form of phosphatides. Pancreatic and intestinal secretions contain phospholipases that hydrolyze the phosphatidylcholine consumed as part of the diet. Intestinal microflora convert some of the ingested choline to betaine and methylamines before the choline is absorbed. However, some of the dietary choline is absorbed in all portions of the small intestine as choline. Estimates of choline bioavailability are not available. Choline is found in high concentrations in the brain and nerves, liver, kidneys, mammary glands, and placenta. Choline may be oxidized in the kidney and excreted as betaine, though some is also excreted as choline.

Function

Choline functions as a component of acetylcholine and phosphatidylcholine or lecithin. Acetylcholine is a neurotransmitter, and phosphatidylcholine, is a major component of membranes, plasma lipoproteins, and sphingomyelins. Choline, as a component of phospholipids, including phosphatidylcholine, and sphingomyelin has cell signaling functions. Choline also functions as a precursor for the methyl group donor betaine.

Food Sources

Choline is widely distributed in foods. Rich sources of choline include meats, whole grains, egg yolks, peanuts, and legumes. Lecithin, or phosphatidylcholine, is frequently added to foods during processing by the food industry.

Dietary Recommendations

Although choline intakes have not been reported in national surveys, adults have been estimated to consume 700 to 1100 mg choline daily. The Panel on Folate, Other

B Vitamins, and Choline, Food and Nutrition Board, in 1998 stated that "sufficient human data are not available to determine if choline is essential in the human diet and how much is required if essential." However, this Panel did recommend an Adequate Intake for choline for men and women 19 years of age and older of 550 and 425 mg/day, respectively.

The young of all animal species, perhaps even humans, appear to be susceptible to choline deficiency. It is likely that newborns need dietary choline. The American Academy of Pediatrics recommends that infant formula contain 7 mg choline/100 kcal, an amount approximating that found in human milk.

Deficiency

Decreased choline stores and sometimes liver damage have been reported in men fed diets deficient in choline but adequate in methionine, folate, and vitamin B_{12}. Patients on total parenteral nutrition (TPN) solutions devoid of choline but adequate in methionine and folate have been reported to develop fatty liver and liver damage. In many cases, this abnormal liver functioning has been successfully treated with choline or lecithin. Serum alanine aminotransferase activities are elevated in choline-deficient humans and other animals; this parameter is utilized in assessing choline adequacy.

Pharmacologic Doses

Large quantities (~20 g) of choline or lecithin given orally have been reported to result in several adverse effects including nausea, diarrhea, sweating, dizziness, hypotension, fishy body odor (from excessive excretion of the choline metabolite trimethylamine), depression, excessive cholinergic stimulation, and electrocardiographic abnormalities.

Taurine

Taurine, a water-soluble substance, is also known as β-aminoethanesulfonic acid. Taurine has long been considered an end product of S-containing amino acid metabolism (Figure 5.43). Taurine can be synthesized in humans from dietary cysteine or methionine which requires vitamin B_6. Taurine is a vitamin for cats and some laboratory animals. Taurine is abundant in muscle foods of all types including shellfish.

Taurine is found in high concentrations in muscles, the nervous system, and platelets. In humans, taurine is incorporated into the bile acid taurocholic acid. Reports exists, though controversial, that taurine may have other functions.

Plasma and urinary levels of taurine are lower in pre-term and full-term infants fed synthetic formulas without added taurine and in infants maintained by parenteral

$$NH_2-CH_2-CH_2-SO_3H$$

Figure 5.43 Structure of taurine.

nutrition than in breast-fed infants. Cow's milk is much lower in taurine than human milk. However, taurine supplementation of infant formulas has failed to have an impact on growth, nitrogen retention, or serum protein levels. Dietary essentiality of taurine has not been demonstrated in humans.

Carnitine

Carnitine, a water-soluble substance, is known chemically as β-hydroxy-[γ-N-trimethyl-ammonia] butyrate (Figure 5.44). In 1947 G. S. Fraenkel found that the meal worm *Tenebrio molitor* required a growth factor present in the charcoal filtrate of yeast. In 1948 G. S. Fraenkel and H. E. Carter found that vitamin B_T and carnitine were the same.

Carnitine is found primarily in muscle tissues. Rich food sources of carnitine are those of animal origin (particularly meats and dairy products). Carnitine functions in the transport of long-chain fatty acids as acylcarnitine (Figure 5.45) into the mitochondrial matrix for energy production. Carnitine can also function as a non-specific methyl donor, thus sparing other methyl donors such as methionine. Carnitine may be needed for fatty acid synthesis.

The first case of carnitine deficiency in humans was reported in 1973 by A.G. Engel and C. Angelini; a young woman had progressively worsening muscular weakness, and a muscle biopsy showed that there were lipid droplets in abnormal spaces in the muscle fibers. By 1975 six cases of carnitine deficiency had been reported in humans, and two of the patients were treated with oral carnitine and showed improvement. Over 100 individuals have been diagnosed as having a genetic carnitine deficiency. Symptoms of the deficiency include muscular weakness, lipid

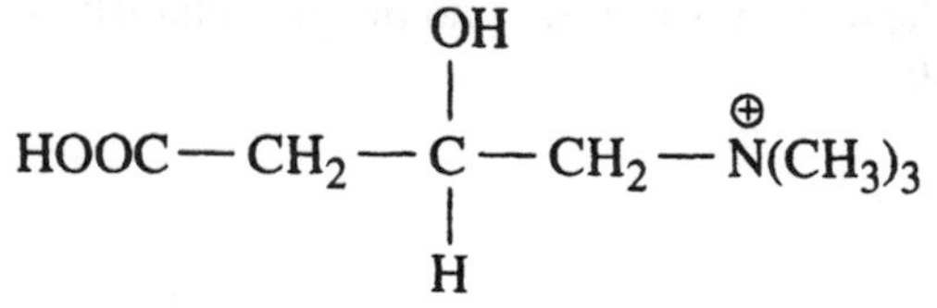

$$\text{HOOC}-\text{CH}_2-\overset{\overset{\displaystyle \text{OH}}{\displaystyle |}}{\underset{\underset{\displaystyle \text{H}}{\displaystyle |}}{\text{C}}}-\text{CH}_2-\overset{\oplus}{\text{N}}(\text{CH}_3)_3$$

Figure 5.44 Structure of carnitine.

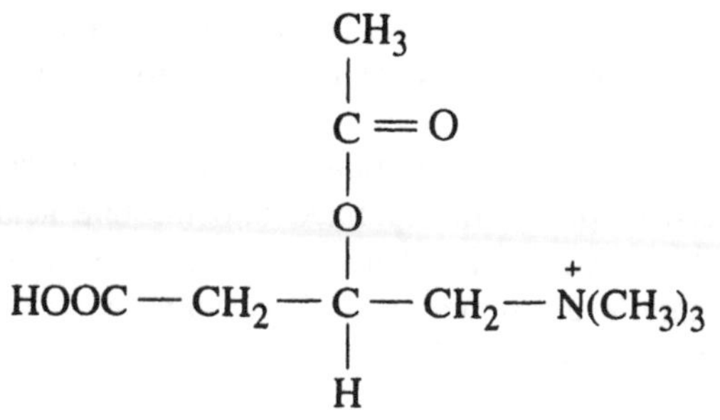

$$\text{HOOC}-\text{CH}_2-\overset{\overset{\displaystyle \text{CH}_3}{\overset{\displaystyle |}{\underset{\displaystyle |}{\text{C}=\text{O}}}}}{\underset{\underset{\displaystyle \text{H}}{\displaystyle |}}{\text{C}}}-\text{CH}_2-\overset{+}{\text{N}}(\text{CH}_3)_3$$

Figure 5.45 Structure of acylcarnitine.

infiltration of skeletal muscle, cardiomyopathy, severe hypoglycemia, lower than normal ability to increase ketogenesis during fasting, and lower than normal concentrations of muscle and plasma carnitine. The deficiency has been reported in individuals on long-term total parenteral nutrition (TPN) and some kidney conditions, such as chronic hemodialysis. Improvement in the symptoms has been reported in some but not all patients given oral carnitine. Some studies indicate that oral carnitine increases oxygen consumption levels in endurance athletes, while other studies report no effects. Occasional diarrhea has been reported in individuals given large amounts of carnitine.

Carnitine deficiency has also been reported in fetal calves, neonatal rats, and guinea pigs. Symptoms include depressed long-chain fatty acid oxidation and excessive triglyceride synthesis. Well-nourished adults can synthesize sufficient quantities of carnitine in their livers and kidneys from the amino acids lysine and methionine. Newborns seem to have reduced reserves of carnitine and a low capacity for synthesizing carnitine. Human milk has been reported to contain enough carnitine to meet the needs of infants. Infants fed soy-based formulas or those on total parenteral nutrition (TPN) receive no exogenous carnitine and have low plasma carnitine levels. Some researchers believe that carnitine is a vitamin for the newborn, particularly the pre-term infant. Currently, carnitine is not considered to be a vitamin for humans.

Myo-inositol

Myo-inositol, or cyclohexanehexol, is a water-soluble substance having a formula similar to glucose (Figure 5.46). Myo-inositol is sometimes called meso-inositol. There are nine isomers of inositol, but only myo-inositol is biologically active. Myo-inositol is found in foods usually as inositol phospholipids (see Chapter 3). Foods particularly rich in myo-inositol include fruits, meats, milk, nuts, vegetables, whole grains, and yeasts. In plants, myo-inositol is part of phytic acid (see Chapter 6) or inositol hexaphosphate, and in animals it is part of membrane phospholipids. Myo-inositol is sometimes referred to as muscle sugar.

Myo-inositol functions as a component of phosphatidylinositol and polyphosphoinositides (cephalins) in cellular and subcellular membranes. Myo-inositol apparently has a lipotropic action via its effects on lipoproteins. Phosphatidylinositol appears to function as a cellular mediator of signal transduction, metabolic regulation, and growth. Myo-inositol triphosphate seems to function in mobilizing intracellular calcium.

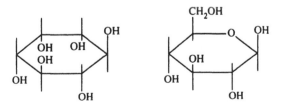

Figure 5.46 Structure of myo-inositol and β-D-glucose.

Myo-inositol deficiency has been demonstrated in mice, gerbils, and chicks where symptoms include intestinal lipodystrophy, alopecia, poor growth and lactation, encephalomalacia, triglyceride accumulation, and abnormal fatty acid metabolism. Deficiency of myo-inositol has not been demonstrated in humans. Myo-inositol is found in many foods, and can be synthesized from glucose by many of the tissues in the body. The kidney seems to be the main regulator of inositol concentrations in humans as it can synthesize as well as degrade myo-inositol. The intestinal microflora can synthesize inositol and contribute to the metabolic pool. Human breast milk and colostrum are rich in myo-inositol. The American Academy of Pediatrics has recommended that myo-inositol be included in infant formulas at levels equal to or greater than those of human milk.

The metabolism of myo-inositol appears to be altered in individuals with diabetes mellitus, chronic renal diseases, respiratory distress syndrome, galactosemia, and multiple sclerosis. Large amounts of myo-inositol given orally seem to be nontoxic, although its use in situations where inositol metabolism is impaired has been questioned. Excess dietary myo-inositol has been shown to reduce motor conduction velocities in rats.

CHAPTER **6**

Minerals

The mineral content of plants, animals, and humans is inorganic and is that material which remains after either thermal (fire or high temperature) or chemical (nitric or perchloric acid) oxidation. The mineral content that remains following oxidation is often called "ash." Minerals are elements. In animals and humans, minerals constitute about 4% of our adult body weight. Minerals are found in the body in combination with organic compounds or as free ionized ions.

Our bodies contain and require several minerals. Essential minerals are part of major organ systems, proteins, enzymes, and hormones, and regulate metabolism. When they are removed from the diet or are absent naturally, a disease often occurs. When the mineral is refed, the disease state goes away — pure cause and effect. In addition, for a mineral to be essential, functionality has to have been demonstrated. The minerals listed in the first two columns of Table 6.1 are classified as being essential for humans. Column 3 lists minerals for which biological function has been demonstrated. Column 4 lists overtly toxic minerals.

Calcium, phosphorus, and magnesium are the minerals that are highly concentrated in bone, and represent about 80% of the total mineral content of the human body. Sodium, chlorine, potassium, and sulfur complete the largest group of minerals, called macrominerals (column 1). Macrominerals are minerals that are required at dietary levels of 100 mg or more daily. Sometimes macrominerals are defined as being the minerals that are present in the body in quantities larger than 5 g. Ionized solutes which serve the body as electrically charged particles are called ions. Sodium, chloride, and potassium are the major electrolytes when in their fully (100%) ionized form as ions. The remaining minerals are the microminerals, most commonly referred to as trace minerals or trace elements (column 2). Trace minerals were so named during the time when analytical procedures and instrumentation were insufficiently sensitive to measure and quantitate accurately minerals found in tissues in very small amounts. Thus, their detection was often quantitatively reported as "trace" amounts. Microminerals are required by the body in amounts of less than 100 mg daily. Sometimes microminerals are defined as being those minerals present in the

Table 6.1 Minerals

Macrominerals	Micro (trace) minerals	Newer trace minerals	Toxic metals
Calcium	Iron	Silicon	Cadmium
Phosphorus	Fluorine	Nickel	Lead
Magnesium	Zinc	Cobalt	Mercury
Sodium	Selenium	Tin	Silver
Potassium	Manganese	Arsenic	
Chlorine	Iodine	Vanadium	
Sulfur	Copper	Boron	
	Molybdenum		
	Chromium		
	Cobalt		

body in quantities less than 5 g. There are a number of trace minerals having general scientific acceptance as being essential trace minerals for humans and other higher animals. These are, in order of descending body concentration: iron, fluorine, zinc, copper, selenium, manganese, molybdenum, iodine, chromium, and cobalt. The newer trace elements (Table 6.1, column 3) are those elements that have been demonstrated to have some biological function associated with them in plants or experimentally in animals, but for which there is no specifically known conclusively proven biological function in humans. The newer trace elements are silicon, nickel, tin, arsenic, boron, and vanadium. Some researchers consider the least concentrated trace minerals to be the ultramicro trace minerals or elements. Cadmium, lead, mercury, and to a lesser degree silver are toxic metals (Table 6.1, column 4).

There are 90 naturally occurring elements in the periodic table, and 78 elements have been reported to occur in animals or human tissues. In light of present knowledge, many of these elements are nonessential. Presently, the list of nonessential elements includes aluminum, antimony, germanium, rubidium, and the remaining elements of the periodic table for which no biological function has been demonstrated.

GENERAL NUTRITIONAL FUNCTIONS OF MINERALS

Minerals are components of or are found in body tissues. The elemental composition of the adult human body is given in Figure 6.1. The macrominerals function to provide (1) strength to the organic endoskeleton through the deposition of calcium, phosphorus, and magnesium in bone, (2) principal electrolytes — sodium, potassium, and chlorine as the chloride anion, and (3) sulfur to provide structure to proteins. Macrominerals have, in addition to these primary functions, other vital metabolic regulator roles in cells.

Micro (trace) elements found in tissues and cells in parts per million (ppm) or parts per billion (ppb) function primarily with enzymes as components of the active site of enzymes or as regulators of enzymatic activity. Enzymes that contain minerals are referred to as metalloenzymes. As components of enzymes and proteins, trace elements are frequent participants in redox reactions, with the metal often function-

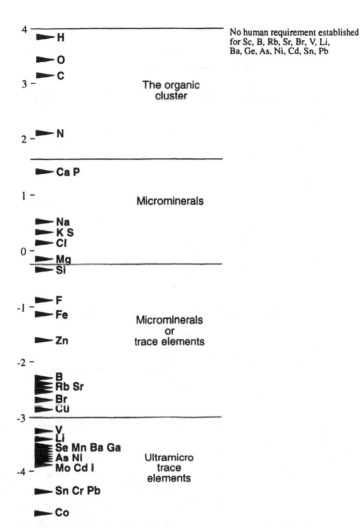

Figure 6.1 Elemental composition of the adult human (log gram-moles for 75-kg man). (Adapted from G. Schrauzer, *Biochemistry of the Essential Ultratrace Elements*, E. Frieden, ed., Plenum Publishing Co., 1984, Chapter 2, p. 18.)

ing as the electron carrier. Several of the earliest evolved proteins of primordial cells may have been metalloproteins and metalloenzymes containing iron, copper, sulfur, or manganese. These minerals, along with selenium and molybdenum, function in a variety of redox and respiratory chain enzymes and proteins. Many of these redox proteins, both in plants and animals and humans, probably came into being when plants, simple at first, began to liberate oxygen from photosynthesis. The other trace elements, such as manganese and zinc, along with the macroelements calcium and magnesium, perform nonredox functions in proteins and enzymes. They evolved with proteins and enzymes by contributing to their structural organization as binding

Table 6.2   Mineral Antagonists and Organic Facilitator
            Compounds

Major Mineral Antagonists

$$
Ca - \begin{bmatrix} P \\ Al \\ Zn \\ Mg \end{bmatrix} \qquad
P - \begin{bmatrix} Ca \\ Mg \\ Mn \end{bmatrix} \qquad
Mg - \begin{bmatrix} Ca \\ P \end{bmatrix} \qquad
Na - \{ K \qquad
S - \begin{bmatrix} Se \\ Zn \end{bmatrix}
$$

$$
Fe - \begin{bmatrix} Mn \\ Cu \\ Co \\ Mn \\ Zn \end{bmatrix} \qquad
Mn - \begin{bmatrix} Cu \\ P \\ Fe \\ Co \\ Mg \end{bmatrix} \qquad
Zn - \begin{bmatrix} Fe \\ Ca \\ Cu \\ Pb \\ Cd \end{bmatrix} \qquad
Cu - \begin{bmatrix} S \\ Ag \\ Cu \\ Fe \\ Mo \\ P \\ Cd \\ Zn \\ Pb \\ Se \end{bmatrix} \qquad
Mo - \begin{bmatrix} W \\ S \\ Cu \\ Mn \end{bmatrix}
$$

$$
Cr - \begin{bmatrix} Zn \\ V \end{bmatrix}
$$

$$
Cd - \begin{bmatrix} Zn \\ Cu \\ Fe \\ Hg \\ Pb \\ Se \end{bmatrix} \qquad
F - \begin{bmatrix} Al \\ Ca \\ Mg \end{bmatrix} \qquad
I - \{ Co \qquad
F - \begin{bmatrix} Al \\ Ca \\ Mg \end{bmatrix} \qquad
Se - \begin{bmatrix} S \\ As \\ Hg \\ Cd \\ Ag \\ Pb \\ Au \end{bmatrix}
$$

$$
Co - \{ Fe \qquad Sn - \begin{bmatrix} Fe \\ Cu \end{bmatrix}
$$

Organic Inhibitors and Facilitators of Mineral Absorption

Organic inhibitors of some minerals for absorption
  Phytic acid, fiber, some drugs
Organic facilitators of mineral absorption
  Vitamin C, citric acid, lactic acid, pyruvic acid, succinic acid, lactose,
  fructose, glucose, histidine, lysine, cysteine, valine

sites for enzymes and/or substrates as well as metabolic regulators of proteins, enzymes, and nucleic acids.

Many of the macroelements and trace elements are antagonistic to one another during absorption from the gastrointestinal tract, in which two or more minerals compete for absorption sites or interact chemically. Many examples of mineral antagonists are well known, both from natural observations and laboratory experimentation with animals. It is known, for example, a high dietary intake of copper reduces absorption of iron, and in principle could lead to an iron deficiency if ingestion of a high dietary copper diet was sustained. Diets also contain organic factors that may either reduce or enhance mineral absorption from the digestive tract. Mineral absorption may be reduced by dietary fiber, oxalic acid, and phytic acid. Oxalic acid, found in spinach, "greens," sweet potatoes, rhubarb, and cocoa, binds with some minerals, such as calcium and iron, and decreases their absorption. Phytic acid, hexaphosphoinositol, found in whole grains where it serves the need of growing plants for phosphate, binds and can prevent the absorption of the minerals calcium, iron, and zinc. There are also those organic factors in the diet that facilitate mineral absorption. Amino acids, organic acids such as citric and lactic acids, and some carbohydrates increase absorption of some minerals. Table 6.2 is a partial listing of mineral antagonists and organic facultative compounds for mineral absorption. Drugs and medicines may also adversely affect mineral absorption (see Chapter 16).

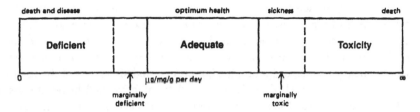

Figure 6.2 Deficiency, adequacy, and toxicity of essential minerals.

ESSENTIALITY AND BIOAVAILABILITY OF MINERALS

Almost all of the macrominerals, the trace minerals, the nonessential minerals, and the toxic metals are supplied to the body through the diet having once originated in soils. The soil's minerals are absorbed from the vegetables, fruits, grains, and animal products eaten. Lesser amounts of minerals are normally ingested in water; still lesser amounts are absorbed by the lungs from air. The elements derived from the soil, passed to us through plants and animals, are essential for humans if a dietary inadequacy results in a physiological or structural abnormality, and its addition to the diet prevents or reinstates normal health. Specific biochemical changes and defined functions for minerals which can be accurately measured lend credence to their essentiality. Lack of dietary adequacy of the essential macrominerals and trace elements results in the classic diseases, conditions, afflictions, and anemias (Cu and Fe), rickets (Ca), goiter (I), and Keshan's disease (Se).

Essentiality is a qualitative feature of all minerals whose dietary deficiency or inadequacy over an extended period results in a disease condition, a feature shared with vitamins. Mineral deficiency, dietary adequacy, and mineral toxicity are quantitative values that can be assigned to each essential mineral over a dietary range beginning with no dietary intake. Each mineral will have its own quantitative range of dietary adequacy and will vary in toxicity when excessive dietary intake exceeds excretory capacity. Almost all minerals can produce some toxicity when consumed in excess. These effects of dietary deficiency, adequacy, and toxicity that almost all essential minerals share are demonstrated in Figure 6.2.

There is some evidence, though not considered conclusive, that other minerals might also be essential for humans. As more people are consuming formulated supplements such as Enfamil, Sustacal, Ensure, Isocale, Osmolite, and individually formulated intravenous parenteral nutrition formulas for several months to several years, researchers are finding that some of the minerals present in foods are missing from these formulas, and that these minerals are essential for good health.

TOXICITY OF MINERALS

Whereas the toxicity of the macrominerals is minimal in all cases, toxicity from some of the micro (trace) minerals can be severe. Toxicity from the trace minerals may occur from both acute and chronic ingestion. Upon metabolic accumulation iron causes hemochromatosis, and copper causes Wilson's disease. Both diseases may be fatal. Another very toxic trace element is selenium. Long known for its toxicity in animals it can be toxic to humans taking supplements. Also toxic are the nonessential heavy metals, cadmium, lead, mercury, and silver. All of the toxicities that arise from the essential trace elements and the nonessential heavy metals are thought to occur because of the generation of free radicals. Such free radicals may be produced through the reaction with cellular thiols (SH compounds) that generate superoxide (O_2^-) or via the generation of the hydroxyl ($\cdot OH$) radical as a result of Fenton chemistry, the scission of hydrogen peroxide by copper or iron (see Chapter 15).

COORDINATION AND CHELATION
OF MINERALS

The key to understanding the general role of many of the macrominerals and the microminerals as metabolic regulators and as catalysts in proteins and enzymes is their ability to form coordination compounds, metal complexes, or what is often referred to as just "complexes." Coordination complexes usually contain a centrally located metal cation, surrounded by negative ions, molecules, or water. Coordination complexes are formed by coordinate covalent bonding (Appendix A), and coordination positions may be from one to six, with two, four, six, and sometimes eight common. Molecules that have two or more coordinate positions or ligands are multidentate or chelating compounds. As the number of ligands increases about the central metallic cation, the stability of the metal complex is usually increased. Thus the stability of metal complexes is usually determined by the number of coordinating ligands about the metal cation, the size and charge of the metal ion, the ligating molecule, and the final structure of the chelate complex.

Surrounding the central metallic cation forming the coordination complex may be found ions, Cl^- (chloride) or PO_4^{2-} (phosphate) and SO_4^{2-} (sulfate), for example, which may be either inorganic or organic in form. Organic compounds forming complexes include $NH_2CH_2CH_2NH_2$ (ethylenediamine) and ethylenediaminetetraacetate (EDTA) (Figure 6.3). Other organic compounds forming a variety of metallocomplexes include various amino acids, disulfides, and tetrapyrroles. Molecules containing amines, carboxyl anions, hydroxyl anions, thiols, sulfate and phosphate anions, and heterocyclic nitrogen compounds may also coordinate metals. Some of these other metal complexes are also shown in Figure 6.3. It is the coordination chemistry of metal ions to ligands, forming either loosely or tightly bound metalloorganic complexes, that accounts for the absorption of minerals and the binding of cation minerals by fiber, by metallothionein, by DNA, by tetrapyrroles, and by the many proteins and enzymes requiring minerals for regulation and catalysis.

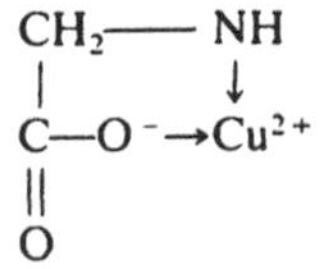

CH$_2$——NH
| ↓
C—O$^-$→Cu^{2+}
||
O

copper glycinate

Nutritional/Physiological Significance
Amino acid metal complexes, especially cysteine and histidine for transport and mineral storage

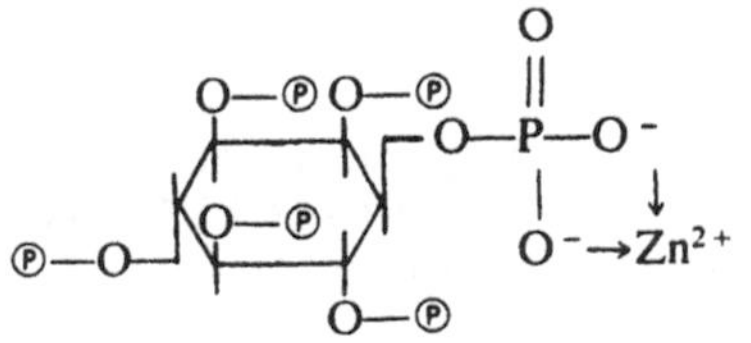

phytic acid
(hexaphosphomyoinositol)

Phytic acids binds Zn^{2+}, Fe^{2+}, Ca^{2+}, and may reduce absorption of these minerals

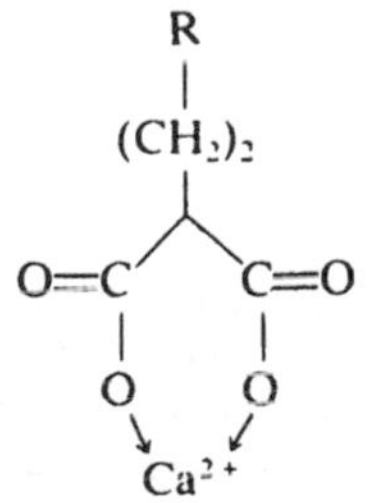

R
|
(CH$_2$)$_2$

O=C   C=O
| |
O   O
Ca^{2+}

calcium γ-carboxyglutamate

Calcium γ-carboxyglutamate binds Ca^{2+} precipitating prothrombins binding to blood platelets [see "Phylloquinone (K$_1$) and Analogs"]

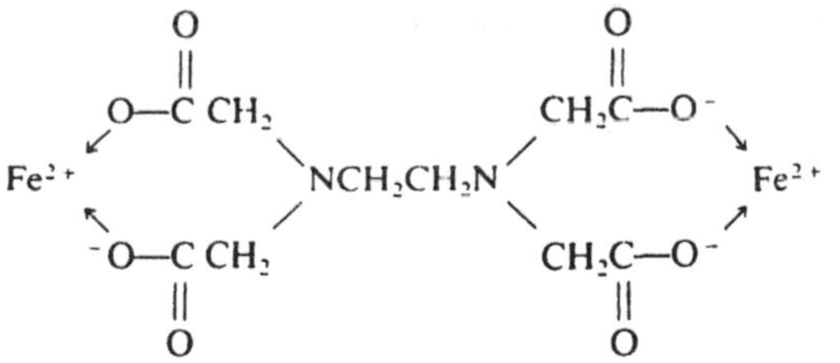

iron–EDTA
(ethylenediaminetetraacetic acid)

EDTA chelates Ca^{2+}, Zn^{2+}, Ca^{2+}, Fe^{2+}, Mn^{2+}, Mg^{2+}, sometimes used as food preservative

Figure 6.3 Nutritional ligands and chelates.

ABSORPTION AND METABOLISM OF MINERALS

All minerals in the diet are not equally absorbed, nor are all different compounds and complexes of the same mineral absorbed with the same degree of efficiency. Such differences in absorption, along with factors such as age, sex, genetic variables, general health, nutritional status, and diet, affect mineral absorption and bioavail-

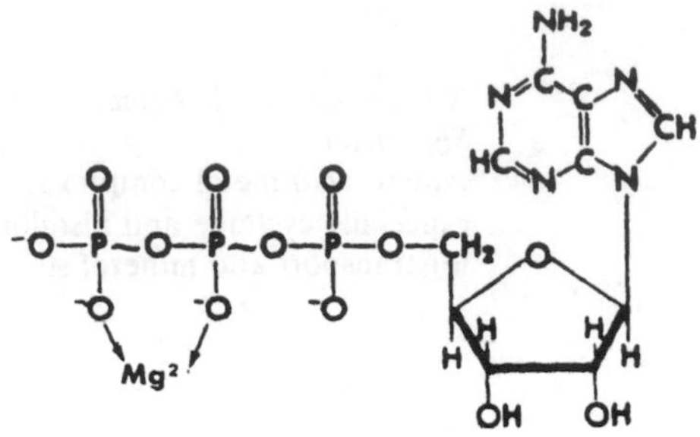

magnesium-ATP
(adenosine triphosphate)

Magnesium-ATP complex for the
hydrolysis of ATP (ATP → ADP
+ P$_i$)

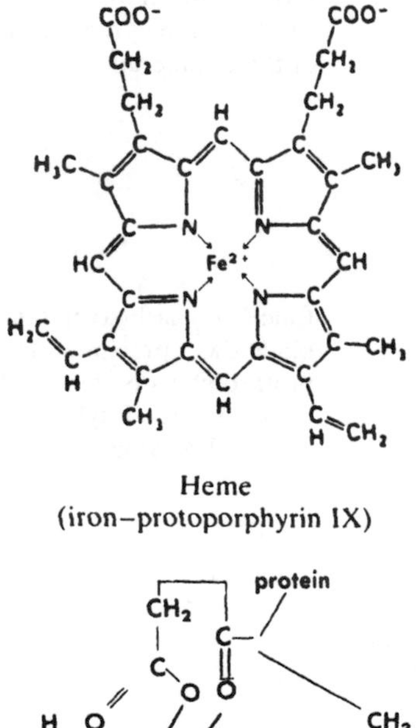

Heme
(iron–protoporphyrin IX)

Heme-tetrapyrrole complex
containing Fe^{2+} in hemoglobin,
myoglobin, and cytochromes.
May complex Zn^{2+} in iron-
deficiency anemia. Similar
coordination complexes contain
Mg^{2+} (chlorophyll) and Co^{2+}
(vitamin B$_{12}$)

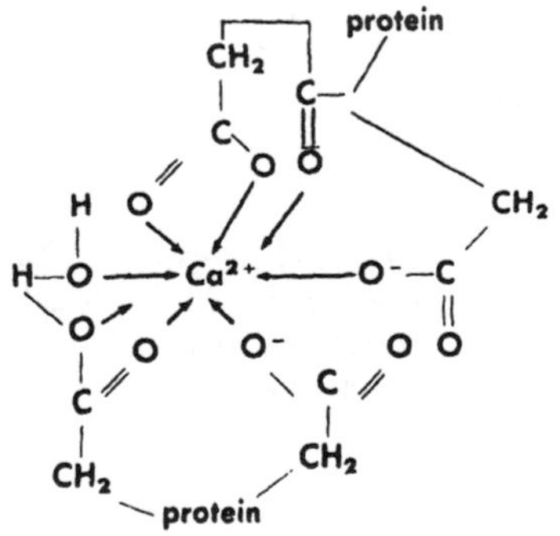

parvalbumin

Parvalbumin—shown is one of
three calcium binding sites of this
protein. Calcium binds to four
acidic amino acid residues, one
ketone, and a molecule of water
occupies the eighth coordinate
position

Figure 6.3 *Continued.*

ability. Minerals become bioavailable from the diet following absorption, the process that predominates in mineral regulation. Following mineral absorption across the intestinal mucosa, they enter their metabolic pool and are transported, often by a specific transport protein, to their storage, physiological, or biochemical site of action.

In the following section on minerals, beginning with calcium, the minerals are presented in decreasing order of abundance in the human body. To each mineral is affixed the date of nutritional recognition, relative atomic size (H = 1.0) to hydrogen, its place within the periodic table, its usual oxidation state(s), and total body burden or content for an idealized 70 kg person. Within the discussion of each mineral, tables have been included listing the known extent to which the mineral interacts with proteins, enzymes, and other molecules. For each mineral (where known) an overview of its absorption, modes of excretion, and metabolism are presented in a figure.

CALCIUM

Date of nutritional recognition: 1842
Relative atomic size: 6.6
Oxidation state: +2
Body burden: 1500 g
Major function: Bone strength

Calcium (Figure 6.4) is the most abundant mineral of animals with a calcified skeleton, including humans, representing 52% of the body's mineral content. Almost all of this calcium is found in insoluble form in bone and teeth (99%) as hydroxyapatite $[3Ca_3(PO_4)_2 \cdot Ca(OH)_2]$ providing the structural support to the endoskeleton and dentition. The remaining 1% of calcium is found bound to proteins and ionized intra- and extracellulary, where it controls a wide variety of physiological and enzymatic controls. This small fraction of calcium is responsible for electrical cell potentials, muscle contraction, cell division, the clotting of blood, and adenyl cyclase formation. In many ways, ionized calcium is almost hormone-like in its varied functions.

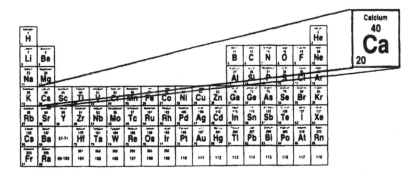

Figure 6.4 Calcium's place in the periodic table.

Calcium is a rather abundant alkaline earth metal, often having been concentrated in deposits of limestone as calcium carbonate. The metal was discovered in 1808 by Sir Humphry Davy, who gave it its name, calcium, after the Latin *calx*, meaning "lime." The nutritional importance of calcium was noted by M. Chossat in 1842, when he recognized the need for calcium for the development of the bones of pigeons.

The dietary absorption of calcium from the gastrointestinal tract is explicably tied to the physiological role of vitamin D (Chapter 5). Indeed, there are at least two calcium deficiency diseases, rickets and osteoporosis. Rickets caused by a lack of bone calcification is in reality a vitamin D deficiency disease which can occur in the face of adequate calcium nutriture. Osteoporosis, "porous bones," is an insidious loss of bone mineralization over a period of years which occurs most often in white, Anglo-Saxon, postmenopausal women of small bone stature. This disease leads to a loss in height, dowager's hump, and frequent fractures of vertebrae, wrists, and hips among the elderly. The course of osteoporosis is not fully understood, but increased calcium intake and exercise beginning early in life is being advocated as a preventative measure to slow or prevent this disease. In spite of recommendations for increasing one's dietary intake of calcium for osteoporosis, there are clearly no calcium deficiency diseases *per se.* Many elderly people do not exhibit fully developed osteoporosis, so it would appear that vitamin D, estrogens, parathyroid hormone, inactivity, and other unidentified factors are contributing to osteoporosis.

Calcium is absorbed from the gastrointestinal tract under control of vitamin D and calcium binding proteins (Figure 6.5). Although it is difficult to measure calcium absorption precisely, estimates of 20 to 30% calcium absorption of the 300 to 1200 mg ingested daily appears reasonable. The main storage site for calcium is bone, which constantly undergoes turnover by osteoclastic and osteoblastic cellular activity, with about 20% of bone being remolded each year. Bone calcium is the reservoir for serum calcium, which is carefully regulated and maintained by hormonal controls at around 10 mg/dl. PTH (parathyroid hormone) secretion controls the synthesis of renal 1,25-dihydroxyvitamin D, affecting intestinal absorption of calcium and osteoclastic activity, effectively raising levels of serum calcium. When serum calcium

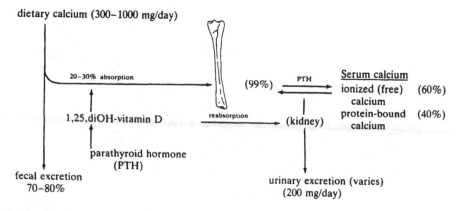

Figure 6.5 Calcium absorption and metabolism.

Table 6.3 Calcium Proteins and Regulated Enzymes

Enzyme/Protein	Ca/Molecule
Troponin-C	1
Parvalbumin	3
Calmodulin	4

Ca^{2+}-regulated enzymes and proteins via
  Ca^{2+} binding proteins
  Phosphorylases
  Adenylate cyclase
  Phosphatases
  Prothrombin
  Vitamin D dependent
  Ca^{2+} binding protein (CBP)

levels are high, PTH secretion is decreased, reducing synthesis of 1,25-dihydrox-yvitamin D and osteoclastic activity. Calcitonin, secreted by both the thyroid and parathyroid glands when PTH secretion is diminished, effectively lowers serum calcium levels. Serum and intracellular calcium bind to several calcium binding proteins, such as troponin-C, parvalbumin, and calmodulin (Table 6.3). Troponin-C within muscle binds calcium ion, permitting the contraction of muscle by the binding of the muscle proteins actin and myosin. Parvalbumin is an abundant calcium binding protein found in the muscle tissue of fish, reptiles, and amphibians. Its function remains unknown, but parvalbumin binds three calcium ions. Calmodulin, present in mammalian cells, binds four calcium ions, suggesting that the protein may have multiple functions when binding one, two, three, or four calcium ions. In cells, calmodulin participates in the regulation of phosphorylation reactions, microtubule formation, and in the regulation of unbound intracellular calcium. The intra- and extracellular concentrations of calcium ions bound to these proteins are important regulators of glycogenolysis, ATPase activity, ATP synthesis, membrane electrical potential, and calcium ion transport. Excretion of dietary calcium is predominately in the feces (unabsorbed) and urine, and lesser amounts are lost through perspiration.

Dairy products are rich sources of calcium. Chinese cabbage, kale, broccoli, "greens," bony fish, and calcium-set tofu are good-to-rich sources of calcium. In recent years the food industry has also produced calcium-fortified orange juices and other beverages.

The 1997 Adequate Intake (AI) for men and women, aged 19 to 50 years, is 1000 mg daily, while that for those 51+ years is 1200 mg. Commercial calcium supplements are used fairly extensively by individuals, particularly women, in the United States. According to NHANESIII data, the median daily calcium intakes of men and women, 20 to 59 years, in the United States were 847 and 617 mg, respectively.

Calcium toxicity, to date, has only been reported in individuals taking nutrient supplements. Hypercalcemia has been reported to result in increased kidney stone formation, adverse interactions with other essential minerals (iron, zinc, magnesium, phosphorus), myopathy, excessive calcification of bone and soft tissues, and the so-called "milk-alkali syndrome." In 1997 the Tolerable Upper Intake Level (UL) for calcium for adults was set at 2.5 g daily as part of the Dietary Reference Intakes.

PHOSPHORUS

Date of nutritional recognition: 1842
Relative atomic size: 3.7
Oxidation states: +3, +5
Body burden: 860 g
Major function: Bone ossification; energy transfer

The element phosphorus (Figure 6.6) was discovered by the German alchemist Hennig Brandt in 1669. The first nutritional reference to phosphorus, like calcium, was made by M. Chossat (1842), who observed bone development in pigeons. Phosphorus is the second most abundant element of the human body, which contains about 860 g or 30% of the total mineral content.

Most phosphorus (80%), like calcium, is stored in the bone and teeth in an inorganic mineral state, the hydroxyapatite. The remaining 20% of body phosphorus is distributed throughout body cells in inorganic and various organic forms of great importance to the metabolic functioning of cells (Figure 6.7). In addition to the structural role of phosphorus in nucleic acids, coenzymes, and phospholipids, the function of phosphorus as phosphate in energy transfer is unique. Inorganic phosphorus within cells is the primary buffer system ($HOP_4^{2-}/H_2PO_4^-$) regulating intracellular pH. Table 6.4 lists some of the known functions of phosphorus.

Phosphorus, being widely distributed in all foods, is ingested in both organic and inorganic forms. Phosphoric acid can be a major dietary source of phosphorus when carbonated beverages are consumed. Most phosphorus is absorbed with 60 to 70% efficiency, while some phosphorus, such as the organic phosphate of phytic acid, may go unabsorbed. Unabsorbed phosphorus is excreted in the feces, and most absorbed phosphorus is excreted in the urine as inorganic phosphate, PO_4^{2-}. Phosphate absorption can be adversely affected by ingestion of high amounts of antacids containing magnesium or aluminum hydroxides. Dietary deficiency of phosphorus

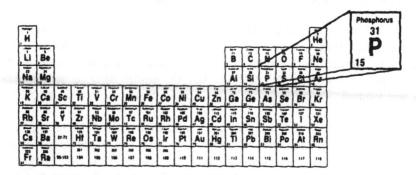

Figure 6.6 Phosphorus' place in the periodic table.

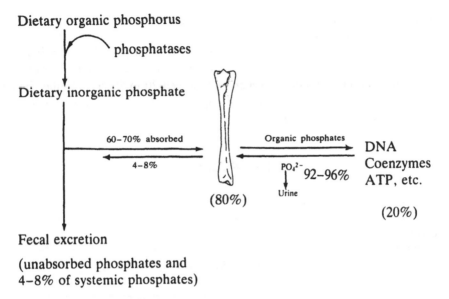

Dietary organic phosphorus

phosphatases

Dietary inorganic phosphate

60–70% absorbed

4–8%

(80%)

Organic phosphates

PO_4^{2-} 92–96%

Urine

DNA
Coenzymes
ATP, etc.

(20%)

Fecal excretion

(unabsorbed phosphates and
4–8% of systemic phosphates)

Figure 6.7 Phosphorus absorption and metabolism.

Table 6.4 Functional Roles of Phosphorus in Living Systems

(Inorganic)	Structural component of mineralized tissues: bones, teeth
	Intracellular buffer: $H_2PO_4 \rightleftharpoons H^+ + HPO_4^{2-}$
(Organic)	Structural component of:
	Nucleic acids
	DNA, RNA
	Structural component of:
	Coenzymes
	$NADP^+$, NAD^+
	FMN, FAD
	Thiamin pyrophosphate
	Pyridoxal phosphate
	Coenzyme A
	Structural component of:
	Lipids
	Lecithin and other
	Phosphatidic acid derivatives
	Energy transfer:
	ATP and other trinucleotides
	ADP and other dinucleotides
	AMP and other mononucleotides
	Creatine phosphate
	Glucose-1-phosphate and other
	Organophosphates

in humans would be a rare event, and most common forms of phosphorus found in food are relatively nontoxic.

The 1997 Recommended Dietary Allowance (RDA) for phosphorus for individuals 19 years of age and over is 700 mg daily. According to NHANESIII data, the median daily phosphorus intakes of men and women 20 to 59 years in the United States were 1466 and 1026 mg, respectively. Most people in the United States consume adequate quantities of phosphorus.

MAGNESIUM

Date of nutritional recognition: 1932
Relative atomic size: 5.3
Oxidation state: +2
Body burden: 25 g
Major function: Component of bone, regulator of enzyme activity

Magnesium (Figure 6.8) is the sixth and least abundant of the macrominerals of the human body. It comprises approximately 1% of the mineral content of the body, most (60%) being stored in bone along with calcium and phosphorus. Magnesium metal was discovered in 1808 by Sir Humphry Davy, and magnesium salts have been used as a medicine since the Renaissance. It was not until this century that H. D. Kruse and colleagues would, in 1932, demonstrate a nutritional need for magnesium in the rat. Experimentally, M. E. Shils was to describe magnesium deficiency in humans in 1964.

Much of the magnesium not associated with bone mineralization is complexed with phosphate or acts as a regulator of enzymatic activity (Table 6.5). It is the second most abundant mineral in cells after potassium. Magnesium participates as an enzymatic regulator of ATPase by complexing with the two terminal phosphates of ATP, forming Mg–ATP and all enzymatic reactions that involve phosphate transfer (see Figure 6.9). Magnesium is responsible for the structural integrity of the subunits forming ribosomes and the maintenance of the double-helical structure of DNA. In

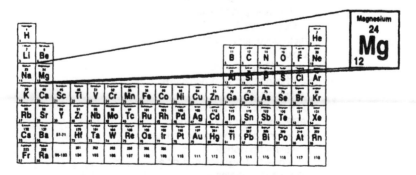

Figure 6.8 Magnesium's place in the periodic table.

Table 6.5 Enzymes/Hormones Regulated by Magnesium

ATPase
Adenylate cyclase
Enolase
Pyruvate kinase
Fructokinase
Creatine kinase
Some peptidases
May regulate insulin function
Thyroxine secretion regulated

plants, magnesium complexes with a tetrapyrrole to form chlorophyll, which is necessary for photosynthesis.

Magnesium deficiency in healthy people is rare, as foods usually contain and provide for a dietary adequacy of the element. Green leafy vegetables, unpolished grains, nuts, and seeds are particularly rich sources of magnesium. Magnesium is absorbed (40 to 45%) in the intestinal tract, is usually excreted in the urine, but may also be lost through perspiration (see Figure 6.9). Excessive intakes of magnesium from magnesium salts, but not food sources, has been reported to be toxic, particularly in individuals who have kidney problems. The 1997 Tolerable Upper Intake Level (UL) for magnesium for individuals nine years of age and older is 350 mg daily.

The 1997 RDA for magnesium is 310 and 400 mg for men and women aged 19 to 30 years, and 320 and 420 for men and women over 31 years of age, respectively. According to NHANESIII data the median daily magnesium intakes of men and women, 20 to 59 years, in the United States were 326 and 230 mg, respectively. Many people in our country consume less than recommended quantities of magnesium.

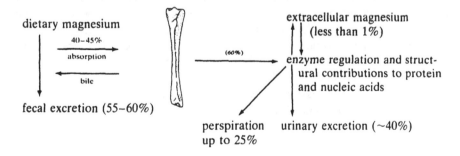

Figure 6.9 Magnesium absorption and metabolism.

POTASSIUM

Date of nutritional recognition: 1926
Relative atomic size: 7.6
Oxidation state: +1
Body burden: 180 g
Major function: Predominant intracellular cation

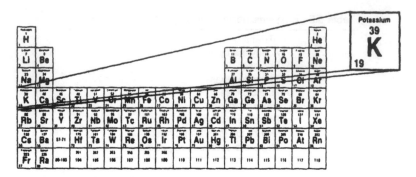

Figure 6.10 Potassium's place in the periodic table.

Potassium (Figure 6.10), the third most abundant mineral within the human body, shares a number of similarities and some differences with its lighter sister mineral, sodium. Potassium was discovered in 1807 along with sodium, by Sir Humphry Davy, in an electrolysis of fused sodium chloride. The nutritional requirement for potassium was first described for the rat by H. G. Miller in 1926.

Potassium is the major intracellular cation, with 90% of all the body's potassium being in the ionized form. The primary functions of potassium are control of muscle (along with sodium and calcium) contraction, enzyme regulation (Table 6.6), nerve excitation, and electrochemical transmission of nerve impulses. Heart muscle is particularly susceptible to hypokalemia (low potassium), and it is for this reason that potassium supplements are often prescribed when diuretics are used or renal or peritoneal dialysis is required. Extended diarrhea may lead to significant losses of potassium. Potassium also contributes to osmolarity and the acid–base balance of cells.

Widely distributed in foods, there is no specific 1989 RDA for potassium, as the diet normally provides 1.8 to 5.6 g daily. The 1989 Recommended Dietary Allowances publication included an Estimated Minimum Requirement of Healthy Persons for potassium which is 2000 mg daily for individuals 18+ years of age. The Committee on Diet and Health, National Research Council, in 1989 recommended a daily intake of 3.5 g and above for potassium. According to NHANESIII data, the median daily potassium intakes of men and women 20 to 59 years in the United States were 3060 and 2230 mg, respectively, which is the suggested intake for the mineral.

Potassium, like sodium, is almost completely absorbed by the intestinal tract, with the majority being excreted in the urine (Figure 6.11). Potassium reabsorption is regulated by aldosterone, and normal renal reabsorption of K^+ is about 20% of total potassium filtration.

All dietary potassium contains a very small proportion (1 in every 104 potassium atoms) of a naturally occurring radioisotope, ^{40}K. Having a half-life of 109 years,

Table 6.6   Enzymes Regulated by Potassium

K^+-ATPase
Acetylkinase
Pyruvate phosphokinase

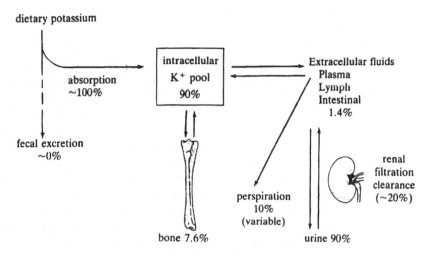

Figure 6.11 Potassium absorption and metabolism.

natural radioactive decay from this isotope can be used to measure total body potassium and can be employed to compute total body lean mass. Such measurement is performed by a whole-body gamma counter.

SODIUM

Date of nutritional recognition: 1847
Relative atomic size: 6.2
Oxidation state: +1
Body burden: 64 g

Sodium (Figure 6.12) was first isolated, along with potassium, by the electrolysis of fused sodium chloride by Sir Humphry Davy in 1807. J. B. Boussingault described the need for sodium by cattle in 1847, but it was not until 1940 that E. Orent-Keiles

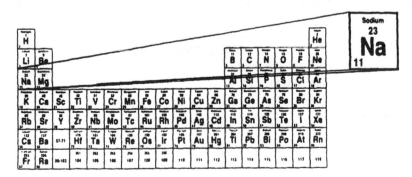

Figure 6.12 Sodium's place in the periodic table.

and E. V. McCollum established a nutritional essentiality for sodium by feeding rats diets extremely deficient in sodium.

The adult human contains approximately 64 g of sodium. Not quite half of this sodium (approximately 40%) is associated with bone, with the remainder mostly in the extracellular fluids. Sodium is the most abundant extracellular cation responsible for the osmolarity and ionic balance of the extracellular fluids, the electrochemical gradient of nerve axions for electrical impulses to be transmitted, and the acid–base balance of cells and their organelles. Sodium is maintained as the primary extracellular cation by ATPase "sodium pumps." General homeostasis of sodium is carefully regulated by the adrenal corticosteroid, aldosterone, which controls renal reabsorption of sodium. Any alteration of the sodium homeostasis adversely affects the state of body hydration. Loss of excess sodium (hyponatremia) by the use of diuretics, diarrhea, vomiting, or perspiration may lead to dehydration, decreased blood pressure, high hematocrits, and possibly death. Sodium retention is thought to be a causative factor in hypertension among some people who are sensitive to salt. For such reasons, restricted-sodium diets are often prescribed to hypertensive persons.

Sodium intake, mainly as table salts of sodium chloride added to prepared foods, is 10 to 15 g per day. Since sodium chloride is 40% sodium, the daily ingestion of sodium is 4 to 6 g per day. Under normal physiologic conditions a sodium balance is sustained with a daily intake of approximately 200 mg of sodium. The 1989 Recommended Dietary Allowances publication listed an Estimated Minimum Requirement of Healthy Persons for sodium of 500 mg daily for individuals 18+ years of age. The Committee on Diet and Health, National Research Council, in 1989 recommended that North American adults and children limit their daily intake of salt to 6 g or less, which is equivalent to ≤2400 mg of sodium. One of the Dietary Guidelines for Americans is to choose a diet moderate in salt and sodium. According to NHANES-III data, the median daily sodium intakes of men and women, 20 to 59 years, in the United States were 3813 and 2641 mg, respectively. Many Americans consume more sodium than is recommended.

Sodium is actively absorbed using ATP from the intestinal lumen with nearly 100% efficiency. In addition to storage in bone (approximately 40%), 30% of the extracellular sodium is in skin; 18% is in muscle, where it counteracts calcium in muscular contraction; 8% is in blood plasma; and 3% is in the brain. The major excretory route is via the urine and secondarily through perspiration during exercise (Figure 6.13).

CHLORINE

Date of nutritional recognition: 1979
Relative atomic size: 3.3
Oxidation state: −1
Body burden: 74 g
Major function: Anion to balance electrical neutrality of cations

The element is chlorine (Figure 6.14), but the nutritional need is for chloride (Cl⁻), a major anion of numerous salts (e.g., NaCl, KCl, $CaCl_2$). Chlorine was

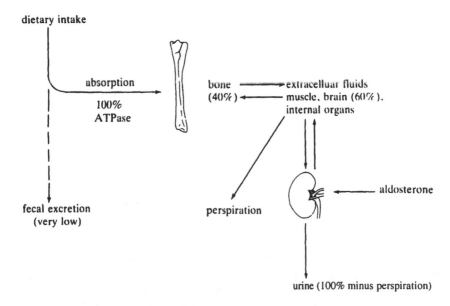

Figure 6.13 Sodium absorption and metabolism.

discovered in 1774 by C. W. Schelle. Chloride was the anion found by Sir Humphry Davy in 1810 in those famous electrolysis experiments.

Since the diet is abundant in chloride, little interest in this element appears to have been expressed by research scientists over time. During the late 1970s, however, chloride-deficient infant formulas were inadvertently manufactured and distributed. Infants consuming only these formula diets developed varied degrees of a chloride deficiency. The deficiency resulted in alkalosis and growth retardation in some infants which was traced to the chloride deficiency of the formulas. This unfortunate event emphasized the nutritional need for chloride. The Recommended Dietary Allowances publication in 1989 listed an Estimated Minimum Requirement of Healthy Persons for chloride for individuals 18+ years of age as 750 mg daily. Daily intakes of chloride for Americans were not estimated in the recent NHANESIII survey.

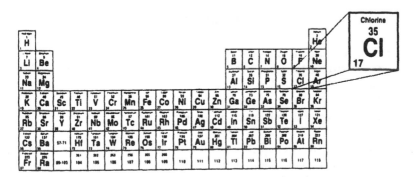

Figure 6.14 Chlorine's place in the periodic table.

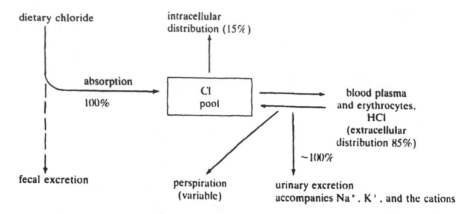

Figure 6.15 Chloride absorption and metabolism.

Chloride is the major extracellular anion which provides electrical neutrality for a multitude of mineral and protein cations. Chloride, together with the carbonic acid/bicarbonate anion, is most important in the maintenance of osmotic equilibria and for buffering the changes in pH (acid–base balance) of the blood. In erythrocytes, carbon dioxide from tissues and plasma is converted to carbonic acid by an enzyme, carbonic anhydrase. Disassociation of carbonic acid and diffusion of the bicarbonate anion (HCO_3^-) from the red blood cell into plasma is replaced by diffusion of Cl^- from plasma into the erythrocyte, contributing to electrical neutrality, referred to as the chloride shift. Large amounts of chloride are used by the chief cells in the synthesis and secretion of hydrochloric acid (HCl) (gastric juice) for the gastric digestion of protein by pepsin. The HCl lowers the pH of the stomach (pH 1 to 2), where pepsin is enzymatically active.

Dietary chloride is nearly totally absorbed, and secretory Cl^- is reabsorbed from the digestive juices of the intestine. The major excretory route of Cl^- is accompaniment of Na^+, K^+, and other cations in urinary excretion (Figure 6.15). Chloride may also be lost in perspiration, during diarrhea, and in vomit (loss of HCl), losses that can vary greatly among individuals according to the severity of the condition.

SULFUR

Date of nutritional recognition: 1932
Relative atomic size: 3.4
Oxidation states: –2, 0, +2, +4
Body burden: 175 kg
Major function: Structural component of protein

Sulfur (Figure 6.16) is uniquely classified within the group of macrominerals, for all but sulfur and chlorine are metals. Chlorine is a halogen, a nonmetal, and sulfur is a nonmetal. All of the macrominerals exist *in vivo* in some inorganic form; whereas sulfur exists predominately in organic molecules, there being only very

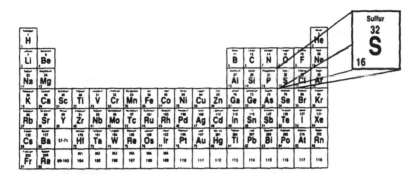

Figure 6.16 Sulfur's place in the periodic table.

small amounts of free metabolic sulfite or sulfate. All of the macrominerals are absorbed from the gastrointestinal tract in their inorganic form, except for sulfur, which is absorbed predominantly as the sulfur-containing amino acids methionine, cysteine, or cystine. There is no known dietary requirement for inorganic sulfur, and sulfates are poorly absorbed when ingested. Sulfites, sometimes used as antioxidants in foods, are absorbed by people sometimes with allergic (sulfite-sensitive) reactions. Warning labels for sulfites are now commonly found on food and beverage labels. Restaurants use sulfites as anti-browning agents for salads (antioxidant) and fruits.

Three forms of organic sulfur compounds exist which predominate in animals and humans. These forms of sulfur include: (1) the thiomethyl of methionine residues in protein; (2) the sulfhydryl disulfides of protein and cysteine–cystine residues in proteins; and (3) a few other sulfur compounds containing ester or amide-bound sulfates of glycosaminoglycans, a few steroids, and xenobiotic metabolites. The dietary requirement for sulfur as methionine was described by R. W. Jackson and R. J. Black in 1932. While methionine is the only essential sulfur amino acid, partial replacement of the methionine requirement can be met by cystine (cysteine). In addition to methionine, the other sulfur-containing dietary nutrients required by humans are the vitamins thiamin and biotin (Figure 6.17).

From methionine is synthesized all the other important sulfur compounds, including cysteine (cystine), glutathione (see "Selenium"), acetylcoenzyme A (see "Pantothenic Acid"), lipoic acid (see "Thiamin"), and taurine (see "Bile Acids and Bile Salts," Chapter 4) used in the synthesis of taurocholate (Figure 6.18). In the synthesis of these compounds methyl groups are donated by S-adenosylmethionine, and the synthesis of sulfated glycosaminoglycans of connective tissues and sulfated xenobiotics is transferred by 3'-phosphoadenosine-5'-phosphosulfate (Figure 6.19).

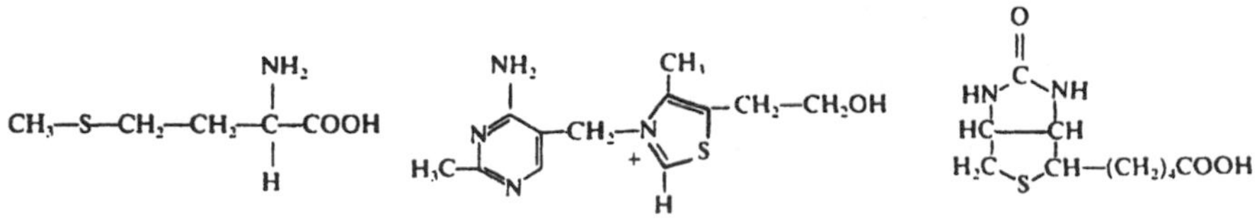

methionine   thiamin   biotin

Figure 6.17 Sulfur compounds required in the human diet.

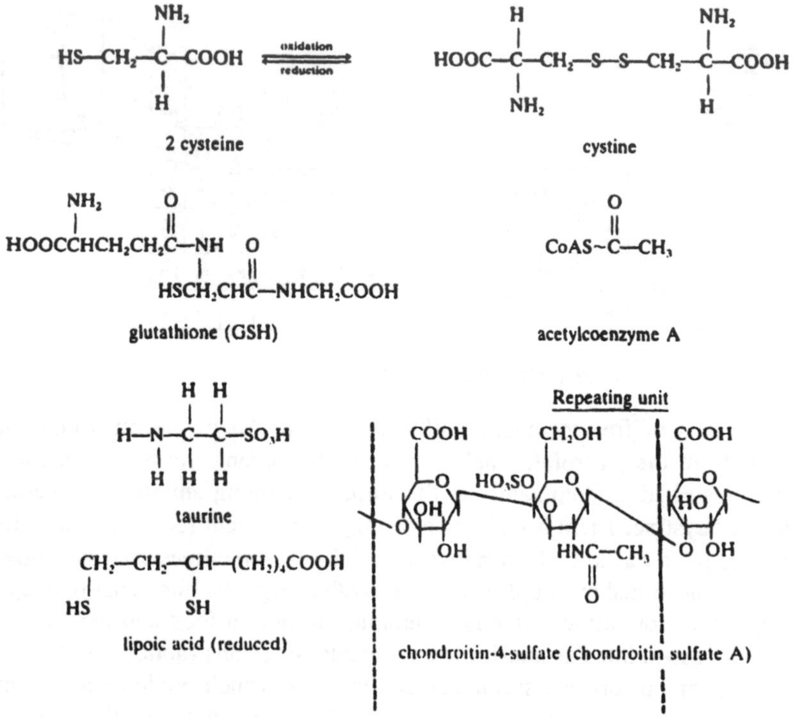

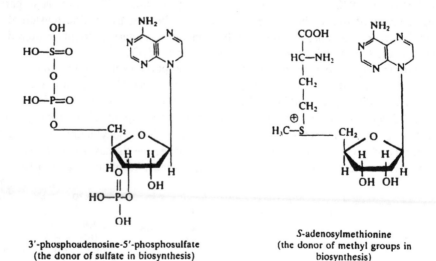

Figure 6.18 Important sulfur compounds not required in the human diet formed from methionine.

3'-phosphoadenosine-5'-phosphosulfate
(the donor of sulfate in biosynthesis)

S-adenosylmethionine
(the donor of methyl groups in
biosynthesis)

Figure 6.19 Metabolic donors of sulfate and methyl groups.

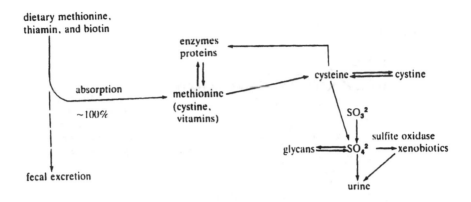

Figure 6.20 Sulfur absorption and metabolism.

During sulfur metabolism, sulfur is oxidized from its organic forms (sulfides, S^{2-}) to sulfites (SO_3^{2-}) and sulfates (SO_4^{2-}). A molybdenum-containing enzyme sulfite oxidase oxidizes the potentially toxic sulfite to sulfate, which is the major excretory form of sulfur found in urine (Figure 6.20).

IRON

Date of nutritional recognition: Ancient Chinese; 1872
Relative atomic size: 4.1
Oxidation states: +2, +3
Body burden: 4.5 g
Major function: Oxygen carrier in blood and muscle tissues, electron carrier in
                    cytochromes, enzyme catalysis

Iron (Figure 6.21) is the most abundant of the trace elements with an estimated body burden of 4 to 5 g and a 1989 RDA of 10 to 18 mg. A dietary need for iron may have been recognized by early civilizations, perhaps during an ancient Chinese

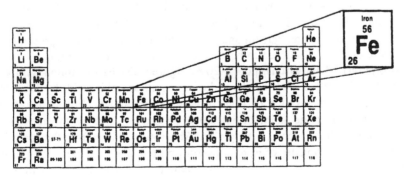

Figure 6.21 Iron's place in the periodic table.

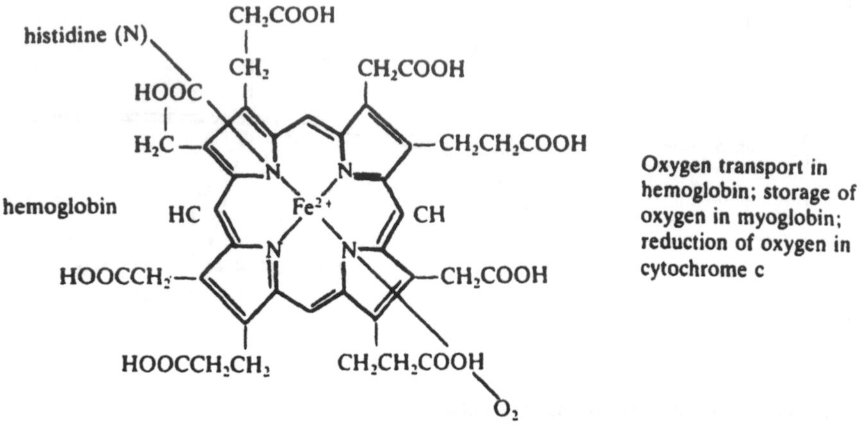

Figure 6.22 Structure of heme-iron in hemoglobin/myoglobin/cytochromes.

dynasty, but such events went unrecorded until 1872, when J. B. Boussingault reported on the importance of iron. Iron is biologically important because its inherent chemical properties, consisting of two oxidation states, Fe^{2+} (ferrous) and Fe^{3+} (ferric), and its ability to complex with organic molecules with a coordination number of 6. Iron's major functions in the body are: (1) the transport and storage of oxygen, (2) the transfer of electrons via the $Fe^{2+} \rightleftharpoons Fe^{3+}$ redox pair and the control of toxic oxygen species such as hydrogen peroxide, H_2O_2. The most important iron-containing protein is hemoglobin, both physiologically as the carrier of oxygen in the erythrocyte, and quantitatively, as it represents about 70% of the body's iron. The iron in hemoglobin is coordinated to four nitrogen atoms of a tetrapyrrole and to a ring nitrogen of a histidine residue within the protein chain. The sixth coordination position is for the free exchange of oxygen, as show Figure 6.22.

Myoglobin, a heme-Fe containing protein similar to hemoglobin, is found in skeletal and cardiac muscle, where it serves as a storage site for oxygen having been transferred from hemoglobin. The iron found in myoglobin is about 3% of total body iron stores. Of the remaining iron in the body, less than 1% is found in the heme-Fe cytochromes a, a_3, b, b_5, c, c_1, located in the mitochondrion as electron ($Fe^{2+} \rightleftharpoons Fe^{3+}$) carriers, microsomal cytochrome P-450, catalase, enzymes, and other iron proteins (Table 6.7). Remaining body iron, about 25%, is found stored principally in two liver proteins, ferritin and hemosiderin. Hemosiderin, representing the major store of iron, is believed to be an insoluble aggregate of ferritin.

Absorption of dietary iron is poor (~20%; Figure 6.23). Its absorption is improved by reduction of Fe^{3+} to Fe^{2+} by the reducing agent ascorbic acid, by HCl of the stomach, or by complexation of iron to organic compounds. Iron homeostasis is tightly controlled at the point of intestinal absorption and by the recycling of degraded iron proteins such as hemoglobin. Absorption of iron from the gastrointestinal tract results in transfer of iron to a serum protein aptly named iron transferrin. The iron is transported in the ferric (Fe^{3+}) state to tissues or is stored as hemosiderin. The oxidation of Fe^{2+} following absorption to Fe^{3+} in transferrin, is accomplished by reduction by the copper-containing protein ceruloplasmin.

Table 6.7   Iron Enzymes and Proteins

Enzyme/Protein	Fe/Molecule
Hemoglobin	4 hemes
Myoglobin	1 heme
Ferritin	20% $Fe(OH)_3$
Hemosiderin	35% $Fe(OH)_3$
Transferrin	2 Fe^{3+}
Cytochrome c	1 heme
Catalase	1 heme
Ferridoxins	1 Fe—S—Fe or 2 Fe—S—Fe
Rubedoxins	1 Fe or 2 Fe
Aldehyde oxidase	1 Fe—S—Fe, Mo, Flavin
Sulfite oxidase	1 heme, Mo

Among bacteria, plants, and animals exist nonheme iron proteins in which iron is coordinated not to nitrogen but to sulfur. These are the iron–sulfur proteins, in which iron is often coordinated to the sulfur of the amino acid cysteine (Figure 6.24). These proteins, the ferridoxins, are important electron carriers in plant chloroplasts during photosynthesis and participate in N_2 reduction by bacteria. Azoferridoxin contains only iron; whereas the bacterial protein molybdoferridoxin contains both iron and molybdenum.

With the many important biological oxidations mediated by iron and the relatively large dietary intake required because of poor absorption, it is perhaps not surprising that iron deficiency is quantitatively the leading trace mineral deficiency. Age, sex, health status, and dietary iron intake are factors contributing to adequate iron status. Under ordinary conditions iron is excreted in very small quantities through the urine, and even smaller amounts are lost through perspiration. Larger amounts of iron are lost by desquamation of intestinal epithelial tissue in feces.

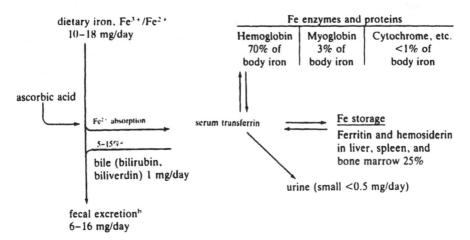

[a] May double during iron-deficiency anemia.
[b] Other variable iron losses from desquamated cells, sweat, and menstrual blood losses, which can be significant for premenopausal women.

Figure 6.23   Iron absorption and metabolism.

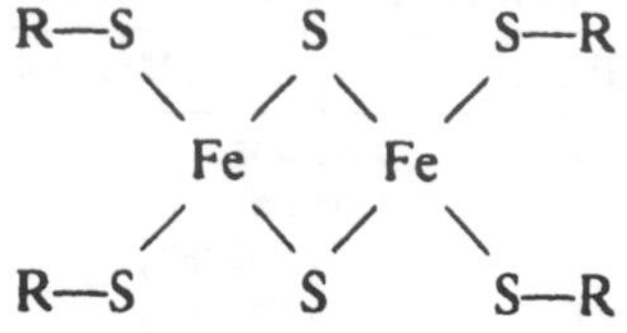

```
R—S        S        S—R
    \   /   \   /
     Fe      Fe
    /   \   /   \
R—S        S        S—R
```

Figure 6.24 Iron–sulfur protein.

Considerable loss of iron occurs during menstruation and when internal or external hemorrhaging is prolonged and protracted.

The best sources of iron are organ meats (especially liver), oysters, clams, and molasses. Rich to good sources include lean meats, spinach, egg yolks, legumes, and some dried fruits. Many processed foods, particularly cereals, are fortified with iron. Ascorbic acid and a factor found in red meats can increase iron absorption, while calcium carbonate, phytates, oxalates, and polyphenols can hinder iron absorption.

The 1989 Recommended Dietary Allowance for iron is 10 mg daily for men and 15 mg for premenopausal women. According to NHANESIII data, the median daily iron intakes of men and women, 20 to 59 years, in the United States were 15.8 and 10.9 mg, respectively.

Iron is one of the least toxic trace metals, with acute and chronic iron toxicity being uncommon events. Mild iron toxicity may occur with the condition hemosiderosis, whereby iron accumulates in the liver, heart, and pancreas. Hemochromatosis is a more severe hereditary condition whereby excessive iron accumulates and can cause death. Toxicity is thought to occur when the accumulation of iron exceeds the storage capacity of the iron-binding proteins and the loss of excretory mechanisms. A metal chelating agent is administered to bind to the iron, facilitating its excretion, or the person is bled to induce iron loss via hemoglobin removal.

Unbound iron, Fe^{2+}, is toxic due to the generation of the hydroxyl free radical, ·OH (see Chapter 15). The hydroxyl free radical is the most reactive and damaging of the free radical species. It reacts rapidly to damage cells and their genetic material, perhaps causing apoptosis, i.e., programmed cell death. The ·OH radical is catalytically generated by Fe^{2+} catalysis of H_2O_2, known as Fenton chemistry. Fenton chemistry due to the saturation of the transport iron protein, ferritin, has recently been suggested to be the cause of cardiovascular disease in men. Women, until the time of menopause, have higher circulating blood levels of apoferritin and thus have a greater capacity to bind any unbound "free" iron providing protection from Fenton chemistry and vascular free-radical damage.

FLUORINE

Date of nutritional recognition: 1968, 1972
Relative atomic size: 2.4
Oxidation state: −1
Body burden: 2.6 g
Major function: Contributes to the hardness of teeth and bone

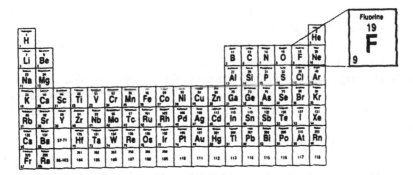

Figure 6.25 Fluorine's place in the periodic table.

Fluorine the element (Figure 6.25) is widely dispersed in biological tissues as the fluoride ion (F^-). Fluoride is found in mostly soft tissues dispersed mostly intracellularly, but it is also in the extracellular fluid space (Figure 6.26). Collectively, the total tissue fluoride represents about 1% of the adult fluorine content of 2.6 g. Most of the fluorine is present in bone and teeth (99%), where it combines with the calcium hydroxyapatite, forming a mixed calcium fluoroapatite. Deposition of fluoride in bone and teeth is dependent on the dietary or supplemental fluoride intake and the age of development of bone or dental enamel. Fluoride incorporated into bone and the dental enamel during development presumably decreases mineral solubility. Fluoridation of public water supplies began in the United States in 1945 (Newburgh–Kingston, New York; Grand Rapids–Muskegon, Michigan) following observations of people living in areas where natural fluorides in water already existed. Observations made in the 1930s suggested that natural fluorides (1 ppm) reduced dental caries, but when natural fluorides exceeded about 3 ppm, mottling of primary and secondary teeth could be expected of children prenatally exposed and postnatally consuming highly fluoridated waters. Use of fluorides to reduce dental cavities has been extended to topical fluoride applications, tablets of sodium fluoride, and inclusion of stannous fluoride and monofluorophosphates in dental pastes.

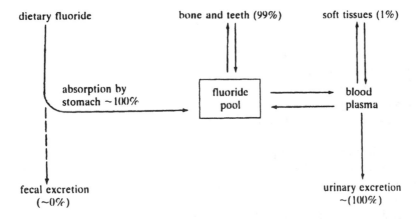

Figure 6.26 Fluoride absorption and metabolism.

Dietary fluoride assists in increasing bone mass (density) and may help to prevent osteoporosis in some individuals. Fluoride supplements, along with vitamin D and calcium supplementation to adult women, decreases their susceptibility to osteoporosis. Fluoride, if ingested in excessive amounts, is toxic, manifested by dental fluorosis (mottling). If ingested in very high amounts, skeletal fluorosis and calcification of tendons, ligaments, and bony erostoses may occur. *Genu valgun* is an endemic crippling fluorosis seen in parts of India. When toxic levels of fluoride are ingested, metabolic disturbances can occur in both lipid and carbohydrate metabolism, owing to enzyme inhibition by the fluoride anion.

Although several reports have suggested that fluoride is essential for animals, the experimental data for this account remain inconclusive, and there is no evidence for a metabolic requirement for fluoride in humans. H. A. Schroeder and co-workers first reported in 1968 that mice given 10 ppm fluoride in drinking water grew better and lived longer than did control animals. During the experimental period, fluoride did not accumulate in soft tissues. In 1972, K. Schwarz and D. Milne observed positive growth responses in rats fed fluoride supplemented up to 7.5 ppm in experimental amino acid diets. The fluoride content of the diet also affected the pigmentation of the rats' incisor teeth. Other data are not supportive of these reported growth effects in animals, and the question of metabolic fluoride essentiality remains open.

Dietary fluoride is rapidly absorbed, probably from the stomach, and is distributed in soft tissues similarly to chloride. Fluoride enters the blood, and excess fluoride appears rapidly in urine (Figure 6.26). There are no known proteins or enzymes that contain fluoride.

The 1997 Adequate Intakes for fluoride for males and females 19 years of age and over are 3.8 and 3.1 mg/day, respectively. The best food sources of fluoride are teas and bony marine fish. Many municipalities in the United States fluoridate their water supply. Fluoridation of public water supplies is recommended if the water's fluoride concentration is <0.7 or 0.8 mg per liter. Fluoride intakes of adults in the United States from food, beverages, and water have been estimated to be about 0.9 mg daily in areas with unfluoridated water and up to about 1.8 mg in areas with fluoridation.

ZINC

Date of nutritional recognition: 1934
Relative atomic size: 4.4
Oxidation state: +2
Body burden: 2 g
Major function: Component of many enzymes and proteins; wound healing

Zinc (Figure 6.27) is a required trace element for all life forms: bacteria, plants, animals, and humans. The presence of zinc detected in terrestrial plants dates from 1869 and in aquatic plants since 1919. A dietary requirement for zinc in the rat was first reported by W. R. Todd and colleagues in 1934. A. S. Prasad was first to report a zinc deficiency in humans in 1961 among people consuming mostly breads and very little animal protein in Middle Eastern countries. Parakeratosis, a disease common to

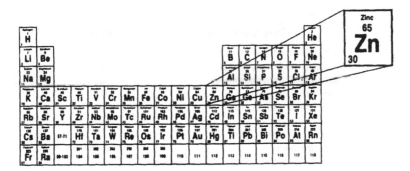

Figure 6.27 Zinc's place in the periodic table.

swine, was prevalent during the 1940s and early 1950s and was prevented by the addition of zinc supplements to diets. This disease was first shown in 1955 to be caused by a zinc deficiency and was aggravated by elevated calcium intake. Human parakeratosis, also caused by a zinc deficiency, was reported in 1976. A genetic human disease, acrodermatitis enteropathica, is corrected by additional dietary zinc supplements.

The formal recognition of zinc as an essential nutrient came in 1974, when dietary allowances for the nutrients were made by the National Research Council, Food and Nutrition Board of the National Academy of Sciences. The 1989 RDAs for zinc for males and females over the age of 11 years are 15 and 12 mg daily, respectively. According to NHANES-III data, the median daily zinc intakes of men and women, 20 to 59 years, in the United States were 12.7 and 9.3 mg, respectively. Many adults have marginal zinc intakes. Zinc absorption is only 20 to 30% of intake, and absorption is reduced further by the dietary presence of phytic acid, fiber, iron II, and various chelates. Zinc is excreted by the pancreas, and a fecal loss of about 1.5 mg of zinc per day is the major excretory route. Additional losses of zinc occur in urine, 0.5 mg/day, and perspiration, 1 to 5 μg/day (Figure 6.28).

All tissues contain zinc, which functions as a prosthetic moiety or regulator of enzyme activity. Carbonic anhydrase was the first enzyme to be recognized as a zinc metalloenzyme. This discovery came in 1940, and by 1960 five more zinc metalloenzymes were known. Over 200 zinc metalloenzymes are now recognized, some of which are listed in Table 6.8.

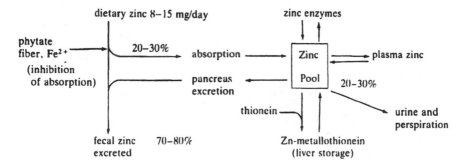

Figure 6.28 Zinc absorption and metabolism.

Table 6.8   Zinc Enzymes and Proteins

Enzyme/Protein	Zn/Molecule
Carbonic anhydrase	1
Carboxypeptidase A and B	1
Liver alcohol dehydrogenase	4
Superoxide dismutase	2
DNA polymerase (*E. coli*)	2
Alkaline phosphatase	2
Leucine aminopeptidase	2
Metallothionein	Many
Glyceraldehyde-3-phosphodehydrogenase	3
Insulin (crystalline)	0.3

Rich sources of zinc include most seafood, lamb, turkey, beans, and mushrooms. Good sources include peanuts, beans, and whole grains. The presence of phytates and oxalates in the small intestine at the same time may decrease the absorption of zinc.

Dietary intakes of 18.5 to 25 mg/day have been reported to impair copper status in adult subjects. Zinc supplements of 80 to 150 mg daily for several weeks reportedly decrease HDL levels. Chronic ingestion of zinc supplements in excess of 15 mg daily is not recommended.

SELENIUM

Date of nutritional recognition: 1957
Relative atomic size: 3.9
Oxidation states: +6, +4, −2
Body burden: 13 mg
Body function: Antioxidant, prooxidant

In 1817 the Swedish chemist J. Berzelius discovered the element selenium (Figure 6.29) in association with the element sulfur. Similar in chemical properties to sulfur, selenium remained for many years an unrecognized nutritional factor.

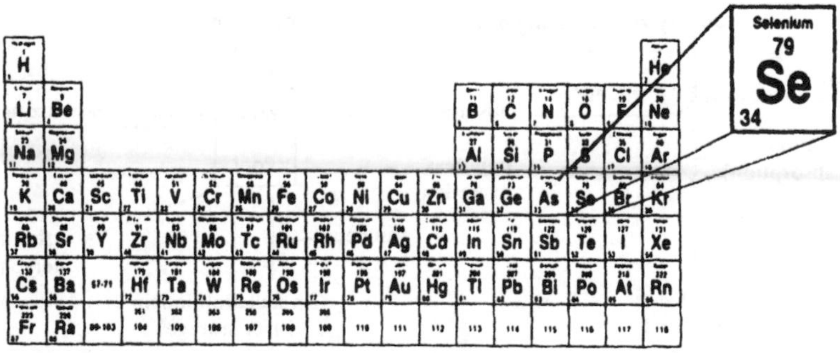

Figure 6.29   Selenium's place in the periodic table.

$$H_2O_2 + 2GSH \xrightarrow{\text{GSHPx}} GSSG + H_2O$$

$$ROOH + 2GSH \xrightarrow{\text{PLGSHPx}} GSSG + ROH$$

Figure 6.30 The reduction of hydrogen peroxide by glutathione peroxidase (GSHPx) and the reduction of organic hydroperoxides by phospholipid hydroperoxide glutathione peroxidase (PLGSHPx).

Selenium was known first, primarily for its toxicity. In the 1930s it was found to be the causative agent of the toxicity diseases "blind staggers" and "alkali disease" among horses and cattle that consumed seleniferous plants, a discovery made by the research staff at the North Dakota Experiment Station of the U.S. Department of Agriculture.

During the 1950s at the National Institutes for Health, German-born physician K. Schwarz discovered that dietary selenium prevented a fatal necrotic liver degeneration in rats fed diets of torula yeast and lacking in vitamin E. This was the first documentation of a biological requirement for selenium in animals, being reported in 1957. This report prompted research that revealed a dietary need for selenium in other animals. More than 40 species of animals are today known to have a biological requirement for selenium. Throughout the 1960s, range animals, cattle and sheep principally, were often found in many parts of the world to have a dietary selenium deficiency. Now, bacteria and algae of several species are also known to need selenium.

In 1973, researchers at the University of Wisconsin discovered that selenium was an integral part of the active site of a widely dispersed enzyme, glutathione peroxidase. It was found that glutathione peroxidase contained four atoms of selenium, each contained within the amino acid selenocysteine at the active site. With its coenzyme glutathione (GSH), glutathione peroxidase (GSHPx) facilitates the reduction of hydrogen peroxide (H_2O_2) to water and organic hydroperoxides (ROOH) to an alcohol (ROH), as in Figure 6.30. In this reaction two molecules of glutathione (GSH) are oxidized to GSSG and hydrogen peroxide or ROOH is reduced to water or the alcohol of the organic peroxide. The enzyme helps to keep to very low levels the cellular levels of peroxides, which damage cell membranes. GSHPx is presently one of several known mammalian enzymes to contain selenium. All but one enzyme, 5′-deiiodinase, are redox enzymes that use glutathione. One enzyme, phospholipid hydroperoxide glutathione peroxidase, catalyzes the reduction of only phospholipid hydroperoxides of the membrane and hydroperoxides of cholesterol. This selenium associated with cell membranes is thought to spare the antioxidant requirement of vitamin E in membranes. Bacteria, insects, nematodes, and many other species of animals possess enzymes involved in redox reactions which contain selenium. Other newer proteins have also been discovered which contain selenium, and their functions are only beginning to become understood (Table 6.9).

In 1979 the first dietary selenium deficiency in people was described to occur in isolated rural populations in the People's Republic of China. The disease, Keshan disease, named for the county where it was first recognized, is a cardiomyopathy affecting primarily children and young women. The disease was often fatal, existing

Table 6.9   Selenium Enzymes and Proteins

Enzyme/Protein	Se/Molecule
Glutathione peroxidase (GSHPx)	4/extensive, including humans
Phospholipid hydroperoxide glutathione peroxidase (PLGSHPx)	1/extensive, including humans
5'-deiiodinase	1/extensive, including humans
Formate dehydrogenase	Bacterial
Selenoprotein-P	10/extensive, including humans
Glycine reductase	Bacterial
Nicotinic acid hydroxylase	Bacterial
Xanthine dehydrogenase	Bacterial
Thiolase	Bacterial
Hydrogenase	4/bacterial; also contains Ni, Fe
B-Hydroxybutyryl-CoA-dehydrogenase	Bacterial
Spermatozoa protein	1/rat, 1/bull

in rural populations where the dietary selenium intake was less than 10 µg per day. A second selenium deficiency, Kashin–Beck disease, known for hundreds of years in China along the Sino–Soviet border, became known in 1980. Also known as "big joint disease," this rheumatoid condition affected children extensively in some areas and was permanently crippling to adults. Both diseases are caused by a primary selenium deficiency of soils or the inability of grains and grasses to assimilate the selenium from soils. These diseases have been essentially eradicated from China's rural populations because of the use of selenium supplements.

The primary form of selenium in plant foods is L-selenomethionine. The dietary need for selenium in people is fulfilled by L-selenomethionine from plants, primarily cereal grains, and from the L-selenomethionine and also selenocysteine found in animal foods in association with protein. The dietary requirement for selenium can also be met by the two selenium salts, sodium selenite (Na_2SeO_3) and sodium selenate (Na_2SeO_4), which are the forms of selenium often found in supplements.

The 1989 RDA for selenium is 70 µg daily for men and 55 µg, for women. The average U.S. diet contains about 80 to 100 µg per day, with dietary intakes being greater for men than for women. A reasonable average absorption of dietary selenium in a mixed diet is 50 to 60%. The absorption and metabolism of selenium is generally understood (Figure 6.31). Whereas sulfur compounds undergo general oxidation, selenium compounds follow metabolic pathways of reduction and methylation. The major urinary metabolite is the trimethylselenonium ion. Selenium is an antagonist of copper, mercury, silver, lead, and cadmium, all toxic metals, and the toxic non-metal arsenic.

MANGANESE

Date of nutritional recognition: 1931
Relative atomic size: 4.6
Oxidation states: +2, +3, +4, +7
Body burden: 12 mg
Major function: Growth, lipid metabolism

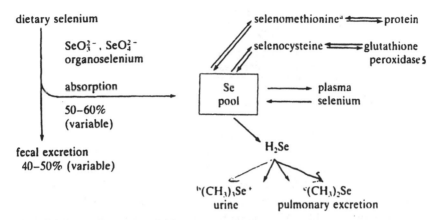

*Not synthesized by animals and humans, dietary source only.
ᵇMajor excretory metabolite, trimethylselenonium ion.
ᶜExcretory metabolite with high selenium (toxic?) intake, dimethylselenide.

Figure 6.31 Selenium absorption and metabolism.

Manganese (Figure 6.32) was discovered by C. W. Schelle in 1774. By 1913, the presence of manganese in the sera of animals was known. The essentiality of manganese was nutritionally demonstrated for the mouse and rat by A. R. Kemmerer and co-workers and by E. R. Orent and E. V. McCollum in 1931. Manganese deficiency in animals retards growth, impairs lipid metabolism, increases susceptibility to convulsions, increases neonatal mortality and ataxia, and in chickens, specifically, causes what is called "slipped tendon disease." Because manganese affects enzyme activity, it exerts metabolic control over various aspects of metabolism. Manganese is a cofactor of at least two enzymes, superoxide dismutase and pyruvate carboxylase (Table 6.10).

Dietary manganese is poorly absorbed by the gastrointestinal tract, with absorption rates being 1 to 4% of dietary intake. Excretion of manganese is almost exclusively via the bile and fecal elimination. Very little manganese appears in urine. Absorption is facilitated by chelating agents, is antagonized by calcium, iron, and

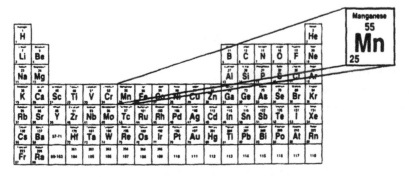

Figure 6.32 Manganese's place in the periodic table.

Table 6.10 Manganese Enzymes

Enzyme	Mn/Molecule
Superoxide dismutase	1
Pyruvate carboxylase	4

phosphorus, and is under some control by ovarian and adrenal corticotrophic hormones (Figure 6.33).

The major depository of manganese is in bone, followed by liver, kidney, and the pituitary gland, with other tissues containing lesser amounts of the mineral. In tissues, subcellular concentration of manganese is in the mitochondrion.

The 1989 Estimated Safe and Adequate Daily Dietary Intake of manganese for adults is 2 to 5 mg. Good to rich sources of manganese are rice, whole grains, nuts, beans, and leafy vegetables. Manganese toxicity is rare except for conditions under which the mineral is mined or through other industrial exposure.

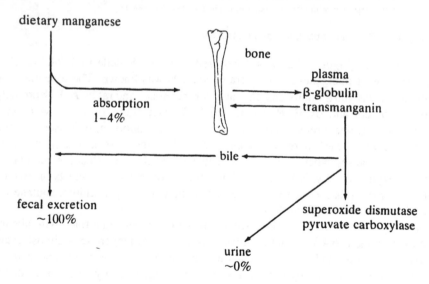

Figure 6.33 Manganese absorption and metabolism.

IODINE

Date of nutritional recognition: 1820
Relative atomic size: 4.4
Oxidation state: −1
Body burden: 11 mg
Major function: Thyroid hormones

Iodine (Figure 6.34) was discovered in burnt seaweed by a Napoleonic munitions manufacturer, M. B. Courtois, in 1812, and was so named by the French chemist J. L. Gay-Lussac. Iodine was found in a sponge ash in 1819 by A. Fyfe. Sponge ash

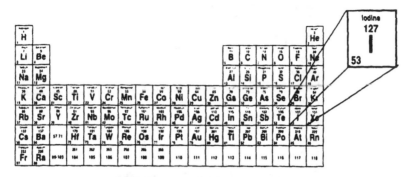

Figure 6.34 Iodine's place in the periodic table.

had long been a treatment for goiter. J. F. Coindet used iodine, believing it to be a drug to treat the disease successfully. Recognition of iodine as a nutrient is attributed to C. A. Chatin, a pharmacist and botanist, who associated traditional goiter with insufficient amounts of iodine in food and water. Chatin's work was poorly accepted until this century, when human experiments with iodine were conducted in the United States among schoolchildren beginning in 1912. Today, goiter is rather a rare disease in developed countries where iodine (as potassium iodide) is added to "iodized salt." Goiter is a very ancient disease, known to the Chinese, Greeks, and Egyptians. Marco Polo on his travels to China in 1271 recorded evidence that describes goiter. In China, as indicated by the following article from the *China Daily* (May 31, 1984, p. 3), goiter has a history as an extensive endemic Chinese disease.

Endemic Disease Reduced

ZHENGZHOU (Xinhua) — Cases of endemic goiter in Henan Province dropped from two million in 1980 to 500,000 in 1983, according to Yang Longhe, director of the provincial public health department.

The province has also set up 3,775 stations to inspect the quality of iodated salt and prevent noniodated salt from entering those regions. In addition, public health departments have injected salt with iodipin in some areas. At present, 47 of the 66 counties and cities that were affected by the disease have managed to control outbreaks of endemic goiter.

In order to control endemic goiter, Henan has expanded its production of iodated salt by constructing 20 iodated salt plants since 1982, bringing the total to 68. These plants now produce 155,000 tons of the substance annually, ensuring an adequate supply for all the 20 million people in areas threatened by the disease.

Almost all (80%) dietary iodine is found concentrated in the thyroid gland, where it is sequestered and covalently stored attached to a glycoprotein, thyroglobulin (TG) (Table 6.11). Oxidation of iodine causes it to become covalently attached to tyrosine residues of TG, forming 3-monoiodotyrosine (MIT) and 3,5-diiodotyrosine (DIT) residues (Figure 6.36). Triiodotyrosine, known as T_3, is formed by linkage presumably between MIT and DIT TG residues. Also found within TG is tetraiodothyronine,

Table 6.11 Iodine in Some Human Tissues

Tissue	µg/g Wet Weight
Thyroid	8000–12,000
Liver	0.20
Ovary	0.07
Lung	0.07
Kidney	0.04
Lymph nodes	0.03
Brain	0.02
Testes	0.02
Muscle	0.01

Reprinted with permission of E. I. Hamilton.

presumably formed between adjacent DIT residues (Figure 6.35). Upon proteolysis of TG, T_3 and T_4 are secreted into the blood plasma. T_3, and T_4, also known as thyroxine, are the thyroid hormones that circulate attached to TBP (thyroxine-binding protein) and serum α-globulin, albumin or prealbumin. The general function of thyroxine is to control basal metabolic rate (BMR) by regulating mitochondrial activity. T_3, arising from the proteolysis of TG or the deiodination of T_4 in the liver or kidney, performs yet unknown functions. Iodine is excreted as reverse T_3 (3′,5′,3-triiodothyronine) or as tetra-iodothyroacetic acid. DIT and MIT released from TG by proteolysis are deiodinated, with the iodide recycled to new TG (Figure 6.36).

Goiter is a direct histological response to the lack of dietary iodine, with a resulting hyperplasia of the thyroid gland (hypothyroidism). Hypothyroidism is prevented by ingestion of about 80 µg of iodide daily. The disease may also be aggravated by goitrogens, natural compounds found in the cabbage family of plants, which inhibit iodination of TG. Ions of thiocyanates and perchlorates, in particular, inhibit the uptake of iodide by the thyroid gland. The 1989 Recommended Dietary Allowance for iodine for individuals 11+ years of age is 150 µg. Iodide is moderately toxic, and toxicity can paradoxically produce hypothyroidism.

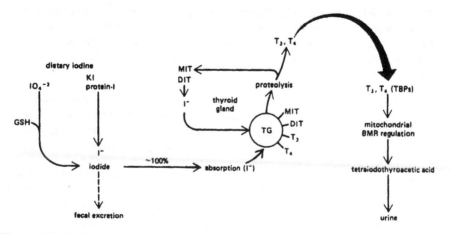

Figure 6.35 Iodine metabolism. (Reprinted with permission of E. I. Hamilton.)

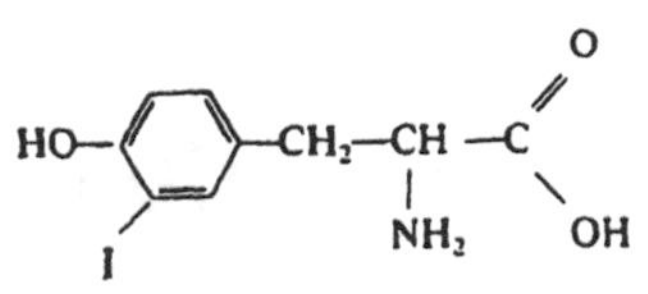

MIT (monoiodotyrosine)

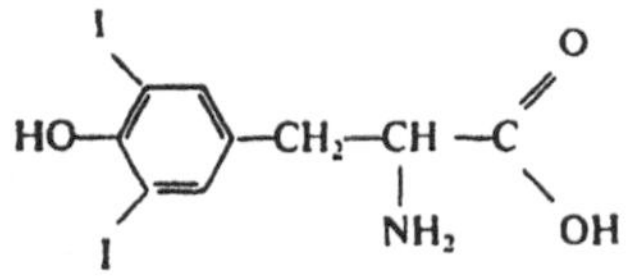

DIT (diiodotyrosine)

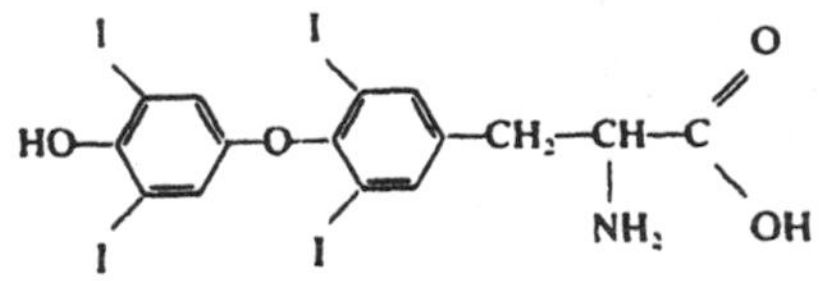

T_4 (3′,5′,3,5-tetraiodothyronine)
(thyroxine)

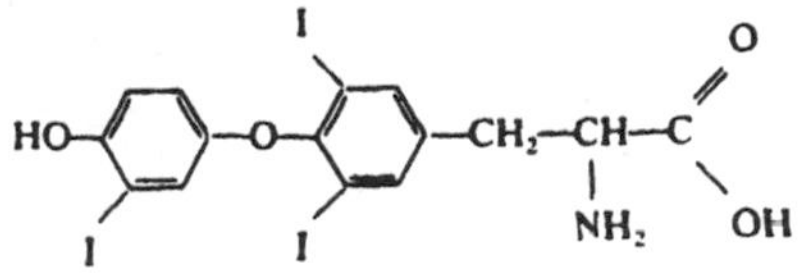

3,5,3′-T_3 (triiodothyronine)

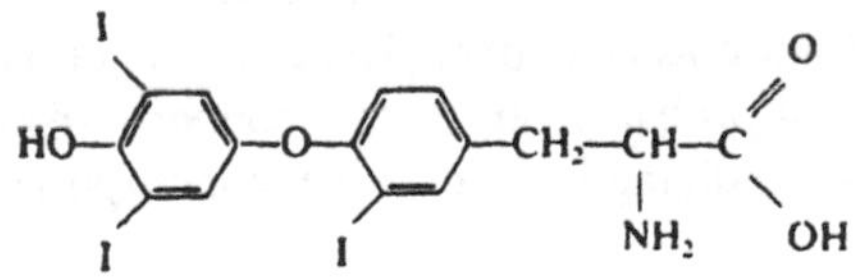

3,3′,5′-T_3 (reverse T_3, excreted)

Figure 6.36 Iodotyrosines and iodothyronines.

COPPER

Date of nutritional recognition: 1928
Relative atomic size: 4.3
Oxidative states: +1, +2
Body burden: 10 mg

Located in the eastern Mediterranean is the island of Cyprus, a most important place in the Mycenaean Bronze Age, for it was here that the finest and largest deposits of copper (Figure 6.37) were to be found. Copper from this island was alloyed with tin to form bronze, and with zinc to form brass.

The use of copper compounds to treat various diseases dates to the time of Hipprocrates. Not until this century, however, was it noticed that animals fed milk diets developed anemia which could not be corrected by dietary iron alone. In 1928, E. B. Hart and co-workers demonstrated that rats which developed the milk diet anemia required copper along with iron to correct the anemia. Copper is required by plants, bacteria, animals, and humans. It is a constituent of several enzymes and proteins in which the copper participates in various redox reactions (Table 6.12).

Absorption of copper occurs in the upper intestinal tract with about 40% efficiency. Unabsorbed dietary copper and copper excreted into the intestinal lumen in bile are excreted in feces. Lesser amounts of copper are lost through urine, perspiration, and menses. Absorbed copper is transported bound to albumin and stored in

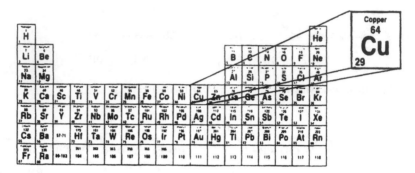

Figure 6.37 Copper's place in the periodic table.

part as copper metallothionein in liver (Figure 6.38). In the liver is synthesized ceruloplasmin, a blue-colored copper protein. Ceruloplasmin circulates in the blood plasma and constitutes about 95% of the total plasma copper. The exact function of ceruloplasmin remains unknown, although it probably serves as a copper transport protein and may have a redox function in oxidizing Fe^{2+} to Fe^{3+} for incorporation into transferrin.

Other copper enzymes and proteins also have important physiological and biochemical roles. Copper is a cofactor of superoxide dismutase; cytochrome oxidase in electron transport; lysyl oxidase, which oxidatively deaminates lysine and hydroxylysine; and tyrosinase, which converts tyrosine to melanin skin pigments. In crustaceans and some invertebrates the copper protein hemocyanin is the principal carrier of oxygen in blood.

Although human copper deficiency is rare, two diseases of copper metabolism are well known. Wilson's disease is a genetic disease characterized by the accumulation of copper in the liver, brain, and cornea. The disease causes a decrease in serum ceruloplasmin, decreased biliary excretion, and increased urinary copper excretion. Treatment in controlling tissue accumulation of copper is via chelation therapy with D-penicillamine and low-copper diets. A second genetic copper disease is Menke's disease, whose primary manifestation is reduced copper absorption. The disease may begin *in utero* and takes on characteristics of a dietary copper deficiency. Loss of hair pigmentation, causing "steely hair," is symptomatic of Menke's disease, which is often fatal by the age of about 45.

Table 6.12 Copper Enzymes and Proteins

Enzyme/Protein	Cu/Molecule
Ceruloplasmin	7–8
Superoxide dismutase	2
Lysyl oxidase	?
Tyrosinase	1–4
Cytochrome c oxidase	2
Dopamine β-hydroxylase	4–7
Hemocyanin	20–200
Erythrocuprein	2

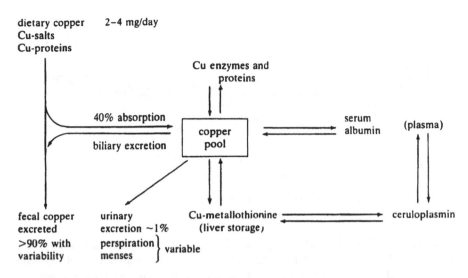

Figure 6.38 Copper absorption and metabolism.

The 1989 Estimated Safe and Adequate Daily Dietary Intake of copper for adults is 1.5 to 3.0 mg. Rich to good sources of copper include organ meats (especially liver), most seafood, nuts, legumes, cereals, dried fruits, and chocolate. According to NHANESIII data, the median daily copper intakes of men and women, 20 to 59 years, in the United States were 1.45 and 1.02 µg, respectively. Copper salts are toxic if ingested in excessive amounts. Copper sulfate has long been used as an algaecide in aquaria. Accumulation of copper in Wilson's disease is one of the causes of liver cirrhosis and neurological dysfunctions in humans.

MOLYBDENUM

Date of nutritional recognition: 1953
Relative atomic size: 4.5
Oxidation state: +6
Body burden: 9 mg

Molybdenum (Figure 6.39), discovered in 1778 by C. W. Schelle, is today known as an important trace element for bacteria, animals, and humans. Initial nutritional interest focused on molybdenum toxicity in the 1930s, with the recognition that a disease in cattle, locally known as "teart" in England, was molybdenosis. Prevention of teart was possible by administering copper salts or sulfates which interfered with the metabolism and absorption of molybdenum. Thus was established the existence of Mo–Cu and Mo–S antagonisms.

The first indication that molybdenum was an essential nutrient came in 1953, when independently, two research groups, E. C. De Renzo and colleagues and D.

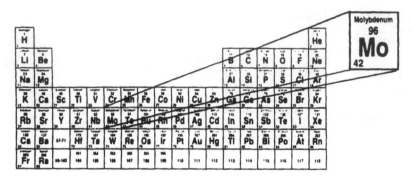

Figure 6.39 Molybdenum's place in the periodic table.

A. Richert and W. W. Westerfeld, reported that the redox enzymes xanthine oxidase and sulfite oxidase contained molybdenum. A third enzyme containing molybdenum, aldehyde oxidase, was discovered in 1954 (Table 6.13). These enzymes contribute to the oxidation of the nucleic acid bases hypoxanthine and xanthine to uric acid, of sulfites to sulfates, and of aldehydes to ketones. In bacteria, molybdenum is required by nitrogenases and nitrate reductases, which provide plants (legumes) with ammonia from nitrogen (N_2) and nitrates from nitrites which are assimilated into protein.

Molybdenum deficiency in animals can be produced experimentally by feeding low-molybdenum diets and an antagonist, tungsten. Molybdenum deficiency in humans is unknown except for rare cases of malabsorption and the use of total parenteral nutrition for extended periods. Metabolic changes with a molybdenum deficiency include abnormal methionine catabolism and low excretion rates of uric acid and inorganic sulfate. These conditions are corrected by administering molybdenum. In a central valley in China (Henan Province), people naturally consuming low-molybdenum diets have been known to have a high incidence of esophageal cancer. Similar observations for esophageal cancer have been made among the Bantu peoples of the Transki, South Africa.

Molybdenum is effectively absorbed from the gastrointestinal tract, from which it is incorporated into the molybdenum enzymes (Figure 6.40). Molybdenum is found in muscle, skin, liver, and spleen, as well as other organs.

Table 6.13 Molybdenum Enzymes

Enzyme	Mo/Molecule
Xanthine oxidase	2
Sulfite oxidase	2
Aldehyde oxidase	?
Formate dehydrogenase	?
Nitrogenase	2
Nitrate reductase	1

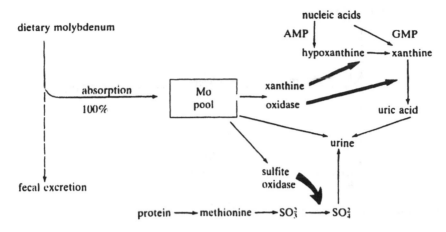

Figure 6.40 Molybdenum absorption and metabolism.

CHROMIUM

Date of nutritional recognition: 1959
Relative atomic size: 4.2
Oxidation states: +2, +3, +6
Body burden: 6 mg

The discovery of chromium (Figure 6.41) as a nutrient is associated with the discovery that selenium prevented dietary liver necrosis in rats. The rats were found to be hypoglycemic and failed to utilize glucose properly, which was corrected by brewer's yeast or pork kidney powder. The factor preventing the hypoglycemia was independent of the protective effects of selenium against liver necrosis and upon partial purification was eventually found to contain traces of chromium. The discovery that chromium affected glucose metabolism was reported by K. Schwarz and W. Mertz in 1959. Believed to contain chromium in an organic complex named the glucose tolerance factor, or GTF, to date it has never been isolated or defined chemically from natural sources. Chromium complexes containing nicotinic acid

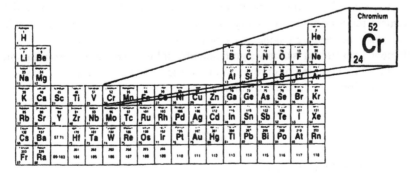

Figure 6.41 Chromium's place in the periodic table.

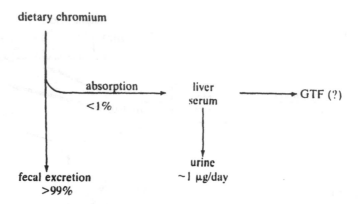

Figure 6.42 Chromium absorption and metabolism.

and coordinated amino acids have been synthetically synthesized and isolated from yeast. None has been determined to be the natural GTF. As it may occur naturally, chromium and GTF, as observed by *in vitro* assays, are believed to enhance the behavior of insulin in improving glucose transport across cell membranes.

One of the complications of chromium analysis is the great difficulty with which it is measured accurately. Since 1964, with greater accuracy in chromium analysis, blood levels of chromium reported to be on the order 1000 ng/ml, are now known to be less than 1 ng/ml. For this reason, analytical data for chromium prior to 1978 for tissues may not reflect true concentrations of chromium. Chromium is believed to be biologically active in the Cr(III) oxidation state. Dietary chromium intake is quite variable, ranging from 11 to 820 μg/day and averaging about 147 μg/day (29 to 455 μg/day with N = 25) for adults. Chromium is poorly absorbed (<1% by the intestinal tract, and urinary excretion of between 1 and 2 μg/day would provide a metabolic balance for an intake of 147 μg per day (Figure 6.42). Urinary excretion of chromium is reported to be about 1 μg per day. At this rate of urinary chromium excretion and with a body burden of approximately 6 mg, it would seem that chromium deficiency for healthy adults would be a rare event. For some people chromium supplementation has been shown to improve glucose tolerance and to reduce cholesterol–HDL ratios, which is an enhanced protective index for the rate of cardiovascular disease. No chromium proteins or enzymes have been specifically identified.

During the 1990s chromium picolinate came into favor as a major dietary supplement reported to reduce body fat and increase lean body mass. In spite of such claims, the research done does not support these widely held views that supplemental chromium is of any significant physiological benefit. Chromium picolinate is a chelate complex of chromium and three picolinates which increases chromium absorption over chromium chloride.

SILICON

Date of nutritional recognition: 1972
Relative atomic size: 3.9

Oxidative state: +4, ±2
Body burden: 24 mg

Silicon (Figure 6.43) is the most abundant element in the earth's crust after oxygen. Silicon is used by plankton to form shells of silica (SiO_2). The element is concentrated by the ancient plants: bryophytes, ferns, and horsetails. Soil bacteria degrade quartz, synthesize organosilicon compounds, and are even known to be able to replace phosphorus with silicon. Even present-day plants contain a fairly high content of silicon, and some varieties contain 15 to 20% silicon by dry weight. Cereals may contain 30 to 40% of their ash as silicon. People consume 20 to 30 mg/day of SiO_2 and about 1200 mg of total silicon per day, yet silicon is present in animal and human tissues to only a slight extent. The question, therefore: Is such a ubiquitous element essential to animals and humans? The evidence to date suggests that it is, but the data are not yet conclusive.

Evidence for the essentiality of silicon originates with E. M. Carlisle, who was able to demonstrate that in the actively growing area of bone (osteoblasts), calcium and silicon are present in almost equal concentrations, but as the bone becomes calcified, the silicon is no longer needed and only participates in the calcification "process." These *in vitro* studies and subsequent *in vivo* experiments have demonstrated the apparent need for silicon for proper calcification of growing bone. In rats and in chicks, low-silicon-containing diets contribute to abnormalities in skull and long bone formation, including formational changes in articulating cartilage and bone density.

Silicon is present in animal and human tissues in probably at least three different forms. These forms include water-soluble orthosilicic acid and silicate anions, organosilicon compounds and silicic esters of carbohydrates, and possibly protein. Steroids, choline, lipids, and phospholipids may contain silicon polymers (—O—Si—O—Si—O—), and insoluble oligo- and polysilicates may be absorbed with other organic molecules. While such compounds are suggested to be present based on silicon analysis of animal and human tissue, their presence in these molecules remains to be confirmed. Human tissues containing high silicon concentration include muscle, kidney, and liver. Especially high in silicon content are lymph nodes and lung tissues, the latter concentrated with silicon due to dust and other inhaled abiotic materials.

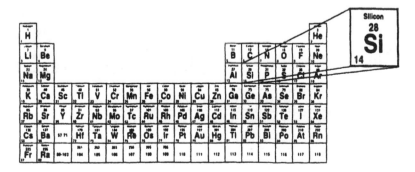

Figure 6.43 Silicon's place in the periodic table.

Dietary silicon is absorbed as silicic acid, silica, and organosilicates by the gastrointestinal tract. Little is known of its metabolism. Silicon is present in blood and urine. Some silica may even be phagositized, the cause of localization of silicon in lymph nodes. From chronic exposure, inhaled silica may lead to silicosis. Some silicates are carcinogenic, as is asbestos, which, when inhaled, in time may cause mesothelioma, a rare cancer of the lung.

NICKEL

Date of nutritional recognition: 1970
Relative atomic size: 4.2
Oxidation state: +2
Body burden: 10 mg

The presence of nickel (Figure 6.44) in plants and animals was initially reported by R. Berg in 1925. G. Bertrand and H. Nakamura made the suggestion in 1936 that nickel might be an essential nutrient. Initial evidence that nickel might be an essential element for the chick was made by F. H. Nielson in 1970. Suboptimal growth, reduced hematopoiesis, and changes in the liver content of iron, copper, and zinc have been the generally observed changes in chicks, cows, goats, guinea pigs, sheep, and rats fed low-nickel diets. Nickel appears to interact strongly with iron to affect its absorption from the gastrointestinal tract as measured by reduced hemoglobin, hematocrits, and erythrocyte counts in rats fed a nickel-deficient diet. Nickel deficiency also reduces a number of enzyme activities associated with carbohydrate digestion and metabolism.

In 1980 a nickel metalloenzyme was discovered in the jack bean, *Conavalia ensiformis*. The enzyme was urease (Table 6.14), responsible for the hydrolysis of urea to carbon dioxide and ammonia. Ureases from other plants and some bacteria have also been identified as nickel metalloenzymes. Other bacterial nickel enzymes have now also been identified. No mammalian nickel enzyme, however, has yet been identified.

Many green leafy vegetables contain 1.5 to 3.0 ppm nickel, and the human intake of nickel varies between 170 and 700 μg per day. Dietary nickel appears to be poorly

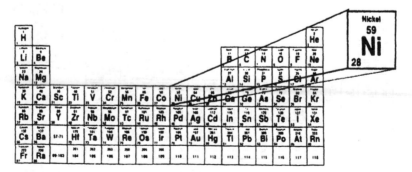

Figure 6.44 Nickel's place in the periodic table.

Table 6.14 Nickel-Containing Enzymes and Proteins

Enzyme/Protein	Ni/Molecule
Jack bean urease	2
Nickeloplasmin	1
Factor 430 (F_{430})	1/1500 daltons

absorbed, with only 1 to 10% being absorbed even at high dietary intakes. The major excretory route for nickel is via the feces, with lesser amounts found in urine and perspiration (Figure 6.45).

Dietary nickel and nickel compounds are normally relatively nontoxic, due in part to poor intestinal absorption. A contact dermatitis to nickel compounds is a common feature of some humans sensitive to nickel. Both the contact dermatitis and a systemic sensitivity to ingested nickel appear possible. Nickel carbonyl, a highly volatile nickel compound, is a known carcinogen.

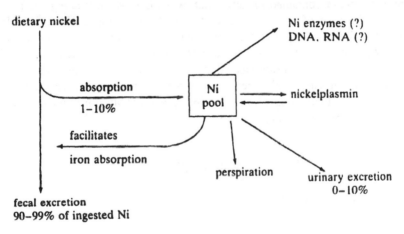

Figure 6.45 Nickel absorption and metabolism.

COBALT

Date of nutritional recognition: 1935
Relative atomic size: 4.2
Oxidation states: +2, +3
Human dietary requirement: As a component of vitamin B_{12}
Body burden: 1.5 mg

The blue glass in the windows of Gothic cathedrals and apothecary jars probably contains cobalt compounds. Nutritionally, cobalt (Figure 6.46) is incorporated into the corrin ring of vitamin B_{12} (see Chapter 5) by the microflora of the gastrointestinal tract. No other nutritional role for cobalt is known with certainty.

The sheep and cattle industry in New Zealand provided the historical setting for the recognition of the dietary essentiality of cobalt. What had been called "bush

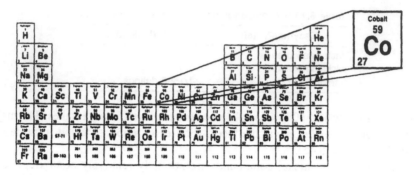

Figure 6.46 Cobalt's place in the periodic table.

sickness" among cattle in New Zealand and "wasting" or "coast disease" in Australia, diseases first attributed to an iron deficiency, were later successfully treated with limonite. Limonite contained nickel, which was effective in treating the animals. Further fractionation of limonite revealed traces of cobalt, and in 1935, E. J. Underwood and J. F. Filmer reported the effectiveness of cobalt salts in eliminating the anemia. Vitamin B_{12} had at this time not been identified, and it was not until 1951 that S. E. Smith showed in ruminants that cobalt deficiency was in effect a vitamin B_{12} deficiency. Humans require dietary vitamin B_{12}, since the intestinal flora do not synthesize adequate amounts of the vitamin if given cobalt. For humans, therefore, cobalt *per se* is not an essential nutrient.

VANADIUM

Date of nutritional recognition: 1971
Relative atomic size: 4.4
Oxidation states: +2, +3, +4, +5
Body burden: 100 µg

The element vanadium (Figure 6.47) was discovered and named by Sefstrom in 1831 after the Scandinavian goddess of beauty, youth, and luster, Vanadis. Vanadium

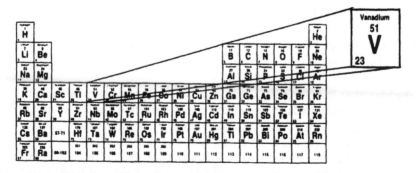

Figure 6.47 Vanadium's place in the periodic table.

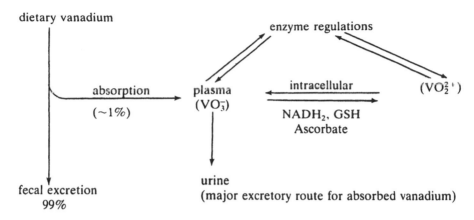

Figure 6.48 Vanadium metabolism.

is thought to be essential for the chick and rat, but experimental data have not been conclusive in reaffirming its essentiality. There is no evidence that vanadium is needed by humans even though the daily intake of the element is estimated to be 10 to 60 µg.

L. L. Hopkins, Jr., and H. E. Mohr, in 1971, reported that chicks fed diets containing 10 ppb vanadium failed to produce normal wing and tail feathers. In the same year, K. Schwarz and D. Milne reported that rats in all-plastic isolators fed purified amino acid diets failed to grow, but that growth improved when the animals were fed the same diet with 10 µg of vanadium as orthovanadate. C. A. Strasia reported similar findings for the rat.

Vanadium appears to be poorly absorbed by the gastrointestinal tract (Figure 6.48). In rats, using $^{48}VO^{2+}$, only 1% of ingested vanadium was absorbed. The principal form of intracellular vanadium *in vivo* appears to exist as the vanadyl $[VO^{2+}(IV)]$ ion maintained by glutathione, $NADH_2$, and perhaps ascorbic acid in the reduced state bound to phosphates. In plasma, vanadium exists as the vanadate $[VO_3^-(V)]$ ion. Vanadium therefore can act as a redox ion and has been reported to facilitate the binding of oxygen to the heme proteins hemoglobin and myoglobin *in vivo*.

Vanadium is a cofactor of only one known protein, hemovanadin (Table 6.15), found in ascidian worms. This protein may function in analogous fashion to hemoglobin, as an oxygen carrier in the ascidians. Vanadium as vanadate is an inhibitor and perhaps a regulator of Na^+-K^+ ATPase, ribonuclease, and other enzymes. Vanadium also has varied physiological effects on the kidney, liver, eye, heart, and nervous system. Because vanadium is so poorly absorbed, most vanadium compounds are not very toxic.

Table 6.15 Proteins and Enzymes Containing Vanadium

Enzyme/Protein	V/Molecule
Hemovanadin	?
Numerous enzymes inhibited or activated by vanadyl or vanadate ions	

The Most Important Nutrient

CHAPTER 7

Water

No other compound is more essential to life than water, for without it there would be no life of any kind. Bacteria, plants, animals, and humans all require exogenous water. Water, H_2O, contains hydrogen and oxygen and is an inorganic solvent. Different life forms contain different anatomical proportions of water. Wheat and corn, properly dried, contain only a small amount of water. Fresh fruits and vegetables may be 80 to 90% water. The water content of a food affects its caloric density. Generally, foods that are high in water are low in calories.

BODY DISTRIBUTION

The human body contains more water than any other component. The water content of the body varies according to age, sex, bone density, lean body mass, and gross body weight. The water content usually varies between 45 and 75% of total body weight. The water content is generally higher in children, in men, and in persons with higher lean body masses. Gender differences in body water content are mainly due to differences in body fat. Most water is localized in cells (55%), particularly those in the muscles and viscera, with the remaining extracellular water (45%) being contributed by interstitial fluids and blood. Smaller amounts of water are found in bone, adipose tissue, the gallbladder (as bile), secretory glands, and spinal, synovial, vitreous, and aqueous fluids. The water content of skeletal muscles is about 65 to 75% by weight. Bone has about the same amount of water as adipose tissue.

FUNCTION

Water is biologically important because of its many unusual physical and chemical properties. It has been called the universal solvent, for it is capable of dissolving not only polar molecules and inorganic salts, but also large organic molecules which may be either polar or contain hydrophobic components. Water has a high specific heat (1 cal/g) and a high heat of vaporization (80 cal/g). These physical properties of water help to prevent rapid fluctuations in body temperature, either hot or cold, and permit small amounts of water (perspiration and transpiration) to remove large amounts of body heat during exercise. Water's large dielectric constant and extensive intermolecular hydrogen bonding relative to other organic liquids (e.g., alcohols) are factors contributing to its special properties. Other characteristics that make water physiologically important include its low viscosity and moderate surface tension, permitting blood flow and lubrication for eyelids, articulating joints, and for peristalsis. Water also permits transmission of light (eye) and sound (ear).

While the primary function of water remains as a solvent for the myriad of biochemical reactions in cells and blood, water also enters directly into some biochemical reactions. Molecular water is consumed during the hydrolysis of proteins, lipids, and carbohydrates undergoing digestion and metabolism. It is also consumed during hydroxylation reactions and is produced as the terminal product of oxidative phosphorylation. It is also consumed in photosynthesis. Water produced in this manner is often referred to as "metabolic water." About 10% of our daily water need is fulfilled by the formation of metabolic water. The remaining 90% of our daily water requirement is ingested in foods and as various liquids (Figure 7.1).

Water helps the body rid itself of waste products. Water is eliminated from the body primarily as urine or as insensible perspiration via epidermal and pulmonary evaporation. Urine is about 95% water by weight. About 5% of the total elimination of body water is contained in feces, providing lubrication and a soft stool. Urinary water provides the solvent for the elimination of the metabolic end products of most nutrients and other substances. Insensible perspiration of skin provides for elimination of some body salts, and insensible perspiration of both skin and lungs carries away body heat by way of evaporation. Diffusion of gases in the body takes place across membranes moistened by water. The evaporation of water as sweat helps the body cool itself. Sedentary adults typically excrete 1000 to 1500 ml of urine, 500 to 700 ml of sweat, 250 to 350 ml of small water droplets in exhaled air, and 100 to 200 ml of water in the feces. Exercise greatly increases the amount of water lost via perspiration and expiration. The amount of water lost in perspiration and expiration is affected by environmental temperature and humidity.

WATER BALANCE

Water intake should approximate the water output on a daily basis. The body has essentially no water reserves. The kidneys along with the gastrointestinal tract and brain homeostatically regulate the amount of water in the body, at least the fat-free components.

When total body water decreases by about 1 to 2%, the normal individual has a sensation of thirst with the message coming from the hypothalamus. The thirst sensation may be blunted in the elderly and in individuals performing vigorous exercise. If individuals become dehydrated, their heat tolerance is affected. The

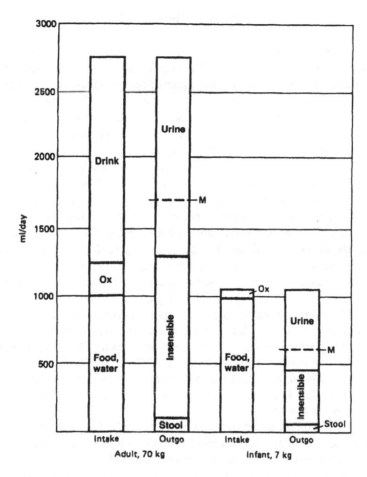

Figure 7.1 Water balance. Routes and approximate magnitude of water intake and outgo without sweating. M is minimal urine volume at maximal solute concentration. Ox is water of oxidation, "metabolic water." [From *Recommended Dietary Allowances*, 9th rev. ed., National Academy of Sciences, New York (1980)].

antidiuretic hormone is released and the kidneys conserve water and electrolytes during dehydration. Due to dehydration an individual could experience a heat stroke or heat exhaustion. The symptoms of heat stroke are headache, nausea, dizziness, clumsiness, stumbling, excessive or insufficient sweating, mental confusion, and loss of consciousness. An individual experiencing extreme dehydration may go into a coma and even die. On the other hand, water intoxication occurs if one is given excessive water or has excessive electrolyte loss, resulting in hyposmolarity. Once again, the antidiuretic hormone and the kidneys try to respond, but if fluid homeostasis cannot be obtained there is headache, nausea, blurring of vision, muscle twitching, gradual mental dulling, convulsion, and even death. Water intoxication is rarely observed in normal adults. Dehydration is frequently observed in the elderly and in individuals participating in vigorous exercise, particularly in hot humid environments.

DIETARY RECOMMENDATIONS

The recommended water intake is 1 to 1.5 ml/kcal expended, or about $^1/_2$ cup/100 kcal. This is equivalent to about 2 to 3 quarts for the person expending 2000 kcal daily. As mentioned earlier, food consumption does contribute to the water intake. Some water, referred to as metabolic water, can also come from metabolism. For a sedentary adult, about 300 to 400 ml of water is provided each day through metabolic reactions. Additional water is needed for extended physical activity. Water is important to athletic performance as well as life itself.

When engaging in strenuous exercise one should drink water before, during (every 15 minutes or so), and after the activity. A typical water intake recommendation for the adult endurance athlete is to drink 2 to 3 cups about 2 hours before an event, 1 to 2 cups 10 to 15 minutes before the event, $^1/_2$ to 1 cup every 10 to 15 minutes during the event, and 1 to 2 cups after the event at about 15-minute intervals. The water should be cool (about 41 to 50°F, or 5 to 10°C). One could consume a beverage containing water, sugar, and electrolytes together as these are all needed in additional quantities during vigorous exercise. The presence of sugar in the beverage slows gastric emptying. The use of glucose polymers, such as maltodextrins, rather than simple sugars reduces the negative effect on gastric emptying. Adult athletes may lose $^1/_2$ to 1 gallon of fluid every hour during heavy exercise. The relative humidity affects the cooling efficiency of sweating. Blood volume becomes reduced when sweating and causes a fluid loss of 2 to 3% of body mass, which puts a strain on the circulatory system which can impair one's capacity for exercise and for thermoregulation. Fluid replacement is important to individuals performing prolonged exercise in the heat.

The consumption of large quantities of protein facilitates water loss through urea production and excretion. This increased excretion of urine can hasten body dehydration. Diarrhea and vomiting can also cause body dehydration.

Bioavailability of Nutrients

CHAPTER 8

Nutrient Digestion

A vigorous and healthy man has just eaten a good meal; in the midst of this feeling of well-being the foods that are at the moment carried to the various parts of the organism are energetically digested, and the digestive juices dissolve them easily and quickly. Should this man receive bad news, or should sad and baneful passions suddenly arise in his soul, his stomach and intestines will immediately cease to act on the foods contained in them. The very juices in which the foods are already almost entirely dissolved will remain as though struck by a moral stupor, and ... digestion ceases entirely... . *Pierre Jean Georges Cabanis, 1802. From Stewart Wolf, The Stomach's Link to the Brain.* Fed. Proc. *44, 2889-2893 (1985).*

THE DIGESTIVE PROCESS

All forms of life must assimilate from their environment a continuous supply of nutrients and energy. Among higher life forms (e.g., animals and humans) nutrients and energy are heterogeneously supplied from a diet containing a great diversity of foods and/or from other substances such as vitamin/mineral supplements that are consumed. Digestion constitutes the physical, chemical, and microbiological process, which begins in the mouth with the mastication of food and ceases with the absorption of individual nutrients across the microvilli of the intestinal mucosa. Digestion of food is foremost a chemical process under physiologic and hormonal controls initiated by the senses: sight and smell. It is a process whereby macromolecules — starch, proteins, and triglycerides and other smaller molecules — undergo hydrolysis and reduction primarily to their monomeric constituent components in preparation for absorption. Other nutrients, vitamins, and minerals, and also drugs, undergo either minor or no chemical change prior to absorption.

Digestion begins in the mouth but may be facilitated by pretreatment of some foods with enzymes, microbiological fermentations, or cooking. Once ingested, foods at various stages of digestion pass through the various anatomical components comprising the gastrointestinal (GI) tract, also known as the alimentary or digestive tract or system (Figure 8.1). The GI tract is lined with tissues of ectodermal origin

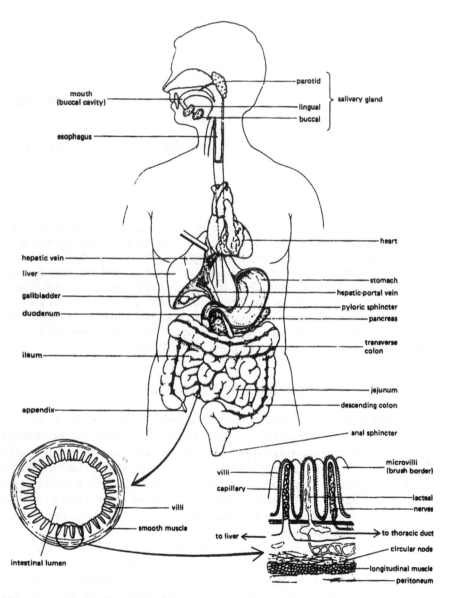

Figure 8.1 The human digestive system.

and lies outside the body proper. For descriptive purposes, digestion of food begins in the oral cavity and terminates with the anal sphincter. The absorption of nutrients is detailed in Chapter 9.

MOUTH

Admittance of food into the buccal cavity (ingestion) invites a series of complex physiological and hormonal events in preparation for the digestion of food. The presence of food in the mouth stimulates the secretion of saliva from the bilateral sets of three salivary glands (buccal, lingual, and parotid). Secreted saliva is mixed during mastication and provides lubrication for swallowing the bolus of food. During mastication, the teeth assist with the mechanical degradation of the food, increasing its surface area. The maintenance of adequate dentition for mastication is most important for proper eating and digestion. Loss of dentition among the elderly often leads to changes in life-long dietary practices, loss of weight from reduction in caloric ingestion, and marginal or severe vitamin and mineral deficiencies. Loss of teeth due to abrasion from dirt and grit in the processed flours of ancient peoples probably contributed to nutritional deficiencies and early death.

Secreted saliva, in addition to providing lubrication for swallowing, contains the enzyme salivary α-amylase or ptyalin. Enzymatically active in the mouth at neutral to slightly acidic conditions, α-amylase [α-(1→4)-glucan-4-glucanohydrolase] hydrolyzes the α-(1→4) glycosides of glycogen and starch, giving rise to maltose, isomaltose, and oligosaccharides (Figure 8.2). The bolus of food is then swallowed. Peristalsis moves the bolus through the esophagus and into the stomach going through the cardiac sphincter. As the bolus of food enters the stomach, hydrolysis of starch continues until the fall in pH and proteolytic enzymes of the stomach inactivate α-amylase, with cessation of carbohydrate degradation.

Hydrolysis of disaccharides, proteins, or triglycerides does not transpire in the buccal cavity. No proteolytic enzymes are present in saliva, and the presence of a buccal lipase becomes active only under the acidic conditions of the stomach.

STOMACH

Food particles move through the stomach, mixed with gastric secretions, by wave-like forward contractions from the fundus to the antrum and pylorus. Concurrent with the ingestion of food, the stomach responds to various stimuli by secreting gastric juice, consisting of mucus secretions, hydrochloric acid (HCl) from the gastric glands, a glycoprotein, the intrinsic factor (IF) for the intestinal absorption of vitamin B_{12}, and pepsinogen, the zymogen precursor of pepsin. HCl kills some of the bacteria present in the food bolus. The stomach is the first organ encountered for protein and triglyceride hydrolysis. The stomach is the major site for protein digestion following the conversion of the enzymatically inactive pepsinogen to the enzymatically active pepsin by HCl and then by pepsin autocatalytically. The pepsin of the stomach rapidly degrades proteins to polypeptides, oligopeptides, and small, limited amounts of amino acids. Proteins are degraded by pepsin primarily by hydrolysis of the peptide bonds of phenylalanine, tyrosine, and tryptophan, and secondarily by bonds of aspartic acid, glutamic acid, and leucine residues. The lipase entering the stomach from the mouth in the bolus of food becomes enzymatically active as the pH falls to between 4.5 and 5.4. As the pH of the food in the stomach continues to fall to approximately pH 2 to 3, which is optimum for the proteolytic activity of pepsin, lipase activity lasts only briefly and triglyceride hydrolysis is restricted. The digestive products from the stomach enter the upper small intestine through the pyloric sphincter as chyme. The stomach is emptied in 1 to 4 hours under normal conditions,

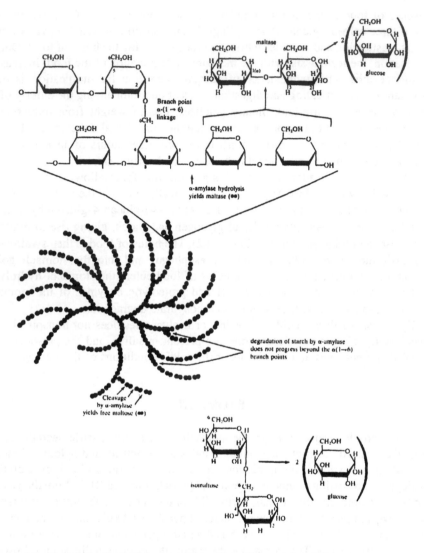

Figure 8.2 Hydrolysis of starch by α-amylase, isomaltase, and maltase.

depending on the amount and kinds of foods consumed. In general, carbohydrates leave the stomach first, followed by protein, and then by fat. Humans usually consume mixed diets that contain more than one of these energy-yielding nutrients. In the case of mixed diets, liquids empty from the stomach before solids and small particles before larger ones.

SMALL INTESTINE

The small intestine is divided into the duodenum, jejunum, and ileum. Most of the digestion takes place in the duodenum. Secretions from the gallbladder (but

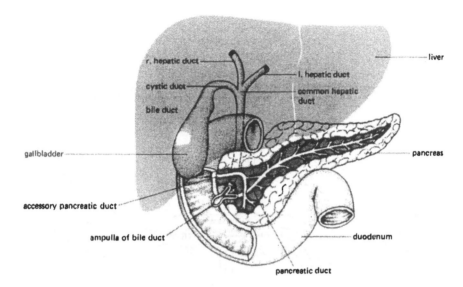

Figure 8.3 Digestion in the small intestine.

synthesized in the liver) and pancreas interact with chyme in the duodenum. The connections of the liver, gallbladder, and pancreas with the duodenum are summarized in Figure 8.3. The intestinal villi secrete mucus that protects the intestinal mucosa and provides lubrication. Food particles move through the small intestine by segmentation. Absorption takes place primarily through the mucosa of the small intestine.

BILE SECRETION

The bile acids are formed by the liver as terminal metabolites of cholesterol metabolism. They are stored in the gallbladder (when anatomically present) and enter the duodenum through the bile duct in the presence of chyme from the stomach. The major human bile acid is cholic acid. The other, less abundant bile acids are formed by the addition of the amino acids glycine or taurine to choloyl-CoA, forming the bile acids, glycocholic and taurocholic acid. The other bile acids are deoxycholic and lithocholic acids. In the intestinal tract, the bile acids (contain Na^+ and K^+) are amphipathic and function to emulsify the luminal lipids, the triacylglycerols, cholesterol, acylcholesterol, phospholipids, and lipid-soluble vitamins. Emulsification of lipids by the bile acids results in the formation of micelles, very small lipid droplets in an aqueous environment similar to formation of a colloid. The result of emulsification is a large expansion of the total lipid surface area exposed to lipase activity. Micellar lipids are then rapidly hydrolyzed to free fatty acids, glycerides, glycerol, free cholesterol, and vitamin A.

The bile acids, having facilitated the digestion and absorption of lipids, may pass through the remainder of the GI tract and be excreted in the feces or they may be reabsorbed by the ileum. Reabsorbed bile acids are returned to the liver by the enterohepatic circulation (Figure 8.4) and are again stored in the gallbladder to

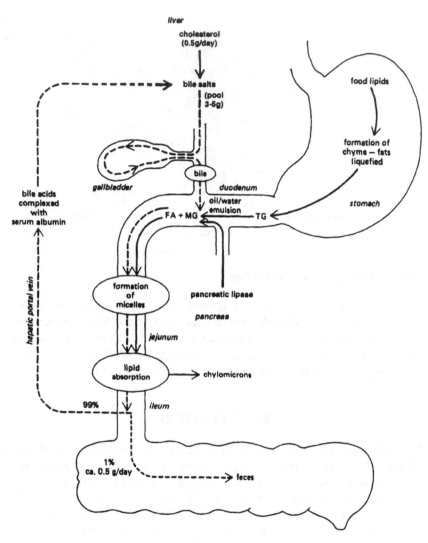

Figure 8.4 Enterohepatic circulation of bile salts and digestion of lipids. Dashes (- - -) indicate
       enterohepatic circulation of bile salts.

repeat their function in lipid digestion. Thirty grams of bile salts may be recycled
in this manner each day through this enterohepatic circulation. Cholestyramine, a
strong anion-exchange resin, is sometimes used medically to bind intestinal bile
acids, breaking the chain of absorption and enterohepatic circulation, facilitating
the excretion of additional bile acids. In this manner, cholestyramine effectively
reduces circulating serum cholesterol by accelerating the excretion of bile acids and
may aid in the control of bile acid-induced diarrhea in individuals who have had
an ileal resection.

Table 8.1   Pancreatic and Intestinal Enzymes and
                    Zymogens

Proteolytic zymogens	Carbohydrate enzymes
Trypsinogen	α-Amylase
Chymotrypsinogen	Sucrase
Procarboxypeptidase	Maltase
	Lactase
Lipid enzymes	Isomaltase
α-Lipase	
Retinyl esterase	Secreted intraintestinal enzymes
Tocopheryl esterase	Aminopeptidases
Cholesterol esterase	Dipeptidases
	Maltase
Proteolytic enzymes	Sucrase
Trypsin	Lactase
Chymotrypsin	β-Lipase
Aminopeptidase	Esterases
Carboxypeptidase	Nucleases
	Nucleotidases
Other enzymes	Phosphatases
Endonucleases	Enterokinases
	Nucleosidases
	Enteropeptidases

PANCREATIC SECRETIONS

Entering the upper small intestine, or duodenum, from the stomach, the chyme (pH 2 to 3) is rapidly neutralized (pH 6 to 7) by the secretions of the pancreas and gallbladder (see Figure 8.3). Entering the duodenum through the pancreatic duct are the enzymes for the continuing degradation of carbohydrates, proteins, lipids, and nucleic acids (Table 8.1). Produced by the cells of the pancreas for the secretion into the duodenum is an α-amylase similar in function to salivary amylase for continued hydrolysis of α-(1→4) glycosides. Glucose, maltose, isomaltose, and mixed oligosaccharides are produced by the pancreatic amylase activity from the remaining starches and glycogen.

In addition to secreting α-amylase, the pancreas synthesizes and secretes several zymogens. These zymogens secreted into the duodenum include two proteolytic zymogens, trypsinogen and chymotrypsinogen, and procarboxypeptidase. Conversion of these zymogens into the active enzymes is initiated by an enteropeptidase synthesized and secreted by cells of the gastrointestinal mucosa. The enteropeptidase hydrolyzes a polypeptide, converting trypsinogen to trypsin. Thereafter, trypsin converts the remaining zymogens to active enzymes. Like pepsin, trypsin and chymotrypsin are proteolytic endopeptidases cleaving proteins inside their amino acid extremities (Figure 8.5). Trypsin hydrolyzes peptide bonds adjacent to lysyl or hystidyl residues, while chymotrypsin hydrolyzes peptide bonds adjacent to phenylalanyl, tyrosyl, or tryptophanyl residues. Trypsin and chymotrypsin are able to degrade proteins and large polypeptides not hydrolyzed by pepsin to even smaller polypeptides, dipeptides, and possibly some free amino acids. Having been activated by trypsin, the procarboxypeptidase hydrolyzes amino acids from terminal carboxyl

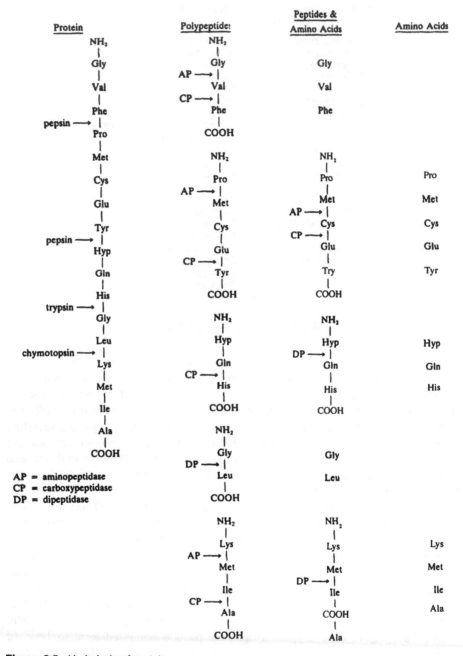

Figure 8.5 Hydrolysis of proteins.

residues of polypeptides. Enzymes that hydrolyze terminal amino or carboxyl residues of polypeptides are classified as exopeptidases and are aminopeptidase and carboxypeptidase. A third class of digestive enzymes secreted in pancreatic juice are the pancreatic esterases, pancreatic lipases, cholesterol, and retinyl esterases.

Pancreatic lipase, in the presence of liver bile acids and lingual and gastric lipases, hydrolyzes emulsified fats and oils, triacylglycerols, principally at the α and α' esters of the triglyceride. The luminal products of pancreatic lipase activity are free fatty acids from the α- and α'-glycerol esters and a monoglyceride, β-monoacylglyceride (Figure 8.6). Cholesterol and retinyl esterases hydrolyze the fatty acid esters attached to cholesterol and vitamin A. Ribonuclease and deoxyribonuclease hydrolyze dietary nucleic acids. Phospholipases hydrolyze the ester bond in the second position of glycerophospholipids.

INTESTINAL MUCOSAL SECRETIONS

The intestinal mucosa secretes enterokinase, an enzyme which converts trypsinogen (produced by pancreas) to its active form trypsin. Secreted by the crypts of Lieberkühn are maltose, lactase, and sucrase. These enzymes promote the hydrolysis of the disaccharides to their constituent monosaccharides. Trehalase, which hydrolyzes trehalose, is secreted by the intestinal mucosa. Aminopeptidases and dipeptidases also secreted by cells of the intestinal mucosa complete the degradation of polypeptides and most dipeptides to amino acids (Figure 8.5). An intestinal β-lipase (Figure 8.6) completes the hydrolysis of most but not all monoglycerides to a free fatty acid and glycerol. A phosphatase removes phosphate from various organic phosphates. Intestinal polynucleotidases and nucleosidases degrade the nucleic acids.

DIGESTION OF VITAMINS AND MINERALS

Unlike the major components of the diet, carbohydrates, proteins, and lipids, which comprise the majority of caloric intake and dietary bulk and undergo extensive chemical degradations, vitamins and minerals are subjected to only minor chemical changes. Vitamins such as riboflavin and biotin, which may be covalently attached to protein, may be hydrolyzed but otherwise are not degraded further. Folic acid, which may contain from two to six additional glutamic acid residues (polyglutamate) is absorbed as the monoglutamyl folate following hydrolysis. Minerals, either ionically or coordinate covalently bonded to proteins or carbohydrates, may be dissociated from proteins or carbohydrates during digestion. Some minerals will undergo redox reactions in the stomach and intestines due to changes in pH as in the case of Fe^{3+} reduction by dietary ascorbic acid and HCl, or have their oxidation state changed by other dietary components prior to absorption.

LARGE INTESTINE

Unabsorbed digestive materials go through the ileocecal valve to the large intestine or colon. The microflora in the colon continue digestion of digestive materials as well as synthesizing some nutrients themselves, particularly vitamins. Vitamin K and biotin synthesized by the microflora can be absorbed. However, the other vitamins are not known to be absorbed to any appreciable extent in the large intestine.

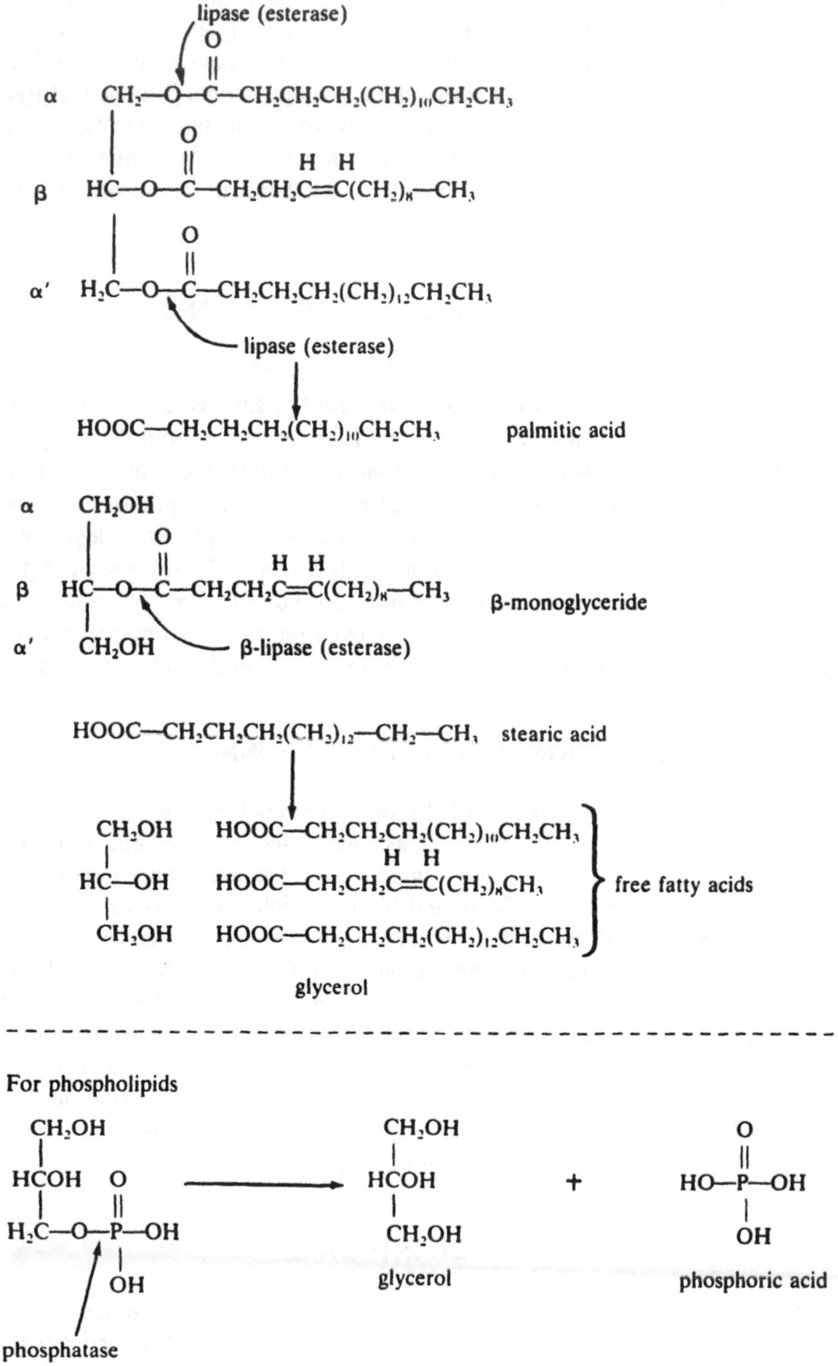

lipase (esterase)

$$\alpha \quad CH_2-O-\overset{\overset{\displaystyle O}{\|}}{C}-CH_2CH_2CH_2(CH_2)_{10}CH_2CH_3$$

$$\beta \quad HC-O-\overset{\overset{\displaystyle O}{\|}}{C}-CH_2CH_2\overset{H}{C}=\overset{H}{C}(CH_2)_N-CH_3$$

$$\alpha' \quad H_2C-O-\overset{\overset{\displaystyle O}{\|}}{C}-CH_2CH_2CH_2(CH_2)_{12}CH_2CH_3$$

lipase (esterase)

$HOOC-CH_2CH_2CH_2(CH_2)_{10}CH_2CH_3$ palmitic acid

$$\alpha \quad CH_2OH$$

$$\beta \quad HC-O-\overset{\overset{\displaystyle O}{\|}}{C}-CH_2CH_2\overset{H}{C}=\overset{H}{C}(CH_2)_N-CH_3 \quad \beta\text{-monoglyceride}$$

$$\alpha' \quad CH_2OH \quad \longleftarrow \beta\text{-lipase (esterase)}$$

$HOOC-CH_2CH_2CH_2(CH_2)_{12}-CH_2-CH_3$ stearic acid

$$\begin{array}{l} CH_2OH \\ | \\ HC-OH \\ | \\ CH_2OH \end{array} \quad \left. \begin{array}{l} HOOC-CH_2CH_2CH_2(CH_2)_{10}CH_2CH_3 \\ \overset{H\ \ H}{HOOC-CH_2CH_2C=C(CH_2)_NCH_3} \\ HOOC-CH_2CH_2CH_2(CH_2)_{12}CH_2CH_3 \end{array} \right\} \text{free fatty acids}$$

glycerol

- -

For phospholipids

$$\begin{array}{l} CH_2OH \\ | \\ HCOH \quad O \\ | \quad\quad \| \\ H_2C-O-P-OH \\ \quad\quad\quad | \\ \quad\quad\quad OH \end{array} \longrightarrow \begin{array}{l} CH_2OH \\ | \\ HCOH \\ | \\ CH_2OH \end{array} \quad + \quad \begin{array}{l} O \\ \| \\ HO-P-OH \\ | \\ OH \end{array}$$

phosphatase   glycerol   phosphoric acid

Figure 8.6 Hydrolysis of triglycerides.

REGULATION OF DIGESTION

Digestion is regulated by the nervous and endocrine systems with enteric nerves existing in the GI tract. The stomach mucosa has neural receptors which respond to the presence of foods and stimulate the secretion of gastric hormones and enzymes causing the muscles of the stomach to contract. As the stomach is emptied, the receptors are no longer stimulated. Neural receptors in the duodenum sense the presence of the acidic chyme causing the pyloric sphincter to close and secretrin to be secreted. Mucosal receptors are sensitive to the composition of the chyme and the lumal stretch (due to fullness) sends impulses to secretory and muscle cells of the GI tract. Neural transmitters known to be involved in the digestive process include enkephalin, somatostatin, serotonin, bombesin, substance P, vasoactive intestinal polypeptide, and neurotensin. The appearance, smell, taste, and even thought of food can affect digestion via the nervous system as can fear, anger, and worry.

Several hormones play a role in the regulation of digestion. Collectively, GI hormones are called enterogastrones. Gastrin is secreted by the antral mucosal cells in the stomach in response to distention of the antrum of the stomach by food, impulses from the vagus nerve, and the presence of secretagogues (partially digested proteins, caffeine, alcohol, and food extracts) in the antrum. Gastrin stimulates the secretion of HCl and pepsinogen by the parietal and chief cells, respectively, of the stomach. Secretin is a hormone released from the duodenum. Secretin is released in response to the presence of the acidic chyme as it enters the duodenum. Secretin stimulates the pancreas to secrete bicarbonate and water into the duodenum which inhibits gastrin secretion. Cholecystokinin is released from the intestinal mucosa in response to the presence of fatty acids and amino acids. Cholecystokinin stimulates the release of pancreatic enzymes (and some bicarbonate and water) and bile (secreted from the gallbladder into the duodenum) as well as the contraction of the colon and rectum. The gastric inhibitory polypeptide, released from the intestinal mucosa in response to the presence of glucose and fat, stimulates insulin release and inhibits HCl secretion. Enteroglucagon, released from the duodenum, stimulates glycogenolysis. Glucagon, released from the jejunum, inhibits the secretion of pancreatic enzymes and intestinal motility. Motilin, released by the intestinal mucosa in response to an alkaline pH, slows gastric emptying and may help to regulate intestinal motility. Somatostatin is released from the hypothalamus and to a lesser extent, the antrum of the stomach and duodenal mucosa. Somatostatin inhibits gastrin release, gallbladder contraction, insulin and glucagon release, and slows the synthesis of pancreatic enzymes.

FECES FORMATION

The feces are formed in the large intestine from water, indigestible and unabsorbed food particles (including dietary fiber), sloughed epithelial cells from the GI tract, and components of digestive secretions (including bile). Feces are excreted or defecated through the anus.

CHAPTER 9

Nutrient Absorption

ABSORPTION OF NUTRIENTS

The principal end products of digestion — glucose, amino acids, fatty acids, monoglycerides, glycerol, nucleic acids, cholesterol, vitamins, and minerals — present in the intestinal lumen are absorbed by the cells of the intestinal mucosa and enter the general circulatory system by way of the capillary beds or lacteals of the villi. Absorption of the nutrients is a process of great complexity, often involving the participation of intracellular enzymes, transport proteins, and ion pumps. Despite the great complexity in each nutrient's individual absorption, absorption of all nutrients can be classified as occurring by either passive diffusion or by an active transport process requiring an expenditure of energy (Figure 9.1).

Passive diffusion from the intestinal lumen across the mucosal cell occurs only for some nutrients and drugs. This process is akin to that of osmosis, whereby selected nutrients move from an area of high concentration (the intestinal lumen) into a lower nutrient concentration in the capillary bed or lacteal, through the semipermeable membrane of the mucosal cells of the intestine. Most nutrients, however, move across the intestinal mucosal cells with great selectivity and expenditure of energy (ATP) despite an often favorable concentration gradient of a nutrient for passive absorption. Here in the mucosal cell, a change in nutrient composition may take place prior to entry into the capillary bed or lymph system. A list of some nutrients and their manner of known absorption is given in Table 9.1.

ABSORPTION OF CARBOHYDRATES

For most people, carbohydrates in the diet provide the largest contribution of total caloric need and singularly account for the largest nutrient mass ingested.

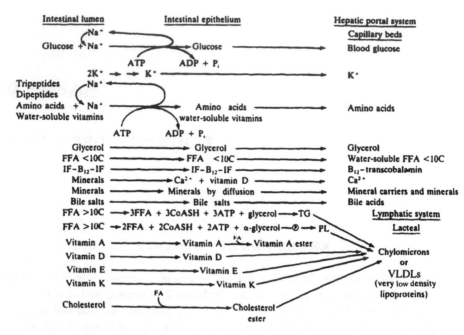

Figure 9.1 Absorption of nutrients.

Table 9.1 Nutrient Absorption[a]

Passive Diffusion	Active Transport
Fructose	Glucose
Mannose	Galactose
Xylose	Fatty acids (long chain)
Fatty acids (short chain)	Bile acids
Monoglycerides	Cholesterol
Nucleic acids	Amino acids
Ascorbic acid (high concentration)	Ascorbic acid
Niacin (high concentration)	Thiamin
Vitamin B_6	Riboflavin
Vitamin A	Niacin
Vitamin D	Folate
Vitamin E	Vitamin B_{12} (intrinsic factor)
Vitamin K	Ca^{2+}
Cholesterol	Fe^{2+}
Bile salts	Zn^{2+}
Water	Na^+
Ca^{2+}	
Cu^+	
K^+	
Cl^-	

[a] Most nutrients are absorbed in the duodenum and ileum. Lipids, subject to the critical micelle formation in the presence of bile salts, are absorbed in the jejunal region.

Glucose is the most abundant dietary monosaccharide, present in mixed diets as a component of di-, oligo-, and polysaccharides. Lesser amounts of fructose, galactose, mannose, and other monosaccharides are to be found in the intestinal lumen. The absorption of glucose and most monosaccharides from the intestinal lumen of the duodenum across the microvilli to the capillary bed is by an active transport process requiring ATP and a sodium (Na^+) ion gradient.

FIBER

One of the largest components of the bulk diet of humans and certainly for animals with a rumen or cecum is cellulose. Like starch and glycogen, cellulose, the major structural component of the cell wall of plants, is a polysaccharide composed of glucose. Cellulose, however, remains indigestible by humans and monogastric animals who lack the enzyme β-$(1\rightarrow4)$ glycosidase, necessary for the hydrolysis of the β-$(1\rightarrow4)$ glycosides of cellulose. Ruminants and animals with a cecum have a digestive system populated with a microflora that synthesizes and secretes the β-$(1\rightarrow4)$ glycosidase, and are thus able to hydrolyze the cellulose and absorb the glucose. In humans cellulose remains mostly nondigestible, is not absorbed, and has little or no caloric dietary value. Cellulose and other nondigestible components of the diet — hemicelluloses, pectin, lignin, gums, mucilages, algal polysaccharides, and others — constitute what has become collectively known as dietary fiber. There is no consensus on a specific definition of dietary fiber. This is because fiber has a diverse chemical composition and some fiber components, such as pectins and gums, are fermentable, yielding absorptive acids, aldehydes, and ketones. Some estimates from animals and human experimentation suggest that 50% of dietary fiber is degradable by bacterial enzymes and may be absorbed. For this reason the author's preferred definition of dietary fiber is "those carbohydrates and lignin remaining for excretion following digestion and absorption."

Dietary fiber has gained a reputation as a significant contributor to healthful dietary practices. Its inclusion in the diet is reported to assist in the prevention of constipation, appendicitis, diverticulosis, hemorrhoids, polyps, ulcers, cancer, and metabolic diseases. Added dietary fiber helps constipation and probably diverticulosis. Other health claims for fiber do not seem to be substantiated. One real beneficial effect of fiber added to the diet is the reduction in caloric density of the diet being consumed (see Chapter 2).

ABSORPTION OF PROTEIN AS AMINO ACIDS, DI- AND TRIPEPTIDES

Gastrointestinal proteins are hydrolyzed to their constituent amino acids, di- and tripeptides. Soluble proteins and proteins that have been denatured are most readily hydrolyzed. All of the digestive enzymes, components of the pancreas, mucosal secretions, and exfoliated tissues of the intestinal lumen are subject to digestion right

188					NUTRITION: CHEMISTRY AND BIOLOGY

along with dietary protein. The amino acids, dipeptides, and tripeptides released
from all these sources are absorbed by an active-transport (ATP) sodium ion (Na⁺)-
dependent system. Passing through the microvilli, the di- and tripeptides undergo
intracellular hydrolysis, and with the remaining amino acids they enter the capillary
bed of the villi. Each amino acid shares its transport system through the microvilli
with other amino acids, based on similarity in structural and chemical characteristics.
Only a small number of basic transport systems are needed for the absorption of
both the D- and L-isomers of the amino acids. Small peptides and, to a very small
extent, proteins may be absorbed. Proteins, as immunoglobulins, may be absorbed
from maternal milk colostrum following birth, and protein absorption may be the
cause of some food allergies.

ABSORPTION OF LIPIDS

The absorption of lipids and the products of lipid digestion from the intestinal
lumen is complex, owing to the variety of lipids in the diet, the participation of the
bile acids in micelle formation, and the intracellular synthesis of triglycerides within
the microvilli (Figure 9.2).

Dietary lipids and the products of lipid digestion, free fatty acids, monoglycerides, cholesterol, phospholipids, and the lipid-soluble vitamins, combine with the
bile acids synthesized in the liver to form round microdroplets approximately 50 Å
in diameter. These microdroplets, called micelles, are formed by the dietary lipids
and bile acids in preparation for absorption by the microvilli. Micelles contain all
the products of lipid digestion, with the exclusion of the shorter-chain free fatty
acids (FFAs) and glycerol, both of which are water soluble. Free fatty acids of 10
or fewer carbons ($\leq C_{10}$), such as in medium-chain triglycerides, and glycerol may
pass directly through the microvilli and into the capillary bed of the villus entering
the general hepatic portal circulation.

Monoglycerides and free fatty acids ($>C_{10}$) entering the microvilli are reassem-
bled into triglycerides. For the synthesis of triglycerides, free fatty acids are activated
by the formation of a fatty acid acetyl-coenzyme A (FA-CoA). The formation of
each FA-CoA requires activation by ATP. This reaction predominates for the long-
chain free fatty acids, which are then esterified with a β-monoglyceride, forming
newly synthesized triacylglycerides.

Free intracellular glycerol may also be esterified with activated (FA-CoA) fatty
acids. In this pathway, glycerol is phosphorylated by ATP, forming α-glycerol-
phosphates. Two FA-CoAs are esterified with α-glycerolphosphate, forming
α-phosphatidic acid. Dephosphorylation and reaction with an additional FA-CoA
completes the synthesis of a triglyceride. Triglycerides assembled within the
microvilli enter the lacteal of the villi as chylomicrons and lipoprotein complexes:
the very light (or low) density lipoprotein (VLDL). From the lacteals the chylomicrons and VLDLs transverse the lymphatic system to the thoracic duct, in which
lymph and lipids enter the general systemic circulation through the left subclavian
vein (Figure 9.3).

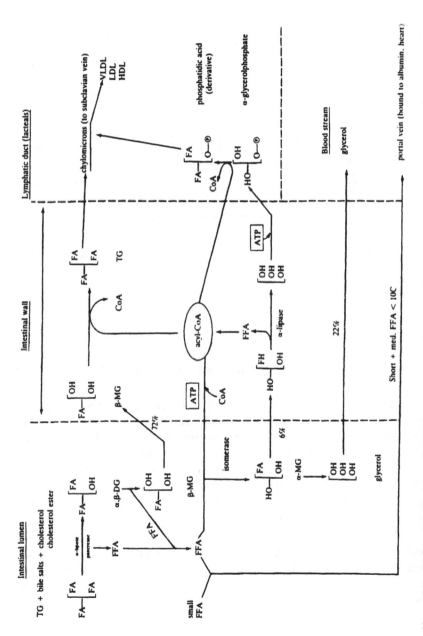

Figure 9.2 Absorption of lipids. (Modified from F. H. Mattson and R. A. Volpenheim. The digestion and absorption of triglycerides, *J. Biological Chemistry* 239, 2722 (1964); and F. J. Stare, Ed., *Atherosclerosis*, Medcom, Inc., New York, 1974.)

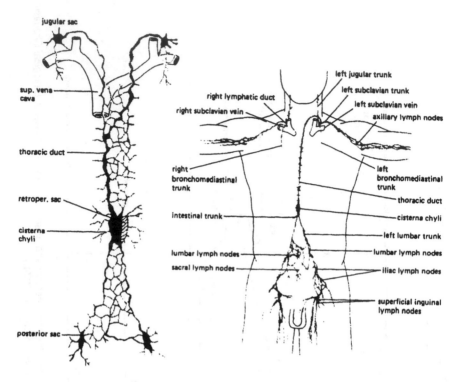

Figure 9.3 The human lymphatic system.

LOW AND NO CALORIE FAT SUBSTITUTES

Food technology is rapidly providing food products which are safe and efficacious. Food products are now available to help those who need to lower their caloric intake from fat which are made from carbohydrate, proteins, and even lipids themselves.

Carbohydrates and protein fat substitutes are made into gels which can have a creamy texture and in the mouth feel similar to natural fats. These products cannot be used for frying foods due to their instability at high temperature, but they can be used in products like frozen desserts, salad dressings, and some baked items. Some carbohydrate-based fat replacers include dextrans, oligosaccharides (1 to 4 kcal/g) (such as Oatrum, Ztrim, and Maltrim MO40), polydextrins (1 kcal/g), modified food starch such as Sta-Slim (94 kcal/g), and gels or gum-type fillers such as Avicel and xanthin gum. Simplesse and K-blazer are protein-based fat substitutes which contain 1 to 2 kcal/g. Some lower caloric products combine both mono- and diglycerides with food starch, gums, and non-fat dried milk to form a fat substitute. One such product is N-flate, which contains 5.1 kcal/g.

Another type of fat substitute is a reduced calorie triglyceride such as Benefat, also known as Salatrim (short- and long-chain fatty acid triglyceride molecule) (Figure 9.4). Salatrim is a triglyceride containing stearic acid and short-chain fatty acids such as acetic, proprionic, and butyric acids. The stearic acid in Salatrim is

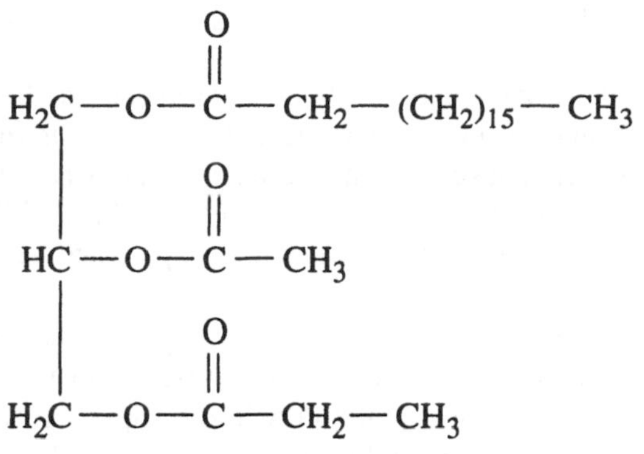

Figure 9.4 Structure of Benefat (Salatrim).

poorly absorbed and the short-chain fatty acids intrinsically have less caloric value following absorption. In total Salatrim has about 5 kcal/g because of these changes in the composition of the triglyceride compared to the normal caloric value of 9 kcal/g of other triglycerides.

Consumption of very large amounts of Salatrim may cause gastrointestinal distress in some rare individuals, but no other side effects have been reported. Salatrim is currently available in products such as candies, reduced-fat baking chocolate chips, and cookies. A similar product is Caprenin, a triglyceride with caprylic, capric, and behenic esterified fatty acids. Behenic acid is only partially absorbed following digestion. Like Salatrim, Caprenin effectively contains only approximately 5 kcal/g.

The fat substitute whose use is most controversial is Olean, also known as Olestra (Figure 9.5). Olestra is a modified sucrose monomer to which fatty acids have been esterified. Containing six to eight esterified fatty acids, Olestra has all the physical properties of normal triglycerides as well as thermal stability. The ester bonds between the sucrose and the fatty acids are inaccessible to pancreatic lipase, and therefore it remains undigested and it is not absorbed. Olestra is also not degraded

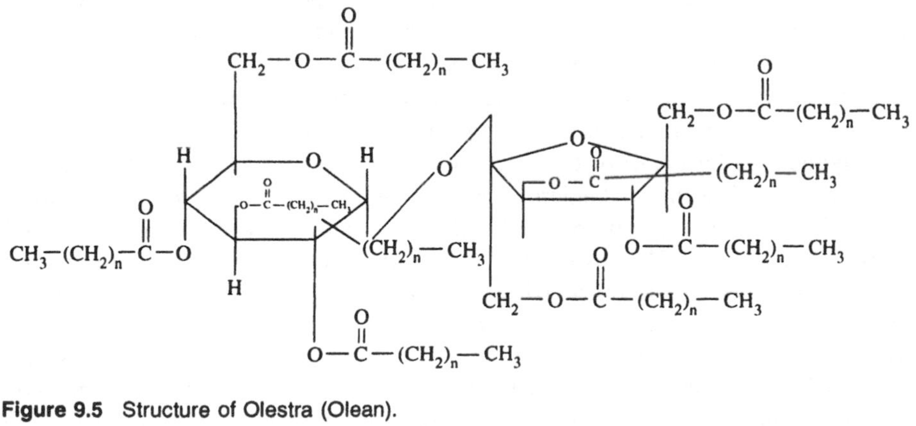

Figure 9.5 Structure of Olestra (Olean).

nor metabolized by the GI microflora of the gut. For these reasons Olestra is effectively non-caloric.

Olestra is one of the most extensively researched food additives and has been found to have both beneficial and problematic dietary effects. Use of Olestra products will lower caloric and fat intake and may reduce total and LDL cholesterol with no effect on HDL cholesterol, triglyceride, or lipoproteins A_1, A_2, or B. On the negative side some individuals who consume Olestra may experience heartburn, flatulence, bloating, and diarrhea.

Olestra also reduces the absorption of the fat-soluble vitamins which is counteracted by the fortification of foods containing Olestra with Vitamins A, D, E, and K. Ingestion of products containing Olestra will also slightly reduce the absorption of the carotenoids, i.e., β-carotene and lycopene, as well as other fat-soluble dietary components. No fortification of Olestra with other than the fat-soluble vitamins is planned.

Other fat substitutes currently in development include dialkyldihexadecylmalonate (DDM), which is composed of malic acid, hexadecane, and fatty acids. DDM is essentially nonabsorbed when ingested. Other products in development are esterified propoxylated glycerol (LEPG) and trialkoxy-tricarballylate (TATCA). DDM is heat stable, and TATCA has properties similar to triglycerides. Esterified fatty acid esters of a trisaccharide of raffinose is also being evaluated as a fat replacement in foods.

As long as the public continues its fixation on no-fat and low-fat foods in order to restrain the problem of obesity as inactivity and age set in, present and newly developed fat substitutes should find a widespread acceptance and growing commercial market.

ABSORPTION OF THE LIPID-SOLUBLE VITAMINS

Vitamins A, D, E, and K, being hydrophobic, are absorbed predominately in association with micelles. Micelles formed in the presence of the bile salts, phospholipids, monoglycerides, free fatty acids, and cholesterol also include in their composition the lipid-soluble vitamins and previtamin A, β-carotene. Carried by the chylomicrons, the fat-soluble vitamins enter the lymphatic system and after joining the circulatory system, are deposited in the liver.

Vitamin A is freed of its esterified fatty acid by retinyl esterase (Figure 9.6) before its inclusion in micellar formation. After entering the microvilli, free vitamin A is reesterified by FA-CoA, forming a new retinyl ester, generally palmitate, and is then included in the chylomicron for lymphatic transport. Approximately 80 to 90% of dietary vitamin A is absorbed in the small intestine, and 75% is reesterified in the mucosal cells. The chylomicrons also carry the remaining 25% unesterified retinol. β-carotene is absorbed with approximately 50 to 60% efficiency in the intestinal mucosa, where it is symmetrically cleaved by a dioxygenase to retinol, and reduced to retinal by an $NADH_2$ or $NADPH_2$ reductase, upon which it is then esterified. Uncleaved β-carotene also enters the chylomicron and the lymphatic system. Vitamin D is absorbed from the intestinal lumen with approximately 50%

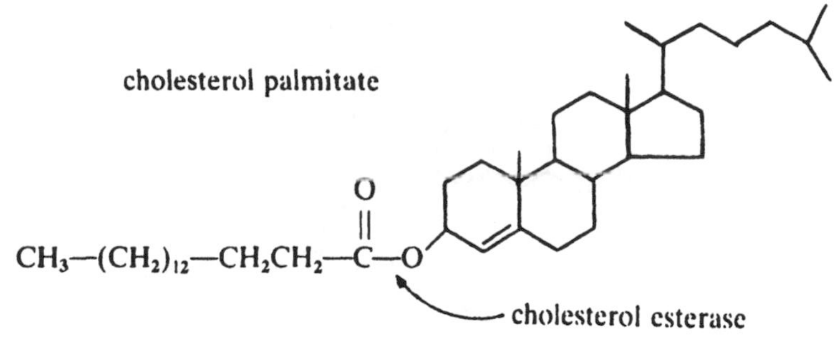

cholesterol palmitate

$$CH_3-(CH_2)_{12}-CH_2CH_2-\overset{\overset{\text{O}}{\|}}{C}-O$$

cholesterol esterase

Hydrolysis by cholesterol esterase yields free cholesterol and palmitic acid

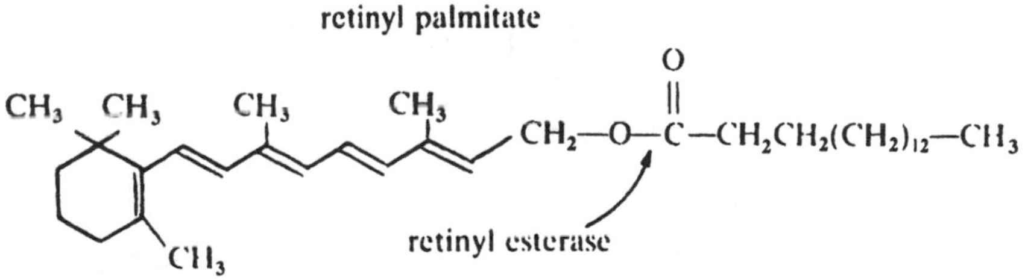

retinyl palmitate

$$CH_2-O-\overset{\overset{\text{O}}{\|}}{C}-CH_2CH_2(CH_2)_{12}-CH_3$$

retinyl esterase

Hydrolysis by retinyl esterase yields retinol and palmitic acid

Figure 9.6 Hydrolysis of cholesterol and retinyl esters.

efficiency. It is incorporated unchanged into the chylomicron prior to entering the lacteal of the lymphatic system.

Vitamin E esters and their isomers (tocopherols) are hydrolyzed by an esterase, producing free succinic or acetic acids and vitamin E prior to absorption by micelles. About 30% of the free tocopheryls are absorbed, and they are not reesterified prior to chylomicron formation.

Like the other lipid-soluble vitamins, vitamin K is absorbed into the mixed micelle. About 50% of the exogenous vitamin K from dietary sources and vitamin K synthesized endogenously by the intestinal microflora is absorbed. Absorption rates and mode of absorption vary considerably depending on the chemistry of the vitamin K analog. Vitamin K is also transported in the lymph by the chylomicron.

ABSORPTION OF CHOLESTEROL

The dietary intake of cholesterol varies considerably between individuals, but averages about 600 mg per day, consisting of free cholesterol and cholesterol esters. In the presence of liver bile and a pancreatic esterase, cholesterol esters are hydrolyzed, producing free cholesterol and a single fatty acid (Figure 9.6). The free cholesterol is incorporated within the mixed-lipid micelles and is absorbed by passive diffusion into the microvilli. About one-half of all dietary cholesterol is absorbed in

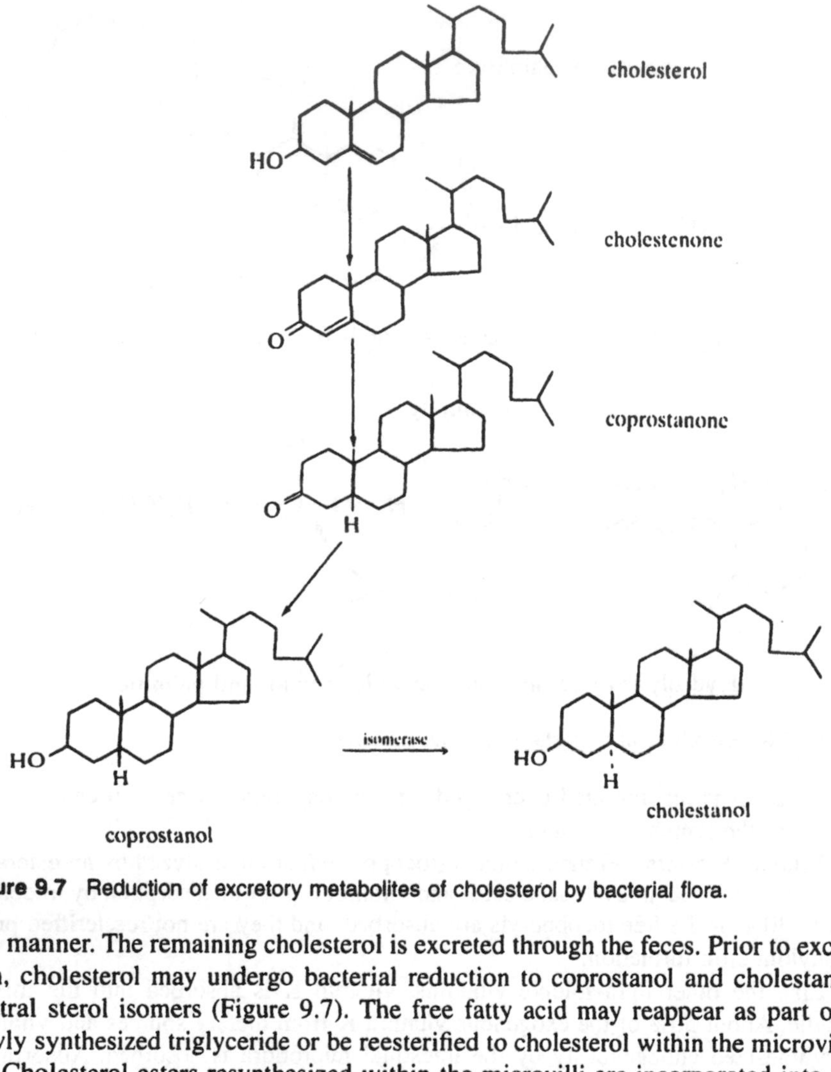

Figure 9.7 Reduction of excretory metabolites of cholesterol by bacterial flora.

this manner. The remaining cholesterol is excreted through the feces. Prior to excretion, cholesterol may undergo bacterial reduction to coprostanol and cholestanol, neutral sterol isomers (Figure 9.7). The free fatty acid may reappear as part of a newly synthesized triglyceride or be reesterified to cholesterol within the microvilli.

Cholesterol esters resynthesized within the microvilli are incorporated into the chylomicrons and VLDLs, and enter the lacteals as described previously. Chylomicrons are comprised of 2 to 7% cholesterol, and VLDLs contain 6 to 12% cholesterol. Approximately 11 g of cholesterol circulates within the lipoproteins found in blood (Table 9.2, Figure 9.8).

ABSORPTION OF THE WATER-SOLUBLE VITAMINS

The water-soluble vitamins, vitamin C and the vitamin B-complex, are efficiently absorbed by the normal gastrointestinal tract. When present in normal physiological concentrations, most B vitamins and vitamin C appear to be efficiently and predominantly absorbed by an active-transport sodium ion (Na^+)-dependent ATPase system.

Table 9.2 Composition of the Lipoproteins[a]

Lipoprotein	Sedimentation Density[b]	Diameter (nm)	Composition (%) Triglyceride	Phospholipid	Cholesterol	Protein
Chylomicron	0.95	100	80–95	7	8	1–2
Very light density (VLDL)	1.00	55	50–80	15–18	10–22	9–10
Low density (LDL)	1.05	22	7–8	18–22	46	21–25
High density (HDL)	1.18	15	2–3	30	20	45–50

[a] Values for sedimentation densities and diameters are approximate averages. Note the relationship of lipoproteins between sedimentation density and diameter; density and triglyceride content. Data compiled from various references showing ranges.

[b] H_2O = 1.0 g/cc.

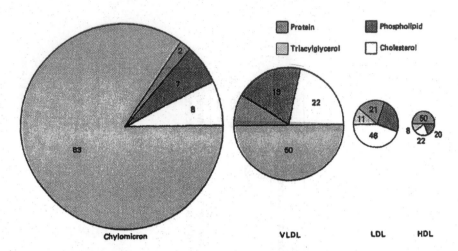

Figure 9.8 Approximate relative size and composition of the chylomicron- and liver-derived lipoproteins.

When present in excessive dietary (pharmacologic) amounts, the vitamin carrier systems appear to become saturated, and absorption is increased by passive diffusion. Under such conditions absorption efficiency is generally decreased, but total absorption of vitamins is enhanced.

Vitamin C is actively transported by an Na^+-dependent ATP system. With dietary intakes of less than 180 mg per day, about 80% of vitamin C is absorbed. When 1 g or more of vitamin C is found in the daily diet, absorption is reduced to 50%.

Thiamin, vitamin B_1, is probably absorbed at physiological concentrations via an ATP-sodium ion (Na^+) transport system. Absorbed as free thiamin, it is phosphorylated *en route* into the epithelial mucosa of the microvilli, appearing as thiamin pyrophosphate (TPP). A pyrophosphatase produces free thiamin again for entry into the hepatic portal circulation.

Riboflavin, vitamin B_2, present in FMN or FAD in the intestinal lumen, must be freed from its coenzyme by enzymatic hydrolysis prior to absorption. In the microvilli, absorbed free riboflavin is phosphorylated by ATP, forming FMN just prior to entering the hepatic portal circulation.

Niacin and NAD^+, vitamin B_6, biotin, and pantothenic acid appear to easily enter the microvilli and hepatic portal circulation system by passive diffusion. An active transport mechanism, however, could be operative for these vitamins at very low vitamin concentrations.

Folic acid absorption is by an active transport process at low luminal concentrations. Prior to absorption by the microvilli, folic acid is present in the intestinal lumen as dietary pteroylpolyglutamic acid. Folate polyglutamate (containing several glutamic acid residues in peptide linkage) must be hydrolyzed to a folate monoglutamate prior to absorption. Folic acid (5-methyl-tetrahydro-pteroylglutamate) in the reduced form (5-methyl-tetrahydro-folic acid) is released into and circulates in blood plasma.

Vitamin B_{12}, cyanocobalamin, absorption is unique among the water-soluble vitamins in that active transport requires a glycoprotein (MW 50,000) to bind vitamin

B_{12} (intrinsic factor, IF) and absorption occurs in the ileum, whereas all other vitamins are absorbed predominantly in the duodenum and jejunum. Absorption of vitamin B_{12} may occur by diffusion if luminal concentrations are high. Prior to combining with IF, vitamin B_{12} is hydrolyzed from its attachment to protein. The binding of vitamin B_{12} to IF and its demethylation renders the vitamin B_{12}-IF complex resistant to proteolytic enzymes. With the assistance of Ca^{2+}, the vitamin B_{12}-IF complex binds to ileal receptors and vitamin B_{12} enters the microvilli. Vitamin B_{12} transverses the microvilli and then enters the plasma of the hepatic portal system, where it circulates bound to specific proteins, the transcobalamins.

ABSORPTION OF MINERALS

Minerals are absorbed by either passive or active transport systems through the intestinal mucosa often using specialized transport proteins, as in the case for Fe^{3+}-ferritin and the hormonal control of Ca^{2+} absorption by vitamin D. Absorption of various metal ions is often competitive, as they compete for transport ligands (see Chapter 6, Table 6.2). Such is the case for zinc and copper, whose absorption is mediated by a primary intestinal metallothionin protein. Absorption of minerals is also affected by a variety of antagonists, ionic state, organic molecules, and fiber. For additional information on mineral absorption, the reader is referred to sections on the various minerals in Chapter 6.

Cellular Metabolism

CHAPTER 10

Body Energy

Energy is the capacity to do work. In nutrition, energy expenditure refers to the manner in which the body utilizes the energy obtained via the metabolism of the energy-yielding nutrients carbohydrates, lipids, and proteins. The body is about 40% efficient in capturing the energy from the catabolism of the energy-yielding nutrients. Food energy must be supplied regularly to individuals for their survival and is necessary for the maintenance of human life. The cells of the body do not use the energy-yielding nutrients in the diet for their immediate energy supply. Rather, adenosine triphosphate (ATP), a high-energy compound, is the fuel for energy-requiring reactions. The potential energy stored in ATP molecules provide the chemical energy for biological work. Energy released during ATP hydrolysis activates other energy-requiring molecules. ATP is the "energy currency" of the cell. Slightly over 85 grams of ATP are present in the adult body at any one time.

AEROBIC AND ANAEROBIC ENERGY RELEASE

Aerobic means oxygen-requiring, while anaerobic reactions do not require oxygen. Energy (ATP) can be released by the cell both aerobically and anaerobically. Energy produced anaerobically can be immediately utilized by the cell and is important in such activities as sprinting and surviving underwater submersion.

ENERGY RESERVOIR

Creatine phosphate, a high-energy compound, serves as an energy reservoir for the body. Anaerobic hydrolysis of creatine phosphate provides energy for the resynthesis of ATP from adenosine diphosphate (ADP) and inorganic phosphate (P_i) forming creatine plus inorganic phosphate (P_i). Both of the these reactions are reversible. The cells of our bodies, particularly those of skeletal muscles, are able to store creatine phosphate in larger quantities than ATP. All-out exercise, such as swimming or running, can be maintained for about 6 to 8 seconds utilizing the energy released from creatine phosphate and ATP. Over time, the body can be resupplied with creatine phosphate and ATP. Through appropriate physical training, individuals can slightly increase their storage capacity for creatine phosphate.

ANAEROBIC AND AEROBIC ENERGY FROM FOODS

Glucose undergoes glycolysis when it is to be used for energy formation. Glycolysis is an anaerobic pathway. Two molecules of ATP (net) are obtained via glycolysis of one molecule of glucose under anaerobic conditions. The by-products of glycolysis can be completely catabolized to CO_2 plus H_2O in subsequent aerobic reactions. The ATP produced in glycolysis provides a rapid source of energy for muscular activity that is particularly useful in short-duration, high-intensity physical activities.

Over 90% of the total ATP produced metabolically comes from the aerobic pathways within the mitochondria. The Krebs cycle (also called tricarboxylic cycle, tricarboxylic acid cycle, and citric acid cycle) and the electron transport system (also called electron transport chain and oxidative phosphorylation) take place in the mitochondria. If oxygen is not available, the pyruvic acid, produced primarily by glycolysis, is converted to lactic acid. Lactic acid may be reconverted to glucose under aerobic cellular conditions. These cellular anaerobic and aerobic pathways are discussed in more detail in Chapter 12.

CALORIES

A calorie is the amount of heat needed to raise the temperature of one gram of water 1° Celsius. Likewise, one kilocalorie is the amount of heat needed to raise the temperature of 1 kg water 1° Celsius. In nutrition, Calorie (or calorie, cal) is used to mean a kilocalorie (kcal), so calorie is really a misnomer. The joule (J) is the accepted international unit of energy. Energy measured in kcal is multiplied by 4.2 (actually 4.184) in converting kcal to kJ (kilojoules). The energy content of diets are generally given in calories or in megajoules (MJ), which is 1,000 kJ.

Calories may be measured either directly or indirectly. The calories present in foods are measured directly by the amount of heat produced when a food is completely burned in a bomb calorimeter. The heat that is released as the food is burned is called the heat of combustion. The heat of combustion values for the energy-yielding nutrients are as follows: 1 g of carbohydrate yields 4.20 cal, 1 g of protein yields 5.65 cal, and 1 g of lipid yields 9.45 cal. The body must expend energy in converting the amino groups from amino acids to urea so that amino acids can be used for energy production. Thus, the energy yield from protein is reduced to 4.35 cal/g. Typically, 97% of carbohydrates, 92% of proteins, and 95% of lipids are digested and absorbed. After digestive efficiencies have been taken into consideration, the net caloric yield values are as follows: carbohydrates, 4 cal/g; proteins, 4 cal/g; and lipids, 9 cal/g. Most foods contain varying portions of these three energy-yielding nutrients as well as water.

Caloric intakes of an individual can be estimated by adding up the calories of each food item consumed by that person. Food composition tables and computerized programs are available which list the caloric (food energy) value and selected nutrient content of various food items. These composition values are estimations at best.

BODY CALORIMETRY

Direct and indirect calorimetry are used to determine the amount of energy being expended by the body. A human calorimeter is an air-tight chamber with an oxygen supply in which an individual can live and work. The heat produced and radiated by that person can be measured. The human calorimeter is expensive and involves subjects not participating in their regular lives. Generally human energy expenditure is measured by indirect calorimetry in which oxygen utilization is measured either as oxygen consumption or carbon dioxide production or both. Approximately 4.82 kcal of heat is produced when one liter of oxygen is consumed by an individual metabolizing a mixture of carbohydrates, proteins, and lipids. A value of 5 kcal/L O_2 is used for calculations.

COMPONENTS OF ENERGY EXPENDITURE

The three components of human energy expenditure are basal metabolism, thermic effect of food (also known as specific dynamic effect, specific dynamic action, and diet-induced thermogenesis), and thermic effect of exercise (also known as physical activity). Frequently, resting metabolism is measured rather than basal metabolism. For most individuals, basal or resting metabolism constitutes the largest portion of the total energy expenditure (also known as gross energy expenditure).

BASAL AND RESTING METABOLISM

Basal metabolism is the minimum amount of energy expenditure needed to maintain the vital activities of life. The basal metabolic rate (BMR) is determined by measuring the oxygen intake of a fasting individual at physiological and psychological rest. The subject arrives at the testing site in the early morning and lies quietly in a dimly lit room (comfortable temperature and humidity) with oxygen uptake being measured after about 30 to 60 minutes. The subject is relaxed, but not asleep. The resting metabolic rate (RMR) is measured at any time of day, but at 3 to 4 hours after the last meal. BMR and RMR generally differ by less than 10% in healthy individuals. Frequently these two terms are used interchangeably.

Several factors affect basal and resting metabolism. On the average, the BMRs of women are 5 to 10% lower than those of men. In most cases, women have a larger percentage of body fat and smaller proportion of lean body (muscle) mass than men. Body surface area also affects the BMR as it is related to the amount of heat lost via evaporation from the skin. Body composition also affects the BMR as the amount of actively metabolizing tissue correlates with BMR. The BMR decreases as individuals age, perhaps because of the shift in proportion of muscle to fat. Some research suggests that exercise may help maintain a higher BMR. The quantities of thyroxine and norepinephrine in the body affect the metabolic rate. Cortisol, growth hormone, and insulin, to a lesser extent, also affect the metabolic rate. The metabolic rate decreases by about 10% during sleep as compared to when a subject is awake but reclining. Physical stresses, such as trauma, burns, and fevers increase the metabolic rate. Environmental temperature, both hot and cold, increase metabolic rate. The metabolic rate is also increased during pregnancy and lactation as well as during growth in children.

THERMIC EFFECT OF FOOD

Energy is expended during the digestion, absorption, and metabolism of nutrients. This diet-induced thermogenesis reaches a maximum within about an hour after a meal. The thermic effect of food usually accounts for 6 to 10% of the total energy expenditure. Some research indicates that exercising after eating increases a person's normal thermic response to food intake.

THERMIC EFFECT OF EXERCISE

The contribution of the thermic effect of exercise to the total energy expenditure varies greatly from individual to individual. According to several surveys, about a third of most individuals' time is spent in resting activities and the rest is spent in a wide range of physical activities. Researchers have measured the energy expended in various types of activities by individuals by indirect calorimetry. Tables have been constructed for total energy expenditure and for thermic effect of exercise for various specific or general physical activities; expenditure values are given on a body weight basis (cal/kg) or a total body basis depending on the tables utilized. Body size affects energy expenditures due to physical activity. The energy expended during weight-bearing activities increases as body mass increases. Little relationship is observed between body mass and energy expended due to exercise in non–weight-bearing activities. The level of physical fitness also affects the energy expended due to exercise with regard to voluntary activities, most likely due to increased muscle mass.

ESTIMATING ENERGY EXPENDITURE

Several tables have been developed for estimating energy expenditures. Tables suggested for use by a committee of the Food and Nutrition Board, National Research Council, National Academy of Sciences are included in this chapter. The first step in estimating total energy expenditure is to calculate the resting energy expenditure using values given in Table 10.1. Table 10.2 lists approximate energy expenditures for various activity categories as multiples of resting energy expenditure. The number of hours that one participates in each activity category should be multiplied by the activity category factor as multiples of REE (resting energy expenditure) accounting for all 24 hours of the day. An example of this calculation step is shown in Table 10.3. Then the weighted REE factors are added together and the mean weighted REE factor calculated (as shown in the example in Table 10.3). The total energy expenditure is calculated by multiplying the REE by the mean

Table 10.1 Equations for Predicting Resting Energy
Expenditure (REE) from Body Weight
(BW in kg)

Gender	Age Range (y)	Equation to Derive REE in kcal/day
Males	0–3	$(60.9 \times BW) - 54$
	3–10	$(22.7 \times BW) + 495$
	10–18	$(17.5 \times BW) + 651$
	18–30	$(15.3 \times BW) + 679$
	30–60	$(11.6 \times BW) + 879$
	60+	$(13.5 \times BW) + 487$
Females	0–3	$(61.0 \times BW) - 51$
	3–10	$(22.5 \times BW) + 499$
	10–18	$(12.2 \times BW) + 746$
	18–30	$(14.7 \times BW) + 496$
	30–60	$(8.7 \times BW) + 829$
	60+	$(10.5 \times BW) + 596$

From *Recommended Dietary Allowances.* ©1989 National
Academy of Sciences. Courtesy National Academy Press.

weighted REE factor and then multiplying the answer by 1.1 (thus accounting for
the thermic effect of food).

If details as to the number of hours a person spends doing various physical
activities are not available, then the total energy expenditure can be roughly estimated
using values given in Table 10.4. Values are given in the table for individuals having
light to moderate physical activity levels. Most Americans have light to moderate
levels of physical activity.

A committee of the Food and Nutrition Board, National Research Council,
National Academy of Sciences has recommended average energy allowances for

Table 10.2 Approximate Energy Expenditure for Various Activities in Relation to
Resting Energy Expenditure (REE)

Activity Category	Representative Value for Activity Factor per Hour
Resting	REE ×1.0
Sleeping, reclining	
Very light	REE ×1.5
Seated and standing activities, painting trades, driving, laboratory work, typing, sewing, ironing, cooking, playing cards, playing a musical instrument	
Light	REE ×2.5
Walking on a level surface at 2.5 to 3 mph, garage work, electrical trades, carpentry, restaurant trades, house-cleaning, child care, golf, sailing, table tennis	
Moderate	REE ×5.0
Walking 3.5 to 4 mph, weeding and hoeing, carrying a load, cycling, skiing, tennis, dancing	
Heavy	REE ×7.0
Walking with load uphill, tree felling, heavy manual digging, basketball, climbing, football, soccer	

From *Recommended Dietary Allowances.* ©1989 National Academy of Sciences. Courtesy National Academy Press.

Table 10.3 Example of Calculation of Estimated Daily Energy Allowances for Exceptionally Active and Inactive 23-Year-Old Adults

Step 1: Derivation of Activity Factor

Activity	Multiple of REE	Very Sedentary Day Duration (h)	Very Sedentary Day Weighted REE Factor	Very Active Day Duration (h)	Very Active Day Weighted REE Factor
Resting	1.0	10	10.0	8	8.0
Very light	1.5	12	18.0	8	12.0
Light	2.5	2	5.0	4	10.0
Moderate	5.0	0	0.0	2	10.0
Heavy	7.0	0	0.0	2	14.0
TOTAL		24	33.0	24	54.0
MEAN			1.375		2.25

Step 2: Calculation of Energy Requirement (in kcal/day)

Gender	Resting Energy Expenditure[a]	Very Sedentary Day (REE×1.375)	Very Active Day (REE×2.25)
Male, 70 kg	1.750	2,406	3,938
Female, 58 kg	1.350	1,856	3,038

[a]REE was compuited from equations given in Table 10.1.

From *Recommended Dietary Allowances.* ©1989 National Academy of Sciences. Courtesy National Academy Press.

individuals having light to moderate physical activity levels (Table 10.5). These recommended allowances should be adjusted for increased physical activity and larger or smaller body size.

Table 10.4 Factors for Estimating Daily Energy Allowances at Various Levels of Physical Activity for Men and Women (Ages 19 to 50 Years)

Level of Activity	Activity Factor (× REE)	Energy Expenditure[a] (kcal/kg BW/day)
Very light		
Men	1.3	31
Women	1.3	30
Light		
Men	1.6	38
Women	1.5	35
Moderate		
Men	1.7	41
Women	1.6	37
Heavy		
Men	2.1	50
Women	1.9	44
Exceptional		
Men	2.4	58
Women	2.2	51

[a] REE was computed from equations given in Table 10.1.

From *Recommended Dietary Allowances.* ©1989 National Academy of Sciences. Courtesy National Academy Press.

Table 10.5 Median Heights and Weights and Recommended Energy Intake

Category	Age (y) Condition	Weight (kg)	(lb)	Height (cm)	(in)	REE[a] (kcal/day)	Multiples of REE	Per kg	Per day[c]
									Average Energy Allowance (kcal)[b]
Infants	0.0–1.5	6	13	60	24	320		108	650
	0.5–1.0	9	20	71	28	500		98	850
Children	1–3	13	29	90	35	740		102	1300
	4–6	20	44	112	44	950		90	1800
	7–10	28	62	132	52	1130		70	2000
Males	11–14	45	99	157	62	1440	1.70	55	2500
	15–18	66	145	176	69	1760	1.67	45	3000
	19–24	72	160	177	70	1780	1.67	40	2900
	25–50	79	174	176	70	1800	1.60	37	2900
	51+	77	170	173	68	1530	1.50	30	2300
Females	11–14	46	101	157	62	1310	1.67	47	2200
	15–18	55	120	163	64	1370	1.60	40	2200
	19–24	58	128	164	65	1350	1.60	38	2200
	25–50	63	138	163	64	1380	1.55	36	2200
	51+	65	143	160	63	1280	1.50	30	1900
Pregnant	1st trimester								+0
	2nd trimester								+300
	3rd trimester								+300
Lactating	1st 6 months								+500
	2nd 6 months								+500

a Resting Energy Expenditure.
b In the range of light to moderate activity, the coefficient of variation is ±20%.
c Figure is rounded.

From *Recommended Dietary Allowances.* ©1989 National Academy of Sciences. Courtesy National Academy Press.

CHAPTER **11**

Components of Cells

THE MAMMALIAN CELLS

The products of animal and human digestion are required for the synthesis of new biomolecules, the replacement of excreted essential nutrients, and the energy (calories) for all cellular and organ functions. The nutrients encounter their final barrier, the cell plasma membrane, prior to entering major metabolic pathways. The variety and function of cells within the human body is extensive, with most cells highly specialized to perform specific functions. Each cell has its specific metabolic activity for its own specialized function. There is no cell that performs all metabolic processes. The human liver cell, however, performs a great many metabolic functions and contains the major metabolic pathways for the synthesis and degradation of carbohydrates, proteins, fats, and nucleic acids. The liver degrades heme and metabolizes cholesterol, synthesizing the bile acids, which become bile salts. It converts ammonia to urea and detoxifies drugs. The liver, in addition to its other specialized metabolic functions, stores nutrients such as glycogen, vitamins A and D, and iron. Better than any other cell, the liver cell typifies a general metabolic cell.

Figure 11.1 is a representation of a general mammalian metabolic cell, such as a hepatocyte, which would contain the major cellular organelles and metabolic pathways. Each cell is surrounded by a plasma membrane, the final barrier to the nutrients prior to their metabolism. The plasma membrane is a lipid bilayer with the inclusion of proteins and enzymes. Proteins, carbohydrates, and metals comprise and serve as membrane receptors for hormones, nutrients, and metabolites. Like the plasma membrane of the microvilli of the small intestine, nutrients and metabolites move into and out of metabolic cells by passive and facilitative diffusion or an active transport system requiring ATP. In maintaining electrical neutrality, ions, particularly Na^+, K^+, and Cl^-, are moved in and out of the cell, sometimes with an expenditure of energy from ATP. Organelles, components of the cell that comprise the microanat-

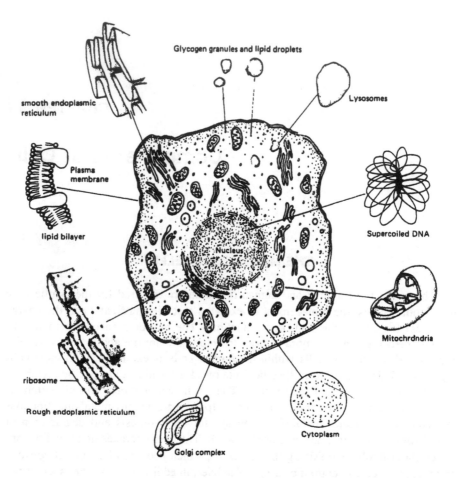

Figure 11.1 Microanatomy of a typical mammalian cell. (Adapted from *Biochemistry*, 2nd ed.,
A. L. Lehninger, Worth Publishers, Inc., 1975. Reprinted with permission.)

omy, carry out the specialized functions within the cell. All of the organelles bathe
in the fluid portion of the cell, the cytoplasm. Contained in the cytoplasm are the
aqueous nutrients, ions, and enzymes of glycolysis and the gluconeogenic pathway,
the hexosemonophosphate (HMP) shunt, and the enzymes for the synthesis of fatty
acids from acetyl-CoA. The enzymes of the citric acid cycle, β-oxidation, fatty acid
elongation, and the electron transport system are located within the mitochondrion.
It is within mitochondria that most ATP is synthesized. Mitochondria are abundant
and metabolically active in cells requiring ATP and are few in number in metabolically less active cells.

Both the smooth and rough endoplasmic reticula of cells are metabolically active.
Within the channels of the smooth endoplasmic reticulum are synthesized lipids:
cholesterol and steroids. The rough endoplasmic reticulum is recognizable by the
presence of ribosomes. Here in the ribosomes are assembled the proteins from amino
acids. The Golgi complex of the cell appears to "package" enzymes and zymogens
for secretion and is highly concentrated in specialized secretory cells. The Golgi

inclusions are often associated with the rough endoplasmic reticulum "packaging" and modify proteins by the addition of lipids (lipoproteins) and carbohydrates (glycoproteins) prior to secretion. In addition, the Golgi apparatus may assist in the synthesis and formation of new plasma membrane.

Some cells may contain lysosomes. Lysosomes contain lysozyme and other degradative enzymes. The function of lysosomes is the digestion of foreign debris that may be engulfed by the cell during phagocytosis. Lysosomes have been called "suicide sacs," for upon cell death (i.e., apoptosis), lysosomal enzymes are released and autodegradation of cell material ensues.

Governing the totality of cellular activity is the cell's nucleus. Isolated from the cytoplasm by its nuclear membrane, the nucleus contains all the genetic material, deoxyribonucleic acid (DNA), except for a small amount of DNA found in mitochondria. Within the nucleus, replication and transcription take place. Replication of DNA takes place during cell division, and transcription yields ribonucleic acids (RNA) for protein synthesis. Also located within the cytoplasm are storage depots of energy which are mobilized as required. Glycogen granules and droplets of lipids, triglycerides, are present in highly active mammalian metabolic cells.

PLANT CELLS

There also exists no one typical plant cell, yet there is less diversity and specialization of cell function within plants than within the cells and organs of the animal kingdom. Plants generally possess much of the same metabolism that many animal cells perform and do so with an architectural array of similar organelles. Figure 11.2 is representative of a typical plant cell from a soybean leaf. The plant cell contains organelles similar to the mammalian cell, including cytoplasm, mitochondrion, rough endoplasmic reticulum, Golgi complex, and nucleus. The plant cell may also contain inclusions of lipid droplets and carbohydrate (starch) granules. The plant cell is not equivalent to any mammalian cell and differs by synthesizing specialized pigments, plant hormones, metabolites, and macromolecules.

Structurally, the plant cell is different from mammalian cells in possessing a rigid cell wall, glyoxysomes, vacuoles, and chloroplasts. The plant's cell wall is rigid, to withstand the hydrostatic pressures of turgor. Much of the plant's cell wall is comprised of cellulose, the most abundant biomolecule. Much of the remaining structural content of the mature plant cell wall is lignin, a major component of wood. Pectins, methylated polymers of glucuronic acid and galacturonic acid, and hemicelluloses, polymers of arabinose, galactose, mannose, and xylose, comprise the cell walls. These components of the cell wall, it may be recalled, constitute dietary fiber (see Chapter 2).

The glyoxysome is a plant organelle not found in mammalian cells. When found in plant cells, the glyoxysome contains the enzymes of the glyoxylate cycle, which converts fatty acids into acetate and oxaloacetate by β-oxidation. Oxaloacetate is then converted to phosphoenolpyruvate, which leads to glucose (gluconeogenesis).

The predominant feature of plant cells that sets them apart from mammalian cells is the presence of cellular chloroplasts, the synthesis of photoreceptive pig-

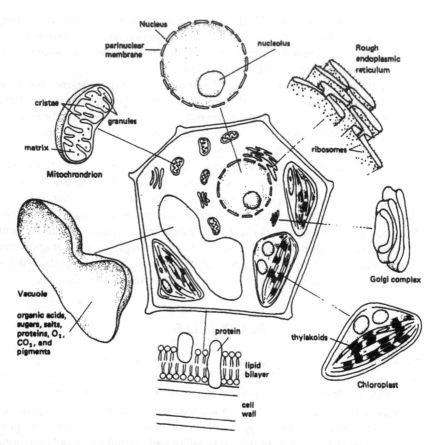

Figure 11.2 Microanatomy of a typical plant cell. (Adapted from *Biochemistry,* 2nd ed., A. L. Lehninger, Worth Publishers, Inc., 1975. Reprinted with permission.)

ments, and direct utilization of light energy for the synthesis of ATP. The chloroplast is an assembly of photoreceptive stacks, or grana, composed of thylakoid discs. The stacked thylakoids contain chlorophyll, the primary photoreceptive pigment, secondary photoreceptive pigments, and the components and enzymes of cyclic phosphorylation. Acyclic phosphorylation is thought to be located on the lamellae between thylakoids. The chloroplasts of algae and plants and the mitochondria of plants, animals, and humans are functionally alike in their synthesis of ATP, and function differently only with respect to their source of energy for phosphorylation of ADP.

ANIMAL AND PLANT METABOLISM

The sum of all chemical events within a living animal or plant cell is what is referred to as metabolism. Cellular metabolism has the purpose of maintaining the homeostasis of the cell within a population of other cells. Metabolism occurs in a freely open system with an active exchange of energy, essential nutrients, metabolites, and metabolic waste materials between the cell and its environment.

Metabolism can generally be subdivided into anabolic and catabolic metabolism. Anabolic metabolism, anabolism, is the building up of macromolecules, e.g., protein synthesis from amino acids. Anabolic metabolism generally requires an expenditure of energy (ATP), which results in increased cellular organization and a decline in internal entropy (S). Catabolic metabolism, catabolism, is the degradation of large and small biomolecules, e.g., proteins to amino acids. Catabolic metabolism generally results in the cellular synthesis of ATP and an increase in the entropy (S) of the molecules that are undergoing catabolism.

Anabolic and catabolic metabolic pathways are generally determined by their biosynthetic or degradative activity and whether ATP is consumed or generated in the process. As a general condition, anabolic processes require energy (ATP) and catabolic processes yield energy (ATP). The names of the major anabolic and catabolic metabolic pathways and the relationships between oxidation, reduction, energy utilization, and entropy is shown in Table 11.1.

Anabolic pathways generally consume ATP and contribute to a decreased net cellular entropy at the expense of an increase in environmental (external) entropy, and such chemical processes utilize and consume $NADPH + H^+$. Anabolic pathways are generally pathways of reduction. Quantitatively, the largest reductive pathway is the reduction of carbon dioxide by the Calvin cycle in photosynthesis. For plants, ATP synthesis can be considered anabolic, for the energy for most of plant ATP synthesis originates with the solar energy falling on plant leaves.

Catabolic pathways in both plants and animals yield a net synthesis of ATP at the expense of an increase in the internal cellular entropy and in total environmental entropy. Major catabolic pathways produce $NADH + H^+$, $FADH_2$, or $FMNH_2$ from the oxidation of substrates, generally carbohydrates and amino and fatty acids. For the biological world as a whole, the overall process of photosynthesis is shown in Equation 11.1. Photosynthesis may be viewed as the major anabolic process whereby CO_2 is reduced by $NADPH + H^+$ to form carbohydrates, to be followed by the synthesis of proteins and lipids. This process is carried out only by phototrophs and is accomplished extensively by algae, plankton, and higher plants.

Animals and humans, the chemotrophs, utilize the energy stored in plants — carbohydrates, proteins, and lipids — by oxidizing these organic compounds, with the concurrent release of energy, which is partially conserved and transferred to ATP. The oxidation of carbohydrates, proteins, and lipids in Equation 11.2 is a summation of the respiratory process of either plants, animals, or humans. Respiration and oxidative phosphorylation is the metabolic opposite of photosynthesis and reduction of CO_2 by plants. The only thermodynamic difference between photosynthesis and respiration is the liberation of heat in Equation 11.2. Heat is liberated because respiration and oxidative phosphorylation is not 100% efficient in converting food energy into ATP energy. As previously noted in Chapter 10, humans are about 40% efficient in our conservation of food energy in metabolically synthesizing ATP. The summation of energy on both sides of Equations 11.1 and 11.2 is, however, equal. The metabolic and energy relationships between phototrophs (plants) and organic chemotrophs (humans) are shown in Figure 11.3.

Table 11.1 Major Metabolic Pathways of Plants and Animals and their Relationship to Energy, Entropy, and Reductive Capacity

Pathway	ATP	S (internal) cell	S (environment)[a]	NADPH + H[-b]	NADP + H[+], FADH2 FMNH2[b]
Anabolic					
Glycogenesis	Consumed[c]	–	+	Used	
Gluconeogenesis	Consumed[c]	–	+	Used	
Fatty acid synthesis	Consumed[c]	–	+	Used	
Protein biosynthesis	Consumed[c]	–	+	Used	
Sterol biosynthesis	Consumed[c]	–	+	Used	
Cyclic phosphorylation	Generated[c,d]	–	+	Produced	
Noncyclic phosphorylation	Generated[c,d]	–	+	Produced	
Calvin cycle	Consumed[c]	–	+	Used	
Catabolic					
Glycogenolysis	Generated[e]	+	+		Produced
Glycolysis	Generated[e]	+	+		Produced
β-Oxidation	Generated[e]	+	+		Produced
Oxidation deaminations	Generated[e]	+	+		Produced
Citric acid cycle	Generated[e]	+	+		Produced
Electron transport	Generated[e]	+	+		Produced

a NADPH + H[+] → NADP[+].
b NAD[+] + 2H → NADH + H[+]; FAD + 2H → FADH$_2$; FMN + 2H → FMHN$_2$.
c ATP → ADP + P$_i$.
d Cyclic and noncyclic phosphorylation is anabolic at the expense of solar energy and increased solar entropy.
e ADP + P$_i$ → ATP.

$$6CO_2 + 6H_2O + (N) + \text{solar energy (hv)} + ATP \rightarrow$$

$$C_6H_{12}O_6 \text{ (proteins (N); lipids)} + 6O_2 \uparrow + ADP + P_i$$

Equation 11.1   General photosynthesis/energy equation.

$$C_6H_{12}O_6 \text{ (proteins; lipids)} + O_2 + ADP + P_i \rightarrow$$

$$6CO_2 + 6H_2O + (N) + ADP + \text{heat}$$

Equation 11.2   General oxidation/energy equation.

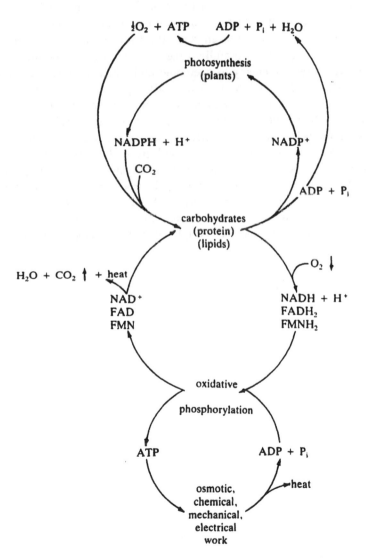

Figure 11.3   Interrelationship of photosynthesis with animal/human respiration.

METABOLIC MAPS

Highway maps produced by cartographers are necessary when driving into unfamiliar country. National maps show the federal interstate highway system and its interchanges at major cities, and state highway maps reveal only a state's portion of the interstate highway system. You do see on state highway maps, detail of primary and secondary state roads, and additionally, smaller cities and towns are located on these maps. Maps of cities, both large and small, provide detailed information on local travel and often provide the names of individual streets. Metabolic charts, which are found on office walls in nutrition and biochemistry departments, are cellular road maps. They show us where metabolic trips begin and end. They take us through both the major and less important metabolic cities. They show metabolic crossroads and side trips to be taken, and major routes may have to be examined carefully to be navigated successfully. Like real highways, some metabolic roads have hills which require energy to overcome and which we can coast down later. Some metabolic roads even have two-way traffic, properly separated, of course.

In the following chapters, we hope you will view the metabolic pathways as highway maps. Major cities on our map are glucose, triglyceride, ribulose-5-phosphate, the amino acid cities (i.e., valine, tyrosine, lysine, etc.), α-ketoglutarate, cholesterol, oxaloacetate, the tri-city ketones, and glycerol, among others. These metabolic cities are found on the major metabolic highways: glycolysis, β-oxidation, Calvin and citric acid cycles, sterol synthesis, electron transport, and so on. Metabolic road highways are serviced by ATP, $NAD^+/NADH_2$, $NADP^+/NADPH_2$, vitamins B_6 and B_{12}, and so on. Major interchanges are to be also found, and none is more important on our metabolic map than acetyl coenzyme A. Happy metabolic motoring!

Energy Utilization

CHAPTER 12

Catabolic Pathways

Energy stored by plants by the reduction of CO_2 in the Calvin cycle is transferred to animals and humans as carbohydrates, lipids, and proteins. Carbohydrates in the typical American diet contribute 51% of the total dietary calories consumed; lipids, typically fats and oils, contribute 34% of total calories; and protein contributes the remaining 15% of calories consumed. In our "Western" American diet, much of the carbohydrate is refined sugars, lipids are animal fats and refined vegetable oils, and protein is usually of high quality, derived principally from animal sources. Throughout much of the world, human diets are much different from the Western diet. In the diets of people from the developing countries, most calories are supplied by naturally occurring sugars and complex carbohydrates. Calories supplied by animal fat and refined oils are greatly reduced. Calories from protein are lessened and the quality of the protein consumed is often much lower.

It makes little difference, calorically speaking, whether dietary energy is obtained from high- or low-carbohydrate diets, from plant oils or animal fats, from high- or low-quality proteins. The need for energy is constant for all living beings, and most people require 1200 to 4000 calories per day, which varies from person to person depending primarily on age and level of physical activity. This chapter examines the major catabolic pathways, with a primary focus on the conversion of food energy into ATP and the synthesis of NADH + H$^+$. The major anabolic pathways are then examined from the viewpoint of NADPH + H$^+$, ATP utilization, and ATP's ability to both receive and transfer energy. We also examine why lipids possess a greater number of calories on an anhydrous basis than do either carbohydrates or proteins. Such insight should prove valuable in understanding the caloric density of foods.

CATABOLIC PATHWAYS OF CARBOHYDRATES

Glycolysis

For many animals, especially the herbivores and many people in developing countries, carbohydrates supply the majority of caloric needs. Glucose, the end

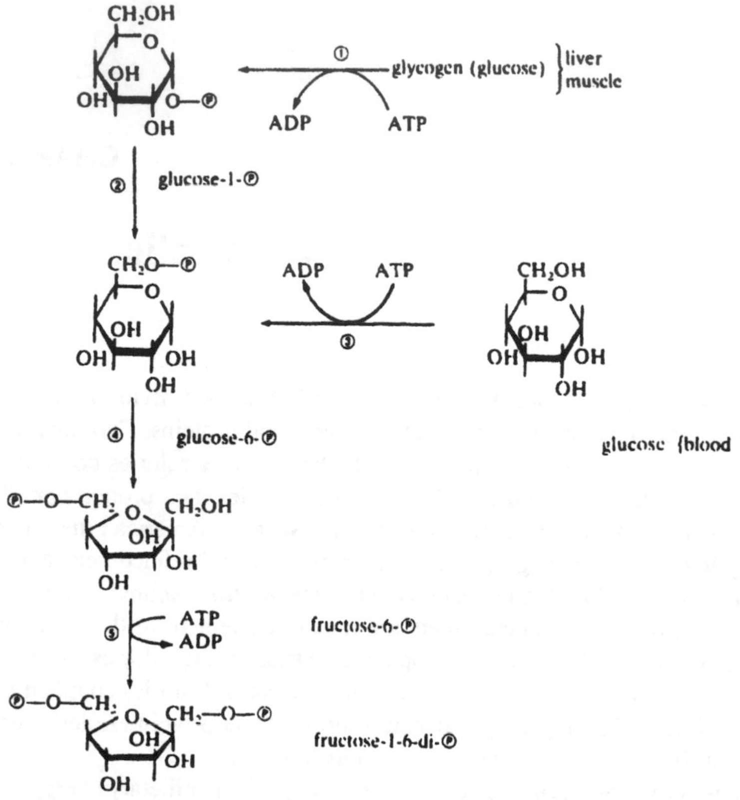

Figure 12.1 Glycolytic pathway. 1. Phosphorylase b 2. Phosphoglucomutase 3. Glucokinase 4. Phosphoglucoisomerase 5. Phosphofructokinase 6. Aldolase 7. Glyceraldehyde-3-phosphodehydrogenase 8. Phosphoglycerolkinase 9. Phosphoglycerolmutase 10. Enolase 11. Pyruvate kinase 12. Pyruvate decarboxylase.

product of cellulose digestion in some animals and starch digestion in humans, is stored in muscle (particularly skeletal muscle), heart, or liver as the polysaccharide glycogen. Glycogen is a ready store of energy and it or glucose can be rapidly degraded to either pyruvate or lactate by the enzymes of the cytoplasm with the concomitant synthesis of ATP. The glycolytic or Embden–Meyerhof pathway is shown in Figure 12.1. Glycolysis occurs *in vivo* under either aerobic or anaerobic conditions. Aerobic glycolysis, beginning with the phosphorylation of glucose by ATP, activates glucose as either glucose-1-℗ (from glycogen) or glucose-6-℗ (from blood). This six-carbon molecule is isomerized and phosphorylated with a second molecule of ATP to form fructose 1,6-di-℗. This hexose is then divided into two three-carbon molecules — dihydroxyacetone-℗ and glyceraldehyde-3-℗ — by an aldolase. Both three-carbon molecules transverse the remaining intermediate steps of glycolysis (one step of which requires niacin as NAD), being transformed into pyruvic acid. Conversion of 1,3-diphosphoglycerate to 3-phosphoglycerate and phosphoenolpyruvate to pyruvate (one-half of the glucose) yields one molecule each of ATP. These steps are repeated again for the remaining one-half of the original glucose

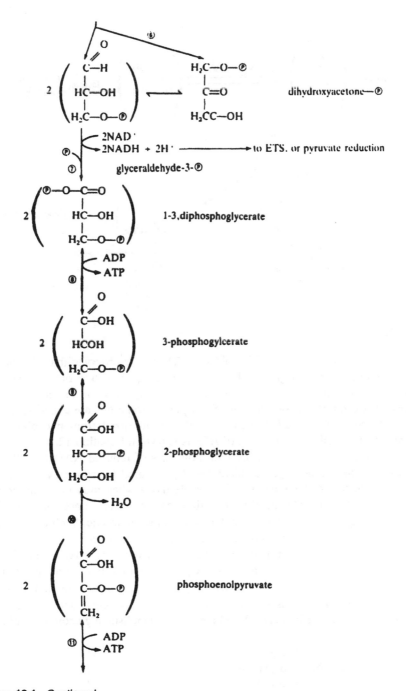

Figure 12.1 *Continued.*

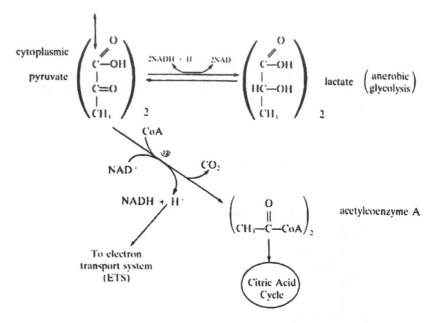

Figure 12.1 *Continued.*

molecule, yielding two more ATP molecules. Thus, it is observed that phosphorylation of one molecule of glucose by ATP, forming glucose 6-℗ or glucose-1-℗,
results in a net yield of two ATP molecules during glycolysis in the conversion of
glucose to two molecules of pyruvate. Such phosphorylations are called substrate-
level phosphorylations (SLPs) because ATP is synthesized from phosphorylated
metabolites and ADP. The net yield of ATP is shown in Equation 12.1.

Under anaerobic conditions, the two molecules of reduced NADH + H⁺ (produced by the oxidation of glyceraldehyde-3-℗) are used to reduce two molecules
of pyruvate to lactate. This happens in muscle tissue when muscular contractions
are rapid under persistent anaerobic conditions and pyruvate cannot enter the citric
acid cycle (Figure 12.2) because of a deficiency of oxaloacetate. Such events cause
lactic acid to accumulate and produce a respiratory oxygen debt.

With purely aerobic conditions, pyruvate is oxidatively decarboxylated and transformed into acetyl-coenzyme A (acetyl-CoA), the most important metabolic intermediate common to the catabolism of carbohydrates, fatty acids, and amino acids.
Acetyl-coenzyme A condenses with oxaloacetate, forming citric acid in the initial
metabolic step of the citric acid cycle, whereby the catabolism of glucose is continued.

1.	Phosphorylation of glucose	= −1 ATP
2.	Phosphorylation of fructose-6-℗	= −1 ATP
3.	1,3-Diphosphoglycerate × 2 (SLP)	= +2 ATP
4.	Phosphoenolpyruvate × 2 (SLP)	= +2 STP
	Net yield of ATP from SLP	= +2 ATP

Equation 12.1 Net yield of ATP by substrate-level phosphorylation in glycolysis.

The Citric Acid Cycle

From glycolysis, two molecules of pyruvate are decarboxylated and are condensed with coenzyme A, forming two molecules of acetyl coenzyme A. Thiamin (as thiamin pyrophosphate), lipoic acid, niacin (as NAD), and pantothenic acid (as a component of coenzyme A) function in the conversion of pyruvate to acetyl-coenzyme A as well as later in the cycle in the conversion of α-ketoglutarate to succinyl-coenzyme A. In this reaction the carboxylic moiety of pyruvate is lost as respiratory CO_2 and the remaining acetyl, a two-carbon unit, is metabolized through the citric acid cycle.

The citric acid cycle (CAC), or tricarboxylic acid cycle (TCA), is also known as the Krebs cycle, bearing the name of Sir Hans Krebs, who elucidated the details of this metabolic pathway within the mitochondria. For this remarkable accomplishment, Krebs received the Nobel Prize in Medicine in 1953.

Acetyl-coenzyme A (acetyl-CoA), in the first reaction of the CAC, condenses with oxaloacetate, a four-carbon dicarboxylic acid, forming the six-carbon tricarboxylic acid, citric acid (Equation 12.2). The complete CAC is shown in Figure 12.2. The six carbon atoms of citric acid then pass through a series of CAC metabolic intermediates. Four of citric acid's six carbons are retained throughout the CAC and reappear as oxaloacetate, completing one turn of the cycle. The two carbon atoms unaccounted for are lost in thiamin-mediated oxidative decarboxylations of the CAC intermediates, oxalosuccinate and α-ketoglutarate. During each turn of the CAC, one ATP equivalent is made in a substrate-level phosphorylation (SLP) of GDP $\rightarrow$ GTP, guanosine diphosphate to guanosine triphosphate. While glycolysis yields four equivalent ATPs from substrate-level phosphorylations of glucose metabolites, the CAC yields only two equivalent ATPs through the synthesis of GTP. The net reactions of one turn of the CAC can be summarized as in Equation 12.3.

Two turns of the CAC are necessary to fully oxidize the equivalent of one molecule of glucose (6C). The equivalent of these six carbon atoms are lost as CO_2; two are lost in the oxidative decarboxylations of pyruvate and its conversion to acetyl-CoA, and four are lost in the oxidative decarboxylations during two turns of the CAC.

Oxidation of one molecule of glucose has now been followed through glycolysis and the CAC. Six molecules of CO_2, equivalent to all the carbon atoms of one glucose molecule, have been lost along with the oxygen atoms of glucose. What remains metabolically unaccounted for in the glucose molecule ($C_6H_{12}O_6$) are the atoms of hydrogen. These hydrogen atoms in glucose were used to reduce NAD^+ (containing niacin) and FAD (containing riboflavin) to $NADH + H^+$ and $FADH_2$,

$$CH_3-\underset{\substack{\| \\ O}}{C}-CoA \; + \; \underset{\substack{| \quad | \\ COOH \; COOH}}{H_2C-\underset{\| }{C}} \quad \xrightarrow{\;CoASH\;} \quad H_2C-\underset{\substack{| \quad | \quad | \\ COOH \; COOH \; COOH}}{\underset{OH}{\underset{|}{C}}}-CH_2$$

Equation 12.2 Condensation reaction of acetyl-CoA and oxaloacetate.

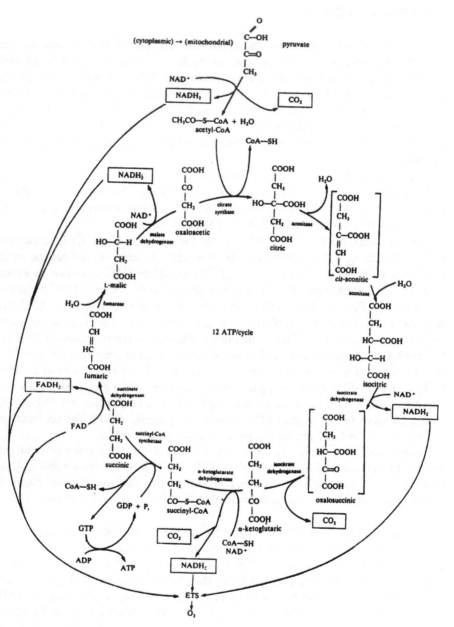

Figure 12.2 Citric acid cycle.

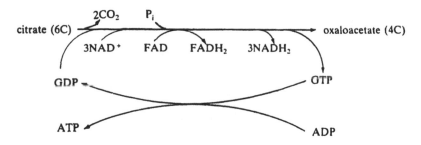

Equation 12.3 Chemical summary of the citric acid cycle.

forming reduced niacinamide and flavin coenzymes. These reduced coenzymes are then oxidized in the mitochondrial electron transport system. The electron transport system (ETS) is also known as the electron transport chain (ETC). The ETS is the fixed common pathway for the oxidation of reduced coenzymes formed in the catabolic pathways of carbohydrates, fatty acid, and amino acid degradation. The ETS provides the majority of newly synthesized cellular ATP by the oxidative phosphorylation of ADP.

The Electron Transport System and Oxidative Phosphorylation

The ETS is found, along with the CAC, within the mitochondria. The ETS is composed of a sequential series of enzymes and membrane-bound proteins, the cytochromes, arranged for the enzymatic coupling of P_i to ADP, forming ATP, and for the reduction of oxygen, forming metabolic water. The ETS, the formation of ATP and metabolic water, is shown in Figure 12.3.

In the first reaction of the ETS, $NADH_2$ formed from the oxidation of glucose, fatty acids, and CAC metabolites is oxidized by FAD, forming $FADH_2$ with the concurrent synthesis of one ATP molecule from ADP and P_i. $FADH_2$ is then oxidized by coenzyme Q (CoQ), also known as ubiquinone. $CoQ \cdot H_2$ gives up two protons ($2H^+$) to the mitochondrial matrix and transfers two electrons ($2e^-$) from the two hydrogen atoms to oxidized cytochrome b (Fe^{3+}). Vitamin C and copper function in conjunction with iron in the ETS. The two electrons, one at a time, are sequentially passed along to each oxidized Fe^{3+} form of the succeeding cytochrome. The final acceptor of the pair of elections is oxygen ($\frac{1}{2} O_2$). Oxygen (O^{2-}) returns the pair of electrons to the two protons discharged from coenzyme Q in combining to form a molecule of water. It is this water that is called metabolic water, for it is formed as a result of metabolism.

In the cascade of the pair of electrons from the discharge of the two protons by coenzyme Q through the sequential array of cytochromes, two molecules of ATP are synthesized from $2ADP + 2P_i$. ATP is synthesized, resulting from the coupling of cytochromes b and c_1 and cytochromes a and a_3 (cytochrome series) with oxygen. From $NADH_2$, arising from the catabolic pathways, hydrogen and electrons flow through the ETS, with the resulting synthesis of ATP. Each $NADH_2$ gives rise to the synthesis of three ATPs in the ETS by oxidative phosphorylation, sometimes referred to as a P/O ratio equal to 3 (ATP formed/oxygen consumed). While $NADH_2$ produces

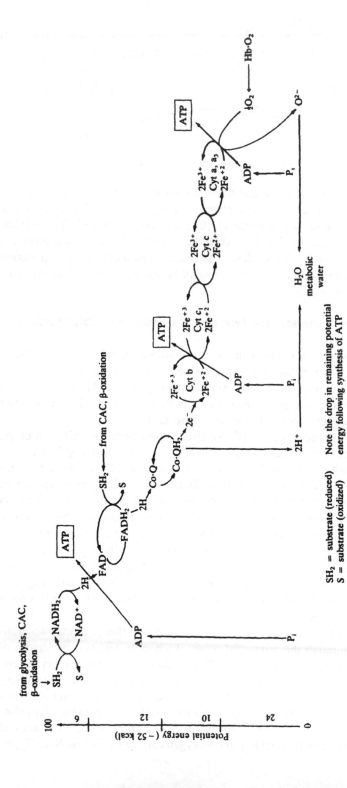

Figure 12.3 Electron transport system and oxidative phosphorylation.

$$NADH_2 + 3ADP + 3P_i + {}^1\!/_2O_2 \rightarrow$$
$$NAD^+ + 3ATP + H_2O \qquad P/O = 3$$

$$FADH_2/FMNH_2 + 2ADP + 2P_i + {}^1\!/_2O_2 \rightarrow$$
$$FAD/FMN + 2ATP + H_2O \qquad P/O = 2$$

Equation 12.4

P/O ratios of 3, $FADH_2$ produces a P/O ratio equal to 2. Why this happens can be seen in Figure 12.3. $FADH_2/FMNH_2$ derived from the β-oxidation of fatty acids, CAC intermediate succinate, or other metabolic oxidations bypasses the synthesis of the first ATP in the ETS, and therefore yields only two ATPs synthesized by the enzymes of cytochromes b and c_1, a and a_3. The net reactions of the ETS from $NADH_2$ and $FADH_2/FMNH_2$ can thus be summarized as in Equation 12.4.

Close examination of glycolysis and the CAC reveals that the metabolism of glucose yields a considerable amount of collective reduced coenzymes, $NADH_2$ and $FADH_2$, which are oxidized by the ETS, producing ATP. From a single molecule of glucose it is possible to ascertain the number of ATPs theoretically synthesized. This summary for the synthesis of ATP from glucose is given in Table 12.1. An examination of the source of ATP from the complete oxidation of glucose reveals that most of the net yield of the 38 ATPs arises from the $NADH_2$ and $FADH_2$ formed by the oxidation of CAC intermediates and the single SLP initiated by succinyl-CoA. Fully 24, or 63%, of the net ATPs synthesized from the oxidation of glucose is from the metabolic operations of the CAC. When reduced coenzymes are included from the oxidation of pyruvate to acetyl-CoA, 79% of the ATP is formed from this reaction and the CAC. Under aerobic conditions, glycolysis accounts for just 21% of the ATP formed from the oxidation of reduced coenzymes produced in this pathway.

Thermodynamics of ATP and ATP Synthesis

We have examined how and where ATP is synthesized in the mitochondria of plants, bacteria, animals, and humans by oxidative phosphorylation. Let us turn our

Table 12.1 Sequential Summary of ATP Synthesis from the Catabolism of Glucose

1. Phosphorylation of glucose: from glycogen −1 ATP or from glucose −2 ATP	−1 ATP
2. Phosphorylation of fructose-6- Ⓟ	−1 ATP
3. Oxidation of 2 glutaraldehyde-3-Ⓟ by 2NAD⁺ (NADH₂)	+6 ATP by ETS
4. Phosphorylation by 2 1,3-diphosphoglycerates	+2 ATP by SLP
5. Phosphorylation by 2 phosphoenopyruvates	+2 ATP by SLP
6. Oxidation of 2 pyruvates by 2NAD⁺ (NADH₂)	+6 ATP by ETS
7. Oxidation of 2 isocitrates by 2NAD⁺ (NADH₂)	+6 ATP by ETS
8. Oxidation of 2 α-ketoglutarates by 2NAD⁺ (NADH₂)	+6 ATP by ETS
9. Phosphorylation of 2GDP by succinyl-CoA (2ATP equivalents)	+2 ATP by SLP
10. Oxidation of 2 succinates by 2FAD (FADH₂)	+4 ATP by ETS
11. Oxidation of 2 malates by 2NAD⁺ (NADH₂)	+6 ATP by ETS
Net ATPs from glycolysis and CAC via ETS	+38 ATP

$$ATP \xrightarrow{\text{Mg}^{2+}\text{--ATPase}} ADP + P_i + (-7.3 \text{ kcal/mol})$$

Equation 12.5 Hydrolysis of ATP.

attention now to the thermodynamics; the energy considerations of ATP synthesis and the metabolic transfer of energy within cells.

In Appendix A the laws of thermodynamics and the relationships between energy, work, and ATP are described. A brief explanation of how energy is "stored" by the ATP molecule is also given. Recapitulating, the amount of energy stored in ATP is equal to a free-energy yield of $\Delta G^{\circ\prime} = -7.3$ kcal/mol under standard conditions. The negative sign signifies that the energy that is "stored" in ATP is released upon hydrolysis as in Equation 12.5.

The reaction in Equation 12.5 can be diagrammed showing the approximate energy content of the reactant (ATP) and products (ADP + P_i) (Figure 12.4). In order to store the −7.3 kcal/mol of hydrolysis in ATP, the drop in potential energy across the point of ATP synthesis (ADP + P_i → ATP) in the mitochondria in the ETS must be greater than −7.3 kcal/mol. In the ETS, the potential drop in energy across all the electron carriers from $NADH_2$ to O_2 is approximately 52 kcal per electron pair. Figure 12.4 demonstrates that approximately 12 kcal of potential energy is used in the synthesis of the first ATP, 10 kcal is used in the synthesis of the second ATP, and 24 kcal is expended in the synthesis of the third and final ATP. The total amount of energy stored by oxidative phosphorylation of ADP per $NADH_2$ is 21.9 kcal. From this value an estimate of overall thermodynamic efficiency can be calculated for a P/O ratio of 3. This efficiency is 21.9 kcal/52 kcal × 100, or about 42%. The ETS is therefore 42% efficient in conserving total potential electron energy as ATP.

Why, one may ask, is ATP synthesized and so important as a carrier of free energy? ATP is an unusual carrier of free energy for anabolic reactions, for its $\Delta G^{\circ\prime}$

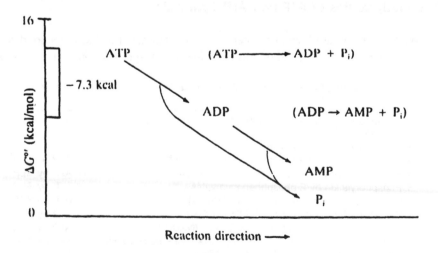

Figure 12.4 Free energy of hydrolysis of ATP and ADP.

Table 12.2 Free Energy of Hydrolysis of Energy-Containing Compounds

Name	$\Delta G^{\circ\prime}$	Direction of Phosphate or Energy Transfer
Phosphoenolpyruvate	−14.8	
α-Glycerol phosphate	−11.8	
Creatine phosphate	−10.3	
Acetylphosphate	−10.1	
ATP (→ AMP + PP$_i$)	−8.6	
Acetyl-CoA	−8.2	
ATP (→ ADP + P$_i$)	−7.3	
Aminoacetyl AMP	−7.0	
PPi (2P$_i$)	−6.7	
Glucose-1-phosphate	−5.0	
Fructose-6-phosphate	−3.8	
Glucose-6-phosphate	−3.3	
3-Phosphoglycerate	−3.1	
Glycerol-1-phosphate	−2.2	

of hydrolysis is of intermediate value among a variety of energetically active compounds. Table 12.2 provides a list of energy-containing compounds ranging from $\Delta G^{\circ\prime} = -14.8$ kcal/mol to −2.2 kcal/mol. The free energy of hydrolysis for the reaction ATP → ADP + P$_i$ (−7.3 kcal/mol) is intermediate among these compounds. Compounds with $\Delta G^{\circ\prime}$ less than ATP can be phosphorylated by ATP as in Equation 12.6. In this equation ATP transferred −5.0 kcal/mol of its −7.3 kcal/mol to glucose. This reaction energy transfer is 68% efficient. It may be recalled from glycolysis that conversion of phosphoenolpyruvate to pyruvate is a substrate-level phosphorylation (SLP) which yields ATP (Equation 12.7). In this reaction phosphoenolpyruvate has a $\Delta G^{\circ\prime}$ of −14.8 kcal/mol and transfers its phosphate to ADP, yielding ATP with a $\Delta G^{\circ\prime}$ of −7.3 kcal/mol. This phosphate transfer shows how ATP is formed only by molecules with a higher $\Delta G^{\circ\prime}$ of hydrolysis than that of ATP. This reaction energy transfer is about 50% efficient.

Creatine phosphate ($\Delta G^{\circ\prime} = -10.3$ kcal/mol) is a high-energy compound found in muscle used in the phosphorylation of ADP for muscular contraction (Equation 12.8). This equation is thermodynamically permissible. During muscular rest, creatine is phosphorylated by ATP, forming creatine phosphate, which seemingly is thermodynamically impossible. This reaction occurs, however, by expending the energy of two molecules of ATP (Equation 12.9). In this equation, the $\Delta G^{\circ\prime}$ of creatine phosphate is restored in a reaction energy transfer that is 70% efficient. These examples of energy transfer from 2 ATPs between molecules which have both

$$\text{ATP + glucose} \rightarrow \text{ADP + glucose-1-®}$$

Equation 12.6   Phosphorylation of glucose by ADP.

$$\text{phosphoenolpyruvate (PEP) + ADP} \rightarrow \text{ATP + pyruvate}$$

Equation 12.7   Phosphorylation of ADP by phosphoenolpyruvate.

$$\text{creatine phosphate} + \text{ADP} \rightarrow \text{ATP} + \text{creatine}$$

Equation 12.8   Phosphorylation of ADP by creatine phosphate.

$$\text{creatine} + 2\text{ATP} \rightarrow \text{creatine phosphate} + 2\text{ADP} + P_i$$

Equation 12.9   Phosphorylation of creatine by ATP.

greater and lesser $\Delta G^{o\prime}$ than ATP should serve to emphasize why coupling energies for the synthesis of ATP in oxidation phosphorylation (plants, animals, and humans) must be larger than +7.3 kcal/mol to form ATP.

CATABOLIC PATHWAYS OF LIPIDS

Lipids, triglycerides principally, provide about 34% of American dietary requirements for calories. Lipids as adipose tissue are also the major store of body energy and possess more than twice the caloric density (9 kcal/g) of carbohydrates or protein (4 kcal/g). In this section we examine the oxidation of triglycerides.

Triglycerides, in comparison to equal anhydrous weights of carbohydrate and protein, contain more calories because they have a higher proportion of total hydrocarbons. Body stores of triglycerides are mobilized in response to low blood glucose and insulin levels by the release of free fatty acids (FFAs) from triglycerides into the blood stream. Bound to serum albumin, FFAs are taken up by the cell's cytoplasm. These cytosolic FFAs undergo an enzymatic activation by ATP and are transferred to carnitine, which acts as a mitochondrial membrane shuttle moving FFAs from the cytoplasm into the mitochondrial matrix, as shown in Equations 12.10 and 12.11. Once transferred by carnitine into the intramitochondrial matrix, the fatty

$$CH_3CH_2(CH_2)_n COOH$$

$$+ \ ATP \xrightarrow{\ \ \text{CoASH (cytoplasmic)}\ \ } CH_3CH_2(CH_2)_n{-}\overset{\overset{\displaystyle O}{\|}}{C}{-}S{-}CoA \ + \ AMP \ + \ PP_i$$

Transfer of Activated Fatty Acid to Carnitine

$$CH_3CH_2(CH_2)_n{-}\overset{\overset{\displaystyle O}{\|}}{C}{-}CoA \ + \ HOOC{-}CH_2{-}\underset{OH}{CH}{-}CH_2{-}\overset{+}{N}(CH_3)_3 \ \longrightarrow$$

$$HOOC{-}CH_2{-}\underset{\overset{\displaystyle |}{O}}{CH}{-}CH_2{-}\overset{+}{N}(CH_3)_3 \ + \ CoASH \ (cytoplasmic)$$

$$O{=}C{-}(CH_2)_n CH_2CH_3$$

Equation 12.10   Activation of cytoplasmic fatty acids.

$$\underset{\substack{| \\ O \\ | \\ O{=}C{-}(CH_2)nCH_2CH_3}}{HOOC{-}CH_2{-}C{-}CH_2{-}\overset{+}{N}(CH_3)_3} + CoASH \xrightarrow{\text{mitochondrial}}$$

$$CH_3CH_2(CH_2)_n{-}\overset{\overset{O}{\|}}{C}{-}S{-}CoA + \text{carnitine}$$

Equation 12.11   Transfer of acylcarnitine to mitochondrial coenzyme A.

acid is reesterified with coenzyme A. This coenzyme A, however, is of mitochondrial origin (Equation 12.11) and provides an activated free fatty acid for β-oxidation.

β-Oxidation

The oxidation of fatty acids was first described by F. Knoop, a German biochemist, in 1904. Oxidation of fatty acids and cleavage of the thioester occurs at the second or β-carbon of the fatty acid, and thus the cyclic process of fatty acid degradation bears the name β-oxidation. β-oxidation, it may be remembered, is initiated by activation of a cytoplasmic free fatty acid by ATP, and it exists as a thioester (Figure 12.5). Equation (1) of Figure 12.5 is the dehydrogenation of the activated fatty acid by a flavoprotein containing oxidized FAD, yielding an unsaturated C:2,3 activated fatty acid. Hydration of either a *cis* or *trans* fatty acid [equation (2) or (2')] produces a stereoisomer which upon dehydrogenation by NAD$^+$ [equation (3)] produces a (C:3)β-ketoacetyl-CoA fatty acid and NADH$_2$. The β-ketoacetyl-CoA fatty acid is cleaved between C:2 and 3, producing acetyl-coenzyme A. The remaining fatty acid fragment, shortened by the loss of two carbon atoms, condenses with another molecule of coenzyme A. This activated free fatty acid [equation (4)] recycles to equation (1) for repetition of the cyclic process. In each repetitive cycle of β-oxidation, the activated fatty acid is shortened by two carbon atoms until butyryl-CoA is cycled. In the final cycle of β-oxidation, this four-carbon fatty acid is symmetrically cleaved to yield two acetyl-CoAs [equation (5)].

Inspection of the β-oxidation of fatty acids reveals that any fatty acid of even carbon number n = 6 or greater undergoes (n/2) – 1 cycles, producing (n/2) per molecule of FADH$_2$ and n/2 molecules of acetyl-CoA. β-Oxidation of stearic acid, a saturated C$_{18}$ fatty acid, would go through eight cycles, producing eight molecules of FADH$_2$ and NADH$_2$ and nine molecules of acetyl-CoA. These reactions can be summarized as in Equation 12.12.

All the acetyl-CoA produced by β-oxidation of fatty acids enters the citric acid cycle. It may be recalled that each turn of the CAC results in the oxidation of two atoms of carbon and the synthesis of reduced coenzymes and GTP equivalent to 12 ATPs per cycle. It should be apparent, therefore, that β-oxidation of cytoplasmic long-chain fatty acids, activated by two ATPs, generates large quantities of FADH$_2$

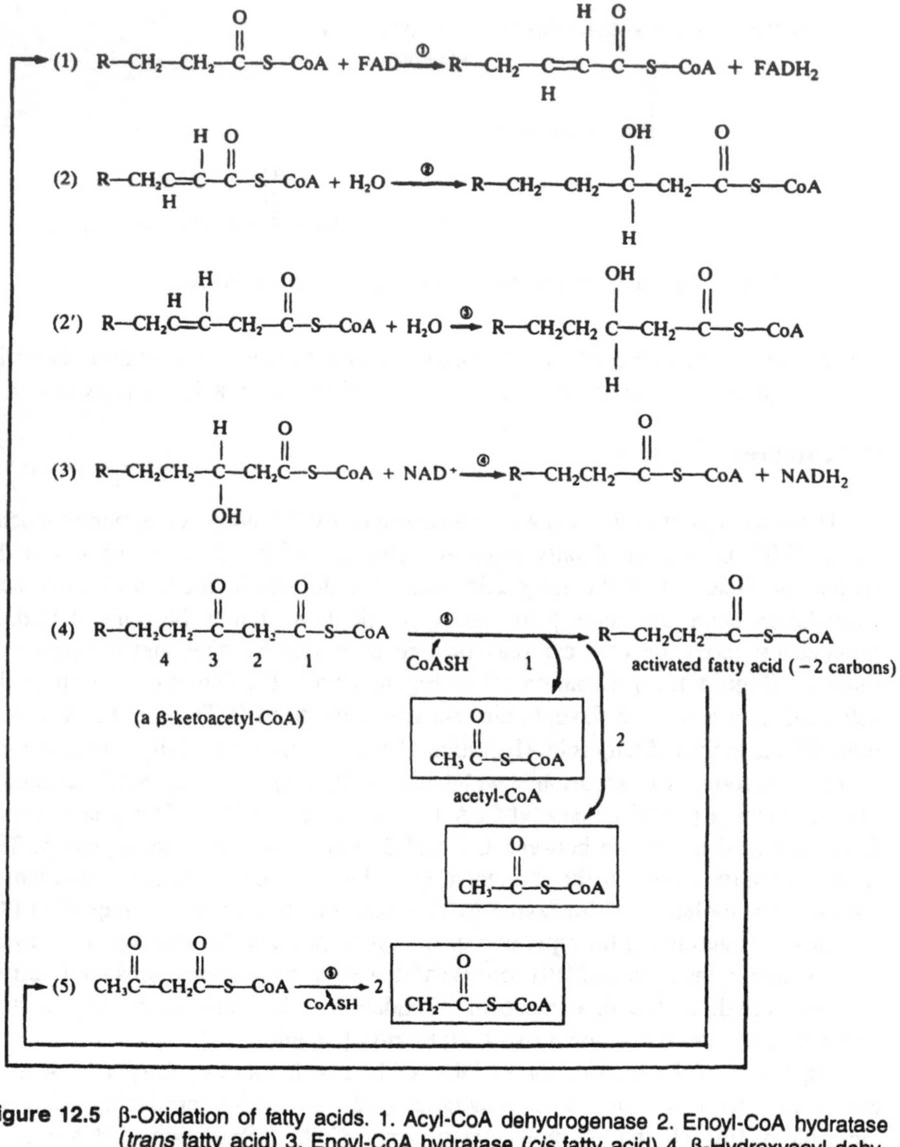

(1) $R-CH_2-CH_2-\overset{O}{\overset{\|}{C}}-S-CoA + FAD \xrightarrow{①} R-CH_2-\overset{H}{C}=\overset{H}{\underset{}{C}}-\overset{O}{\overset{\|}{C}}-S-CoA + FADH_2$

(2) $R-CH_2\overset{H}{C}=\overset{H}{\underset{}{C}}-\overset{O}{\overset{\|}{C}}-S-CoA + H_2O \xrightarrow{②} R-CH_2-CH_2-\overset{OH}{\underset{H}{C}}-CH_2-\overset{O}{\overset{\|}{C}}-S-CoA$

(2') $R-CH_2\overset{H}{C}=\overset{H}{\underset{}{C}}-CH_2-\overset{O}{\overset{\|}{C}}-S-CoA + H_2O \xrightarrow{③} R-CH_2CH_2\overset{OH}{\underset{H}{C}}-CH_2-\overset{O}{\overset{\|}{C}}-S-CoA$

(3) $R-CH_2CH_2-\overset{H}{\underset{OH}{C}}-CH_2C-S-CoA + NAD^+ \xrightarrow{④} R-CH_2CH_2-\overset{O}{\overset{\|}{C}}-S-CoA + NADH_2$

(4) $R-CH_2CH_2-\overset{O}{\overset{\|}{C}}-CH_2-\overset{O}{\overset{\|}{C}}-S-CoA \xrightarrow{⑤} R-CH_2CH_2-\overset{O}{\overset{\|}{C}}-S-CoA$

         4   3   2   1   CoASH   1   activated fatty acid (-2 carbons)

    (a β-ketoacetyl-CoA)

$CH_3 \overset{O}{\overset{\|}{C}}-S-CoA$ 2

acetyl-CoA

$CH_3-\overset{O}{\overset{\|}{C}}-S-CoA$

(5) $CH_3\overset{O}{\overset{\|}{C}}-CH_2\overset{O}{\overset{\|}{C}}-S-CoA \xrightarrow[CoASH]{⑤} 2 \quad CH_2-\overset{O}{\overset{\|}{C}}-S-CoA$

Figure 12.5 β-Oxidation of fatty acids. 1. Acyl-CoA dehydrogenase 2. Enoyl-CoA hydratase (*trans* fatty acid) 3. Enoyl-CoA hydratase (*cis* fatty acid) 4. β-Hydroxyacyl dehydrogenase 5. Thiolase.

$$\text{stearic acid} + ATP + 9CoASH + 8FAD + 8NAD^+ + 8H_2O \xrightarrow{8 \text{ cycles}} 9 \text{ acetyl-CoA}$$
$$+ 8FADH_2 + 8NADH_2 + AMP + PP_i$$

Equation 12.12 β-oxidation of stearic acid.

and $NADH_2$ for ATP synthesis from the electron transport system and oxidative phosphorylation of ADP. Complete oxidation of the C_{18} fatty acid, stearic acid, by β-oxidation nets 146 ATPs or 1066 kcal/mol of stearic acid (calculations shown in Table 12.3). The number of kcal/mol for the complete oxidation of stearic acid by O_2 is shown in Table 12.3.

β-Oxidation of stearic acid results in the conservation of 41% of the total energy of stearic acid, preserved and transferred as ATP equivalents. The efficiency of recovered energy as ATP is reduced for shorter-chain fatty acids, as each requires activation by the equivalent of two ATPs, and short-chain fatty acids contain proportionately less oxidizable hydrocarbon.

Even-carbon-numbered unsaturated fatty acids are metabolized in the same general way as even-numbered saturated fatty acids. Polyunsaturated fatty acids (PUFA) pose some metabolic problems because of the multiple unsaturated double bonds and their location. Nevertheless, these problems are surmounted by enzymes present in the mitochondrial matrix, and polyunsaturated fatty acids also follow the same general pathway of β-oxidation. Monounsaturated and polyunsaturated fatty acids have a slightly lower caloric value than do saturated fatty acids of similar carbon number, as unsaturation results in the reduction of the amount of reduced coenzymes formed and hydrogen traversing the electron transport system for ATP synthesis. Odd-carbon-numbered fatty acids (C:15, 17, 19, etc.) are oxidized in the usual β-oxidation pathway until the three-carbon unit propionyl-CoA (instead of butryl-CoA) is reached. Propionyl-CoA is then carboxylated (involves biotin and vitamin B_{12}) and enters the CAC as succinyl-CoA or succinate.

Table 12.3 Energy Yield and Efficiency of the Complete Oxidation of Stearic Acid (C_{18}:O) by β-Oxidation and the Citric Acid Cycle Through Electron Transport

		P/O Ratio		Total ATP
From β-oxidation of stearic acid	8 $FADH_2$	× 2	=	16
	8 $NADH_2$	× 3	=	24
	From β-oxidation		=	40 ATP
From CAC	9 GTP	× −	=	9
	9 $FADH_2$	× 2	=	18
	27 $NADH_2$	× 3	=	81
			=	108 ATP
	Gross			
	− (activation) 2ATP			148 ATP
	Net yield			146 ATP

β-oxidation of stearic acid $\Delta G^{\circ\prime} = -7.3 \times 146 = 1066$ kcal/mol
Complete oxidation of stearic acid $\Delta G^{\circ\prime}$ by $O_2 = 2596$ kcal/mol

$$\frac{1066}{2596} \times 100 = 41\% \text{ efficient}$$

CATABOLIC PATHWAYS OF PROTEINS

Protein provides about 15% of the average American's dietary requirement for calories. Protein metabolism is continuous and constant in the normal and adequately nourished adult and can be biochemically assessed by measurement of nitrogen balance (nitrogen consumed, nitrogen excreted). In the absence of food (calories) for an extended period, carbohydrates stored as muscle, heart, and liver glycogen are rapidly depleted. This loss of carbohydrate is followed by the hydrolysis of triglycerides, the mobilization of body depot fat, and the oxidation of fatty acids by β-oxidation. In the advent of extended starvation and cacexia, massive amounts of the body's protein stores (e.g., muscle tissue) are mobilized for the body's energy requirements. Such events are serious when they occur and may result in extreme negative nitrogen balance.

Metabolically, proteins are enzymatically converted intracellularly to amino acids. Each of the 20 commonly found amino acids in protein follows catabolic routes after either transamination or deamination. Transamination from one amino acid leads to the synthesis of another amino acid, with the concurrent generation of a new α-keto acid. Vitamin B_6 functions in transamination and deamination of amino acids. In transamination reactions, nitrogen is not lost, only transferred from one amino acid in the synthesis of another amino acid. In deamination reactions, however, the loss of the amino moiety results in the production of ammonia (NH_3) as ammonium ions (NH_4^+), and as in transamination reactions, the synthesis of an α-keto acid. A deamination reaction requiring vitamin B_6 is the initial metabolic reaction common to the elimination of nitrogen from amino acids. Deamination is shown in Equation 12.13 for phenylalanine. The amino acids may be oxidized via amino acid oxidases, requiring the flavoprotein coenzymes FAD or FMN, specific for each amino acid.

The metabolism of the hydrocarbon portion of each of the deaminated amino acids is different and for many amino acids, quite complex. Their ultimate oxidation, however, follows the established final common pathways of the citric acid cycle and the electron transport system. The hydrocarbon portion of all 21 amino acids commonly found in protein enters catabolic pathways as either pyruvate, acetyl-CoA, α-ketoglutarate, succinyl-CoA, fumarate, or oxaloacetate. With the exception of pyruvate, these metabolites are all associated with the citric acid cycle. The hydrocarbon portions of all deaminated amino acids therefore enter common catabolic pathways as either pyruvate or intermediates of the citric acid cycle. Points of entry

phenylpyruvic acid,
an α-ketocarboxylic acid

Equation 12.13 Deamination of phenylalanine.

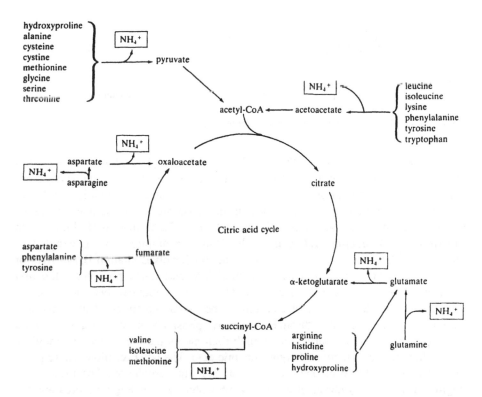

Figure 12.6 Deamination of amino acids and hydrocarbon entry into the citric acid cycle.

of the hydrocarbon portions of the amino acids into the citric acid cycle are shown in Figure 12.6.

It may be apparent from Figure 12.6 that the caloric value and yield of ATP from each amino acid can be somewhat different depending on the point of entry of its hydrocarbon skeleton into the citric acid cycle. Alanine, glycine, lysine, and so on, whose hydrocarbon skeletons become pyruvate, will yield more ATP than will the hydrocarbons of other amino acids, whose entry to the CAC occurs later. The size of the hydrocarbon portion of the amino acid also has a bearing on caloric yield. For example, phenylalanine and tyrosine, larger-molecular-weight amino acids, are divided and enter the CAC as two hydrocarbon fragments, acetyl-CoA and fumarate. Such variations in amino acid metabolism contribute to the average caloric value of 4 kcal/g for proteins.

Elimination of Ammonia: The Urea Cycle

Ammonia produced from the deamination of amino acids and other amines is strongly basic and very toxic. Cells of the liver and to a lesser degree, the kidney and brain, detoxify ammonia by its conversion to the less toxic and water-soluble compound, urea. The conversion of ammonia to urea from amino acids proceeds in

$$\text{NH}_3 + \text{HOOC}-\underset{\underset{H}{|}}{\overset{\overset{NH_2}{|}}{C}}-\text{CH}_2\text{CH}_2-\text{COOH} \xrightarrow[\text{biotin}]{\text{ATP \quad ADP+P}_i} \text{HOOC}-\underset{\underset{H}{|}}{\overset{\overset{NH_2}{|}}{C}}-\text{CH}_2\text{CH}_2-\overset{\overset{O}{\|}}{C}-\text{NH}_2 + \text{H}_2\text{O}$$

glutamic acid   glutamine

Equation 12.14 Conversion of ammonia to glutamate.

the liver, kidney, and brain, predominantly through a single common pathway of a glutamic acid transamination–deamination and the urea cycle. Ammonia arising from deamination reactions in tissues other than the liver, kidney, or brain is coupled to the amino acid glutamate and is carried in the blood plasma to the liver or kidney as the basic amino acid glutamine (Equation 12.14). The formation of glutamine in Equation 12.14 requires ATP and results from the ammonia being coupled to glutamate. Glutamine, via a deamination reaction (involves vitamin B_6) in liver or kidney, yields ammonia, which is converted into carbamoyl phosphate, the first reaction of the urea cycle (Figure 12.7). This reaction requires two molecules of ATP and carboxybiocytin (involves biotin). The remaining amine of glutamic acid enters the urea cycle either through carbamoyl phosphate or via a transamination from glutamic acid to aspartic acid, which then enters the urea cycle via coupling to citrulline in the formation of arginosuccinic acid. The latter reaction also requires an energy expenditure of one molecule of ATP for completion. The urea cycle, beginning with the synthesis of carbamoyl phosphate and ending with urea and the regeneration of ornithine, requires the expenditure of three molecules of ATP per molecule of urea generated. The derived ammonia (amino groups from glutamine, glutamate, and aspartate) in urea is contributed equally from a molecule of carbamoyl phosphate and aspartic acid. Manganese functions as a cofactor of the enzyme arginase with the ketone moiety of urea being derived from CO_2 (C) and water (O).

Energy, ATP, and the Catabolic Pathways

We have examined how the caloric energy of food (starch → glucose; lipids [or fats and oils] → fatty acids and glycerol; proteins → amino acids) is converted in the catabolic pathways to a more useful form of metabolic energy, ATP. The unanswered question throughout this discussion of energy transfer is: Where was the energy in the organic nutrients that was transferred and conserved as ATP? The energy transferred from the organic nutrients to ATP in the catabolic pathways was originally stored by plants during photosynthesis and was retained in the covalent bonds of the starch, lipids, proteins, and other organic molecules. Table 12.4 lists some representative bond energies that are present in organic nutrients. Examination of this table reveals that the organic nutrients of foods, which contain predominately C—C, C—H, C—S, C—N, and C—O bonds, contain a great deal of stored energy expressed as kcal/mol.

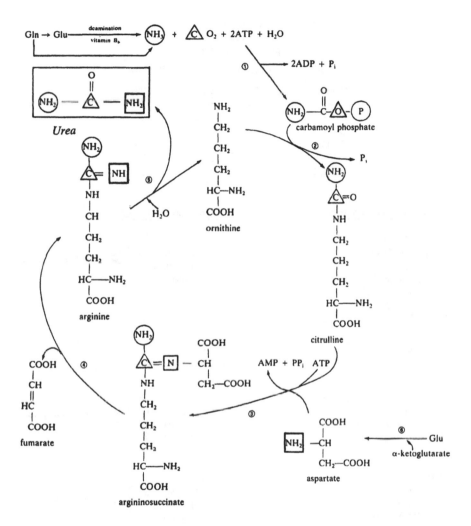

Figure 12.7 Urea cycle. 1. Carbamoyl phosphate synthetase 2. Ornithine-carbamoyl transferase 3. Argininosuccinate synthetase 4. Argininosuccinate lyase 5. Arginase 6.
Transaminase (vitamin B$_6$).

The caloric value of food — carbohydrates, lipids, and proteins — is the amount
of potential energy stored in the molecule's covalent bonds. During catabolic metabolism, the potential energy available for release and transfer to ATP is related to the
total amount of hydrocarbon within molecules. The hydrocarbon content (—CH$_2$—)
of the organic nutrients determines the caloric value of foods. The lipids, i.e., fats and
oils, contain 9 cal/g (actually kcal/g), more than twice the caloric value of carbohydrates and protein (4 cal/g) because they proportionately contain about twice the
amount of hydrocarbon. Figure 12.8 demonstrates the approximate 2.25:1:1 caloric
ratios for lipids, carbohydrates, and protein, respectively, represented by the fatty acids
hexonic and palmitic acids, glucose, and the dipeptide glutamylglycine. These small

Table 12.4 Representative Bond Energies that are Present in Nutrients and Important Biomolecules

Bond	kcal/mol	Bond	kcal/mol
H—C	81	HC—H	108
C—C	144	HO—H	119
C—S	175	OC=O	128
C—N	174	O—O	119
C—O	257	O—P	144
H_2N—H	103	S—S	102
HOH_2C—H	92	N≡N	226

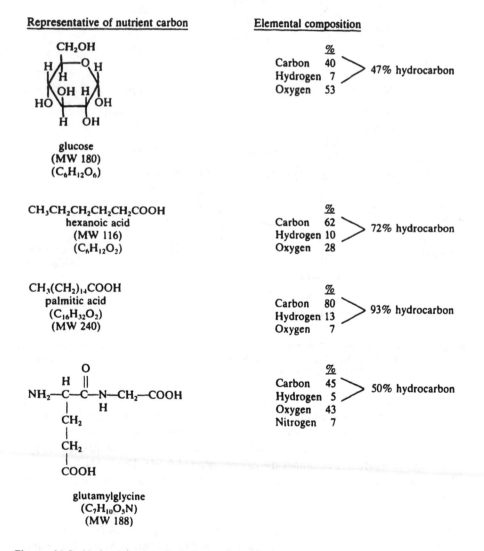

Representative of nutrient carbon

CH₂OH

glucose
(MW 180)
($C_6H_{12}O_6$)

CH₃CH₂CH₂CH₂CH₂COOH
hexanoic acid
(MW 116)
($C_6H_{12}O_2$)

CH₃(CH₂)₁₄COOH
palmitic acid
($C_{16}H_{32}O_2$)
(MW 240)

glutamylglycine
($C_7H_{10}O_5N$)
(MW 188)

Elemental composition

	%	
Carbon	40	
Hydrogen	7	47% hydrocarbon
Oxygen	53	

	%	
Carbon	62	
Hydrogen	10	72% hydrocarbon
Oxygen	28	

	%	
Carbon	80	
Hydrogen	13	93% hydrocarbon
Oxygen	7	

	%	
Carbon	45	
Hydrogen	5	50% hydrocarbon
Oxygen	43	
Nitrogen	7	

Figure 12.8 Hydrocarbon content of organic nutrients.

Table 12.5 Caloric Density of Selected Foods

Food/Nutrient	Percent Water (approx.)	Caloric Density (cal/g)
Water	100	0
Fiber	Varied	0
Diet soda	100	0
Lettuce (iceberg)	96	0.13
Tomato	94	0.20
Orange	86	0.36
Apple	84	0.39
Potato	75	0.76
Egg	75	1.48
Fish (salmon)	71	1.41
Chicken breast	58	1.65
Sirloin steak	44	3.88
Pork chop	42	2.65
Swiss cheese	37	3.75
White bread	34	2.70
Jelly	29	2.78
Margarine	16	7.21
Chocolate	13	5.18
Bacon	8	6.00
Cereals (dry)	4	2.90
Butter	0	7.17
Oils	0	8.84
Lard	0	9.00

molecules approximate the elemental composition of the energy nutrients, the dietary fats, starch, and protein. Figure 12.8 shows the hydrocarbon ratios of palmitic acid, glucose, and glutamylglycine to be 1.98:1:1.2, which approaches the average caloric ratio of 2.25:1:1 for lipids, carbohydrates, and protein. When hexonic acid, with the same number of carbons (six) as glucose, and glutamylglycine are used in such calculations, the energy ratios go down because of a higher percentage of oxygen in hexanoic acid (27.6%) than palmitic acid (13.3%), which does not contribute to caloric value, yet hexanoic acid (MW 116) still has nearly 72% hydrocarbon. As Figure 12.8 indicates, as the molecular weight of fatty acids increases, the percentage of hydrocarbon, and hence calories, also increases. Herein lies the partial reason for the reduced caloric content of triglycerides like Salatrim (see Chapter 9).

Caloric Density of Foods

The proportion of hydrocarbon in molecular structure is but one factor that contributes to the caloric value of foods. The second factor contributing to the caloric value of foods is the proportionate content of water. These two predominant factors then contribute to the caloric density of foods. Foods containing a high proportion of water (also fiber) possess a lower caloric density than that of foods low in moisture and with a proportionately higher content of either fats or oils. Table 12.5 demonstrates that foods high in water content (e.g., lettuce and tomatoes) have a low caloric density (about 0.20 cal/g), whereas butter, oils, and lard, which have essentially no water, have the maximum caloric density of any food (about 9.0 cal/g). Foods with intermediate water content have intermediate caloric densities. The caloric variation between carbohydrates and lipids is seen for dry cereals, white sugar, and the lipids. These foods are all low in water content, but the caloric density of the lipid foods; i.e., butter, oils, and lard, is twice that of sugar and dry cereals, owing to the higher proportion of total hydrocarbon.

CHAPTER 13

Anabolic Pathways

Much of the ATP produced in the mitochondria by the electron transport array of enzymes and cytochromes, the final common catabolic pathway for the oxidation of nutrients, is consumed by the anabolic pathways during biosynthesis. The major anabolic processes that consume ATP energy are the synthesis of glucose and glycogen, gluconeogenesis and glycogenesis, respectively; the synthesis of fatty acids and triglycerides; and the synthesis of the nucleic acids, deoxyribonucleic acid (DNA) and ribonucleic acid (RNA), and proteins. Compounds that contain isoprene, such as cholesterol and its derivatives, also require ATP for their synthesis.

GLUCONEOGENESIS

Of all the nutrient energy stored by the body, carbohydrate constitutes the smallest energy reserve, being found in muscle, heart, and liver. In the face of depleted carbohydrate (glycogen) stores and in the absence of carbohydrate intake, blood glucose levels will be maintained around 80 mg/dl by the synthesis of glucose from noncarbohydrate metabolites. The glycogenic amino acids, glycerol from triglycerides, and pyruvic and lactic acids, all contribute to the synthesis of glucose by gluconeogenesis (Figure 13.1).

Gluconeogenesis occurring in muscle, heart, and liver, beginning with pyruvic or lactic acids, follows nearly the same metabolic pathway as glycolysis but in reverse. It may be recalled that in glycolysis, ATP was made in substrate-level phosphorylations during the conversion of phosphoenolpyruvate to pyruvate. During gluconeogenesis, pyruvic and lactic acids cannot be converted directly to phosphoenolypyruvate because the reaction is thermodynamically "uphill." Thus, direct conversion of pyruvate (or lactate) to phosphoenolpyruvate is circumvented by reactions using carboxybiotin (contains biotin), ATP, and GTP (guanosine triphosphate). In the first reaction pyruvate is converted to oxaloacetate, which in a second reaction (oxaloacetate) is decarboxylated to phosphoenolpyruvate. Both reactions

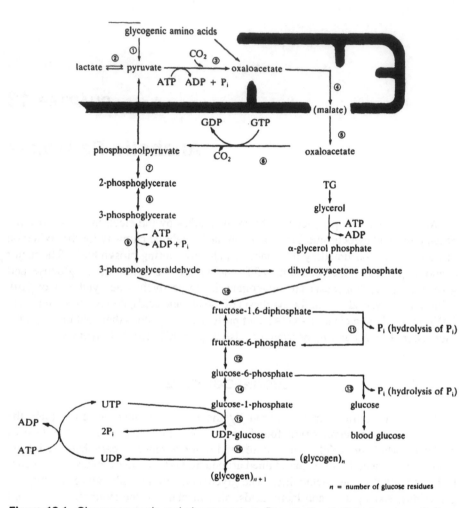

Figure 13.1 Gluconeogenesis and glycogenesis 1. Deamination 2. Dehydrogenase 3. Pyruvate carboxylase 4. Malate dehydrogenase (mitochondrial) 5. Malate dehydrogenase (cytoplasmic) 6. Phosphoenolpyruvate carboxykinase 7. Enolase 8. Phosphoglycerolmutase 9. Phosphoglycerolkinase 10. Aldolase 11. Fructose diphosphatase 12. Isomerase 13. Glucose-6-phosphatase (liver, kidney enzyme) 14. Phosphoglucomutase 15. UDP-glucose pyrophosphorylase 16. Glycogen synthetase (liver, kidney, muscle enzyme).

require the expenditure of high-energy phosphorylated compounds as either ATP or GTP. The conversion of pyruvate to phosphoenolpyruvate is shown in Equation 13.1. Thus, two ATP equivalents (one ATP and one GTP) are expended in gluconeogenesis in converting one molecule of pyruvate (or lactate) to phosphoenolpyruvate. A

$$\text{pyruvate} + \text{carboxybiotin} + \text{ATP} \rightarrow \text{oxaloacetate} + \text{ADP} + P_i + \text{biotin}$$

$$\text{oxaloacetate} + \text{GTP} \rightarrow \text{phosphoenolpyruvate} + \text{GDP}$$

Equation 13.1 Conversion of pyruvate to phosphoenolpyruvate.

$$\text{fructose-6-phosphate} + \text{ATP} \rightarrow$$
$$\text{fructose-1,6-diphosphate} + \text{ADP}$$

Equation 13.2 Phosphorylation of fructose-6-phosphate.

second energy-requiring reaction in gluconeogenesis is the phosphorylation of fructose-6-phosphate, forming fructose-1,6-diphosphate (Equation 13.2). Fructose-1,6-diphosphate may now be converted to glucose-6-phosphate, ending the *de novo* synthesis of glucose from either pyruvate or lactate. In liver, glucose-6-phosphate may be dephosphorylated and enter the blood or be converted to glycogen. In muscle and heart, glucose-6-phosphate is converted only to glycogen. The total requirement for the conversion of either pyruvate or lactate to glucose-6-phosphate (gluconeogenesis) is equivalent to six molecules of ATP (Table 13.1) and it consumes two equivalents of $NADH_2$ (contains niacin). Comparison of the energy requirement for gluconeogenesis with the energy yield of glycolysis shows these two pathways to be thermodynamically very different. The net energy yield from glycolysis is +2 ATP, whereas the net energy requirement for gluconeogenesis is +6 ATP.

Additional energy requirements are needed for the conversion of glucose to glycogen (glycogenesis). For each glucose to be transferred to a growing polysaccharide or glycogen molecule, it must first be activated by the nucleotide uridine triphosphate (UTP) shown in Equation 13.3. The product, uridine diphosphate-1-glucose, results in the activation and specific cofactor configuration for the enzymatic transfer of glucose to glycogen (Equation 13.4). Having transferred glucose, thereby extending the glycogen molecule by one glucose residue, the UDP must again be phosphorylated, forming UTP for activation of an additional glucose molecule. This is accomplished by ATP. One ATP (as UTP) is therefore expended for the incorporation of each glucose residue into glycogen.

$$\text{glucose-1-phosphate} + \text{UTP} \rightarrow \text{UDP-glucose} + 2P_i$$

Equation 13.3 Activation of glucose by uridine triphosphate.

$$\text{UDP-glucose} + (\text{glucose})_n \text{ glycogen} \rightarrow (\text{glucose})_{n+1} \text{ glycogen} + \text{UDP}$$

Equation 13.4 Transfer of glucose to glycogen.

Table 13.1 Energy Requirements for Gluconeogenesis and Glycogenesis from Pyruvate, Lactate, or Glycogenic Amino Acids

	ATP	GTP	UTP
Conversion of pyruvate (lactate) to phosphoenolpyruvate	1	1	—
Reduction of 3-phosphoglycerate to 3-phosphoglyceraldehyde	1	—	—
2 pyruvate (lactate) $\rightarrow$ glucose	4	2	—
Conversion of glucose $\rightarrow$ (glycogen)$_{n+1}$	1	—	1
2 pyruvate (lactate) $\rightarrow$ (glycogen)$_{n+1}$	5	2	1

$$TG \xrightarrow[\text{3 FAs}]{} glycerol \xrightarrow[\substack{NADH_2 \quad NAD \\ ATP \quad ADP}]{} dihydroxyacetonephosphate$$

Equation 13.5 Conversion of glycerol from triglycerides to dihydroxyacetonephosphate.

GLYCOGENIC AMINO ACIDS AND GLYCEROL

Any amino acid that can be converted to an intermediate of the citric acid cycle or pyruvate following either deamination or transamination is a glycogenic amino acid. Each amino acid may become blood glucose or glycogen via gluconeogenesis (glycogenesis). Leucine is the only amino acid that cannot be converted to glucose. Glycerol, from triglycerides, is readily converted to the glycolytic intermediate dihydroxyacetonephosphate (Equation 13.5). Dihydroxyacetonephosphate entering the gluconeogenic pathway may then be converted to glucose-6-phosphate by combining with 3-phosphoglyceraldehyde (see Figure 13.1).

FATTY ACID AND TRIGLYCERIDE SYNTHESIS

Excess nutrient energy intake above and beyond energy requirements is converted to and stored mainly as triglyceride in depot fat. Triglycerides are formed from dietary fatty acids, fats and oils, or from dietary carbohydrates and protein via the cytoplasmic synthesis of fatty acids which are esterified with glycerol within adipose tissue. To a large degree, the synthesis and storage of triglycerides are controlled by the levels of circulating hormones, particularly insulin.

FATTY ACID SYNTHESIS

Fatty acid synthesis begins with acetyl-CoA, which may be formed from carbohydrates (pyruvate), glycogenic or ketogenic amino acids, and fatty acids themselves. Acetyl-CoA formed within the mitochondrion is transported across the mitochondrial membrane to the cell cytoplasm by carnitine. Carnitine combines with acetyl-CoA, forming mitochondrial acylcarnitine (Equation 13.6). Acylcarnitine condenses with another molecule of coenzyme A of cytoplasmic origin and forms cytoplasmic acetyl-CoA (Equation 13.7). The net effect of these reactions is the transfer of acetyl-CoA from the mitochondrion to the cytoplasm with the regeneration of carnitine and mitochondrial Coenzyme A. In the cytoplasm, acetyl-CoA is converted to malonyl-CoA as the initiating step of fatty acid synthesis. This reaction, the synthesis of malonyl-CoA, requires the participation of carboxybiotin (contains biotin) and the expenditure of ATP energy (Figure 13.2, Equation 13.8). Following the synthesis of malonyl-CoA, it is attached to a thiol residue of a protein (1). The protein is known as an acyl carrier protein (ACP). In a separate reaction, (2), a second ACP combines with a molecule of acetyl-CoA which provides the structural framework

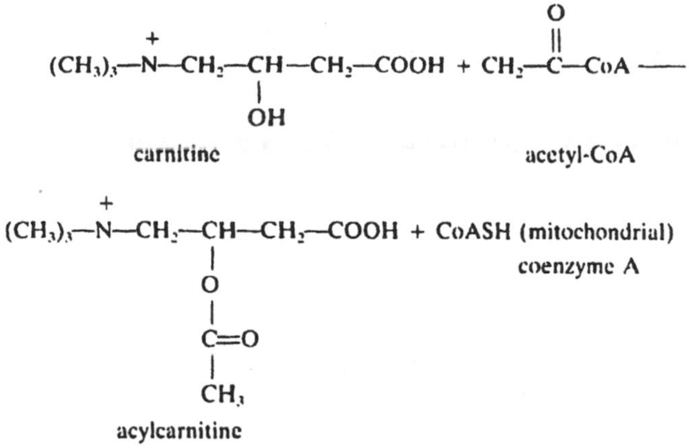

$$(CH_3)_3-N^{+}-CH_2-CH-CH_2-COOH + CH_2-\overset{\displaystyle O}{\overset{\|}{C}}-CoA \longrightarrow$$

$$\underset{OH}{|}$$

carnitine   acetyl-CoA

$$(CH_3)_3-N^{+}-CH_2-CH-CH_2-COOH + CoASH\ (mitochondrial)$$

$$\underset{\underset{\underset{CH_3}{|}}{\underset{C=O}{|}}{O}}{|}$$

coenzyme A

acylcarnitine

Equation 13.6 Transfer of mitochondrial acetyl-CoA by carnitine.

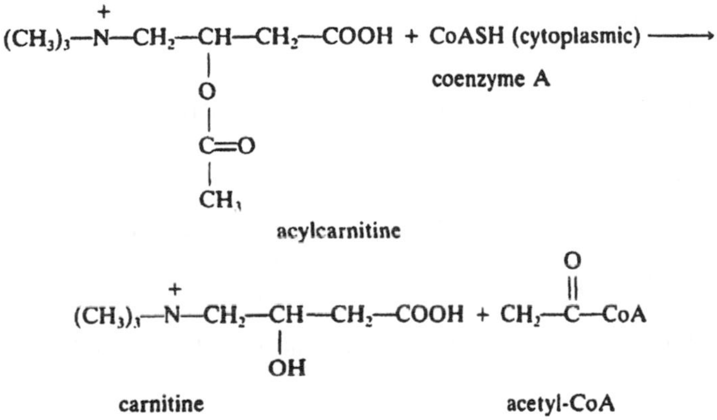

$$(CH_3)_3-N^{+}-CH_2-CH-CH_2-COOH + CoASH\ (cytoplasmic) \longrightarrow$$

$$\underset{\underset{\underset{CH_3}{|}}{\underset{C=O}{|}}{O}}{|}$$

coenzyme A

acylcarnitine

$$(CH_3)_3-N^{+}-CH_2-CH-CH_2-COOH + CH_2-\overset{\displaystyle O}{\overset{\|}{C}}-CoA$$

$$\underset{OH}{|}$$

carnitine   acetyl-CoA

Equation 13.7 Condensation of mitochondrial acetyl-CoA with cytoplasmic CoASH.

for the synthesis of the fatty acid. In step (3), the malonyl-ACP and the acetyl-ACP combine, forming a four-carbon unit, acetoacetyl-ACP. In this reaction, one carbon is lost as CO_2, which had originally been added in the synthesis of malonyl-CoA from acetyl-CoA (Equation 13.8). Acetoacetyl-ACP represents the combining of two molecules of acetyl-CoA and the formation of a four-carbon unit. The remaining steps of fatty acid synthesis (see **Figure 13.2**) consist of reduction reactions by $NADPH_2$, saturating the hydrocarbon. Elongation of the growing fatty acid in two-carbon units is made by coupling a malonyl-CoA to the ACP with simultaneous loss

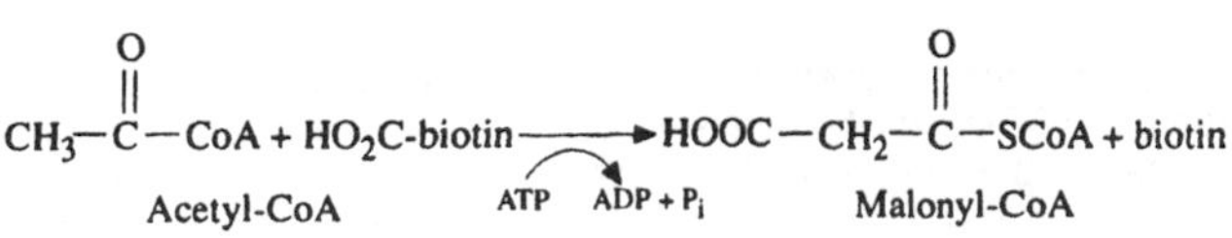

$$CH_3-\overset{\displaystyle O}{\overset{\|}{C}}-CoA + HO_2C\text{-biotin} \xrightarrow[\text{ATP} \quad \text{ADP} + P_i]{} HOOC-CH_2-\overset{\displaystyle O}{\overset{\|}{C}}-SCoA + biotin$$

Acetyl-CoA   Malonyl-CoA

Equation 13.8 Synthesis of malonyl-CoA from acetyl-CoA.

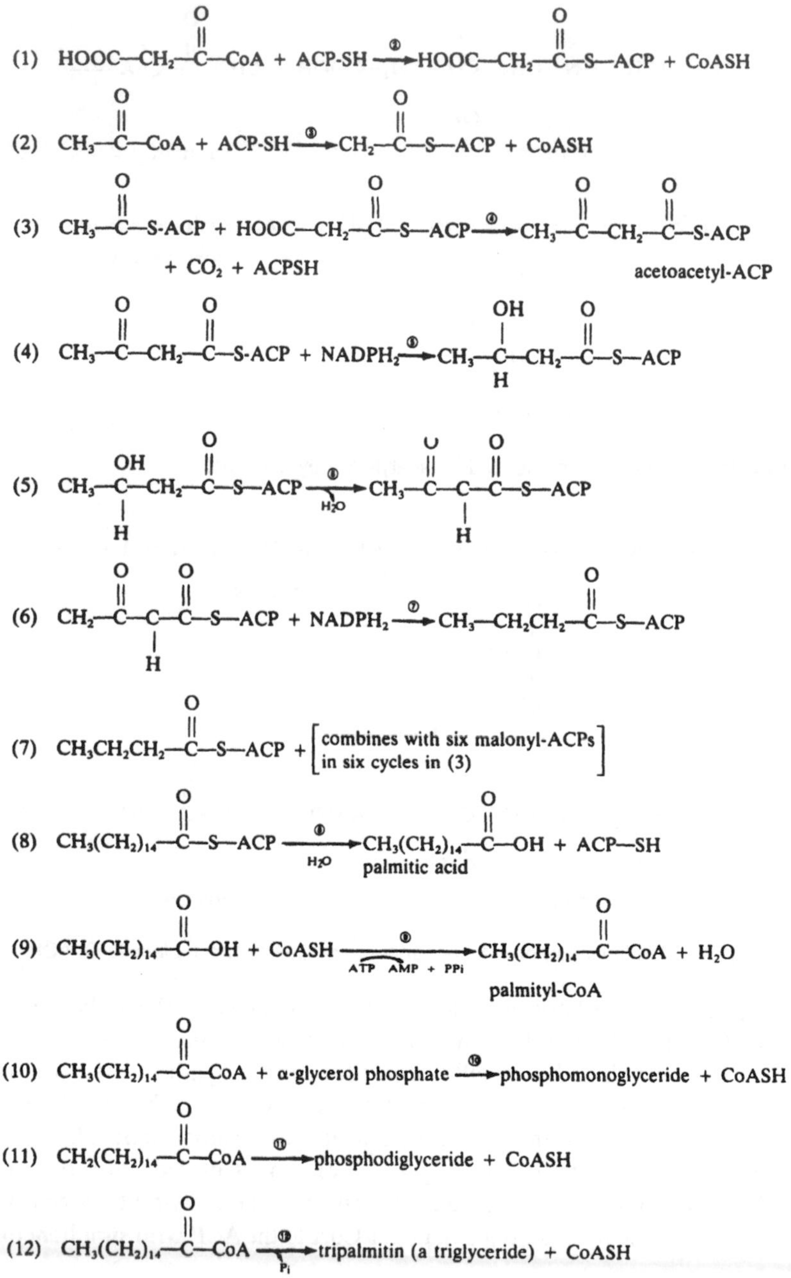

(1) $HOOC-CH_2-\overset{O}{\overset{||}{C}}-CoA + ACP\text{-}SH \xrightarrow{①} HOOC-CH_2-\overset{O}{\overset{||}{C}}-S-ACP + CoASH$

(2) $CH_3-\overset{O}{\overset{||}{C}}-CoA + ACP\text{-}SH \xrightarrow{②} CH_2-\overset{O}{\overset{||}{C}}-S-ACP + CoASH$

(3) $CH_3-\overset{O}{\overset{||}{C}}-S\text{-}ACP + HOOC-CH_2-\overset{O}{\overset{||}{C}}-S-ACP \xrightarrow{④} CH_3-\overset{O}{\overset{||}{C}}-CH_2-\overset{O}{\overset{||}{C}}-S\text{-}ACP$
   $+ CO_2 + ACPSH$ 　　　　　　　　　　　　　　　　acetoacetyl-ACP

(4) $CH_3-\overset{O}{\overset{||}{C}}-CH_2-\overset{O}{\overset{||}{C}}-S\text{-}ACP + NADPH_2 \xrightarrow{⑤} CH_3-\overset{OH}{\underset{H}{\overset{|}{C}}}-CH_2-\overset{O}{\overset{||}{C}}-S-ACP$

(5) $CH_3-\overset{OH}{\underset{H}{\overset{|}{C}}}-CH_2-\overset{O}{\overset{||}{C}}-S-ACP \xrightarrow[H_2O]{⑥} CH_3-\overset{O}{\overset{||}{C}}-\overset{O}{\underset{H}{\overset{||}{C}}}-C-S-ACP$

(6) $CH_2-\overset{O}{\overset{||}{C}}-\underset{H}{C}-\overset{O}{\overset{||}{C}}-S-ACP + NADPH_2 \xrightarrow{⑦} CH_3-CH_2CH_2-\overset{O}{\overset{||}{C}}-S-ACP$

(7) $CH_3CH_2CH_2-\overset{O}{\overset{||}{C}}-S-ACP + \left[\begin{array}{l}\text{combines with six malonyl-ACPs}\\ \text{in six cycles in (3)}\end{array}\right]$

(8) $CH_3(CH_2)_{14}-\overset{O}{\overset{||}{C}}-S-ACP \xrightarrow[H_2O]{⑧} CH_3(CH_2)_{14}-\overset{O}{\overset{||}{C}}-OH + ACP-SH$
   　　　　　　　　　　　　　　　　palmitic acid

(9) $CH_3(CH_2)_{14}-\overset{O}{\overset{||}{C}}-OH + CoASH \xrightarrow[ATP \quad AMP + PPi]{⑨} CH_3(CH_2)_{14}-\overset{O}{\overset{||}{C}}-CoA + H_2O$
   　　　　　　　　　　　　　　　　palmityl-CoA

(10) $CH_3(CH_2)_{14}-\overset{O}{\overset{||}{C}}-CoA + \alpha\text{-glycerol phosphate} \xrightarrow{⑩} \text{phosphomonoglyceride} + CoASH$

(11) $CH_2(CH_2)_{14}-\overset{O}{\overset{||}{C}}-CoA \xrightarrow{⑪} \text{phosphodiglyceride} + CoASH$

(12) $CH_3(CH_2)_{14}-\overset{O}{\overset{||}{C}}-CoA \xrightarrow[P_i]{⑫} \text{tripalmitin (a triglyceride)} + CoASH$

Figure 13.2 Fatty acid and triglyceride (tripalmitate) synthesis from acetyl-CoA, 1. Carboxylase, 2. ACP-malonyltransferase, 3. ACP-acyltransferase, 4. β-Ketoacyl-ACP-synthase, 5. β-Ketoacyl-ACP-reductase, 6. Enoyl-ACP-hydrotase, 7. Enoyl-ACP-reductase, 8. ACP-thiolesterase, 9. Acyl-CoA-synthetase, 10. Glycerolphosphate acyltransferase, 11. Glycerolphosphate acyltransferase, 12. Phosphatase and diacylglycerol acyltransferase.

of CO_2 followed by further reduction of the fatty acid by $NADPH_2$. Thus, each cycle in the synthesis of a fatty acid consumes one ATP in the synthesis of malonyl-CoA, uses two molecules of $NADPH_2$ for reduction of the added hydrocarbon, and results in a two-carbon extension in the *de novo* synthesis of a fatty acid. Seven cycles are completed before palmitic acid ($C_{16}H_{32}O_2$) is formed upon hydrolysis of the hydrocarbon from the acyl carrier protein (8).

Triglycerides may be formed from the fatty acids synthesized *de novo* by activation with ATP and coenzyme A. Activated fatty acids then sequentially combine [(10) through (12)] with α-glycerolphosphate or dihydroxyacetonephosphate, forming mono-, di-, and triglycerides. Addition of choline to the phosphodiglyceride would result in the synthesis of lecithin. Lecithin is not dietarily essential, but controversy exists as to whether choline is dietarily essential.

CHOLESTEROL AND STEROID BIOSYNTHESIS

A third major anabolic pathway that consumes ATP and $NADPH_2$ is the synthesis of cholesterol, principal sterol of animals and humans, and its many derivatives. Blood cholesterol levels are maintained by a combination of dietary cholesterol and endogenous *de novo* synthesis of cholesterol starting from acetyl-coenzyme A (contains pantothenic acid). The *de novo* synthesis of cholesterol by the liver, intestinal epithelium, and skin is affected primarily by dietary cholesterol intake, but it also is affected to a lesser degree by caloric intake, fiber, exercise, and the recirculation of the bile acids via the hepatic portal system. The liver dominates the synthesis and metabolism of cholesterol. Cholesterol synthesis occurs in other tissues, however, as it is a precursor to other important compounds, 7-dehydrocholesterol (vitamin D) in the skin, adrenocorticosteroids produced by the adrenal gland, and the major sex hormones, testosterone and the estrogens.

Cholesterol, $C_{27}H_{46}O$, whose biosynthesis was established by Konrad Block and for which he received the Nobel Prize in 1964, has all of its 27 carbons derived from acetyl-coenzyme A and may be viewed as a polymer of five isoprene units (Equation 13.9). The initial step in cholesterol biosynthesis (Figure 13.3) is the condensation of two molecules of acetyl-CoA to form acetoacetyl-CoA (1), which combines with a third molecule of acetyl-CoA, forming β-hydroxy-β-methylglutaryl-CoA (2). An alternative metabolic route for acetoacetyl-CoA is the formation of acetoacetic acid and the other ketones (Figure 13.4). Reduction of β-hydroxy-β-methylglutaryl-CoA by two molecules of $NADPH_2$ yields a six-carbon molecule, mevalonic acid, which is the reduced product of three combined molecules of acetyl-coenzyme A. (3) Mevalonic acid is synthesized in the cytoplasm and is the immediate precursor of isoprene and ultimately cholesterol and its derivatives. In the synthesis leading to cholesterol, mevalonic acid is sequentially phosphorylated by three molecules of ATP and decarboxylated (involves vitamin B_6) to yield the five-carbon isopentenylpyrophosphate. (4) Through a series of metabolic steps, six isopentylpyrophosphates are combined, forming squalene, a 30-carbon polymer of six isoprene

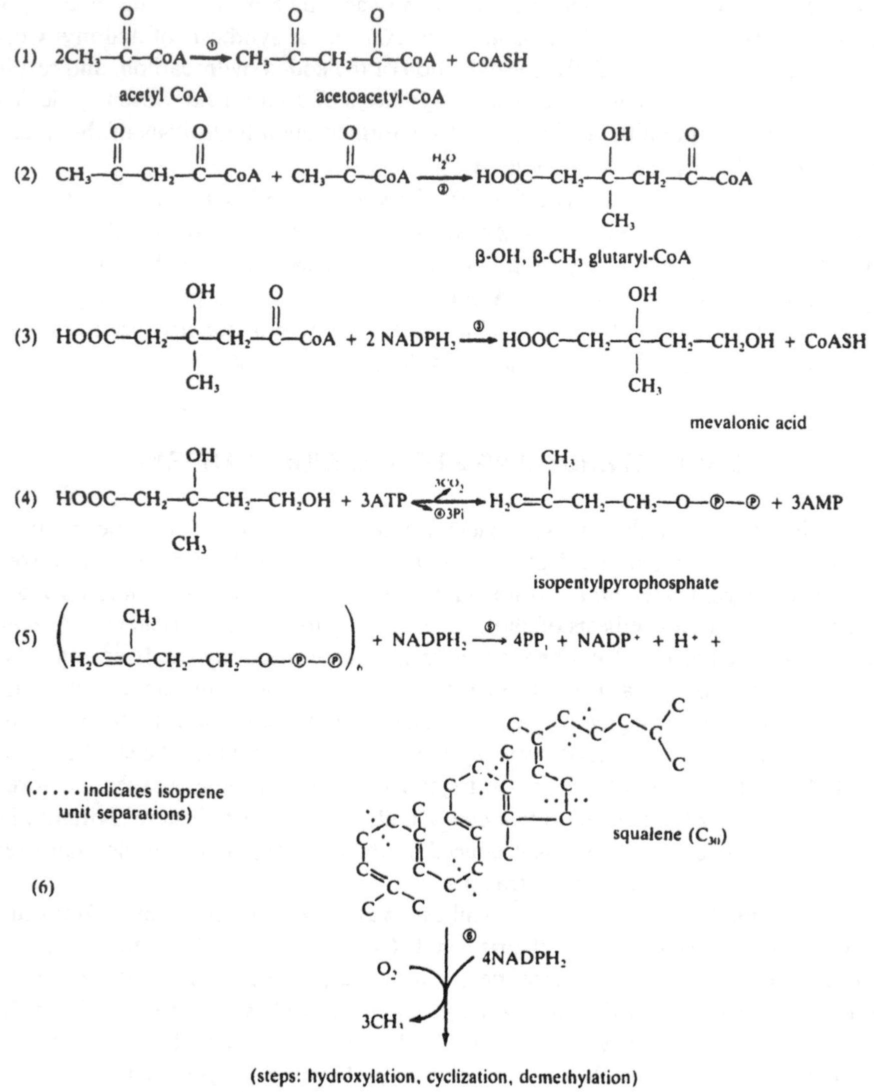

(1) $2CH_3-\overset{\overset{O}{\|}}{C}-CoA \xrightarrow{\text{①}} CH_3-\overset{\overset{O}{\|}}{C}-CH_2-\overset{\overset{O}{\|}}{C}-CoA + CoASH$

      acetyl CoA   acetoacetyl-CoA

(2) $CH_3-\overset{\overset{O}{\|}}{C}-CH_2-\overset{\overset{O}{\|}}{C}-CoA + CH_3-\overset{\overset{O}{\|}}{C}-CoA \xrightarrow[\text{①}]{H_2O} HOOC-CH_2-\overset{\overset{OH}{|}}{\underset{\underset{CH_3}{|}}{C}}-CH_2-\overset{\overset{O}{\|}}{C}-CoA$

                                                β-OH, β-CH₃ glutaryl-CoA

(3) $HOOC-CH_2-\overset{\overset{OH}{|}}{\underset{\underset{CH_3}{|}}{C}}-CH_2-\overset{\overset{O}{\|}}{C}-CoA + 2\ NADPH_2 \xrightarrow{\text{①}} HOOC-CH_2-\overset{\overset{OH}{|}}{\underset{\underset{CH_3}{|}}{C}}-CH_2-CH_2OH + CoASH$

                                                                        mevalonic acid

(4) $HOOC-CH_2-\overset{\overset{OH}{|}}{\underset{\underset{CH_3}{|}}{C}}-CH_2-CH_2OH + 3ATP \underset{\text{①3Pi}}{\overset{3CO_2}{\rightleftharpoons}} H_2C=\overset{\overset{CH_3}{|}}{C}-CH_2-CH_2-O-℗-℗ + 3AMP$

                                                         isopentylpyrophosphate

(5) $\left(\underset{H_2C=\overset{\overset{CH_3}{|}}{C}-CH_2-CH_2-O-℗-℗}{}\right)_n + NADPH_2 \xrightarrow{\text{①}} 4PP_i + NADP^\cdot + H^\cdot +$

(..... indicates isoprene unit separations)

(6)

squalene (C_{30})

$O_2 \searrow \nearrow 4NADPH_2$ ⑥

$3CH_4 \swarrow$

(steps: hydroxylation, cyclization, demethylation)

Figure 13.3 Synthesis of cholesterol from acetyl-CoA.

units. (5) Through a series of metabolic steps, squalene is hydroxylated via formation of a 3,4-epoxide, is cyclized, demethylated, and reduced with four molecules of $NADPH_2$, all of which results in the final synthesis of cholesterol. Equation 13.10 summarized the synthesis of cholesterol from acetyl-CoA. As Equation 13.10 indicates, 18 molecules of ATP and five molecules of $NADPH_2$ (contains niacin) are required to synthesize one molecule of cholesterol *de novo*. The same energy requirement is, of course, expended in the synthesis of adrenocorticoids (C_{21}), androgens (C_{19}), and estrogens (C_{18}), all of which are metabolically derived from cholesterol.

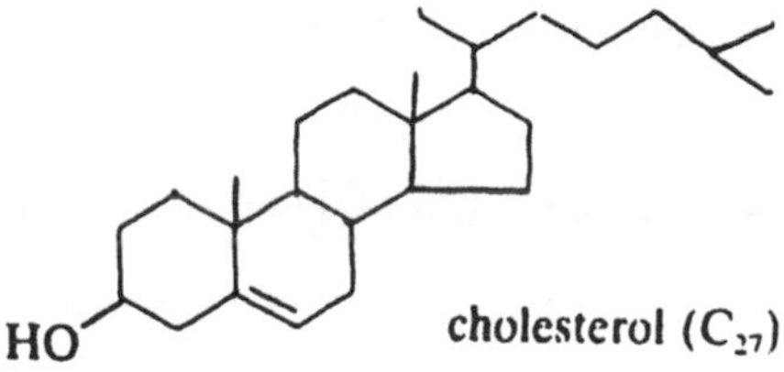

cholesterol (C$_{27}$)

1. Condensation of 2 acetyl-CoA
2. β-Hydroxymethyl-glutaryl-CoA synthase
3. β-Hydroxymethyl glutaryl-CoA reductase
4. Mevalonic kinase
   Phosphomevalonic kinase   } combined reactions
   Phosphomevalonic decarboxylase

5. Isopentyl pyrophosphate isomerase
   Dimethylallyl transferase   } combined reactions
   Squalene synthase

6. Squalene monooxygenase
   Squalene epoxidase   } combined reactions
   Lanosterol cyclase
   7-Dehydrocholesterol reductase

Figure 13.3 *Continued.*

acetyl-CoA   isoprene

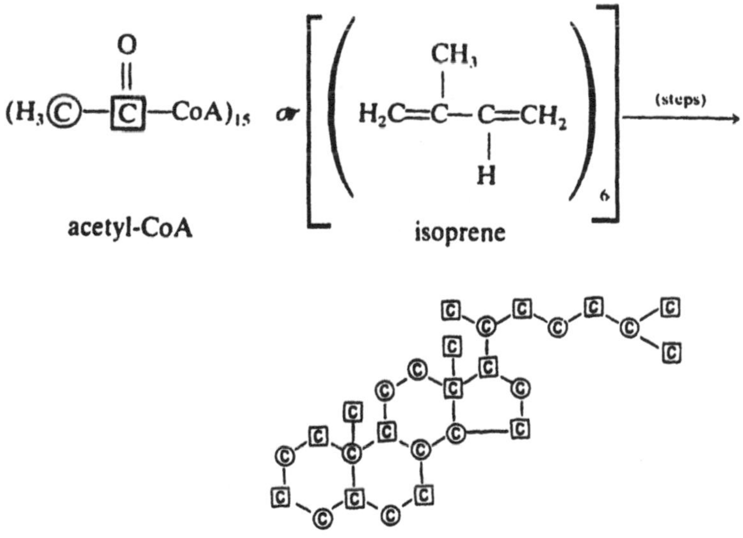

cholesterol carbon skeleton

◯ ☐ : carbons in cholesterol from acetate

Equation 13.9 Acetyl-CoA or isoprene from cholesterol.

$$18\text{acetyl-CoA} + 18\text{ATP} + 5\text{NADPH}_2 + H_2O + O_2$$

$$\xrightarrow[\,+3\text{ADP}+6P_i+6PP_i+5\text{NADP}^+ + (R\!-\!CH_3)_3\,]{\dfrac{6CO_2}{\rule{0pt}{0pt}}} \text{cholesterol}\,(C_{27})$$

Equation 13.10 Chemical summary for the synthesis of cholesterol.

Acetoacetic acid, β-hydroxybutyric acid, and acetone, "the ketones," which normally do not accumulate metabolically, are alternative end products to cholesterol and fatty acid synthesis from acetyl-CoA. In the diabetic, these ketones accumulate, owing to the absence of insulin and excessive β-oxidation. If the diabetic state remains uncorrected, accumulating ketones, acids, and electrolyte abnormalities may lead to ketoacidosis, coma, and death. The ketones are also formed during fasting and starvation states, during gestation, and may occur postsurgically in response to ether anesthesia. Lack of insulin in the Type I diabetic person leads to the lack of glucose in most cells of the body. The cells are therefore dependent on utilization of fatty acids for energy. As the lack of glucose in the cells results in lower levels of citric cycle intermediates, and thus less use of the citric acid cycle, more of the acetyl-CoA enters the alternate metabolic pathway of ketone formation.

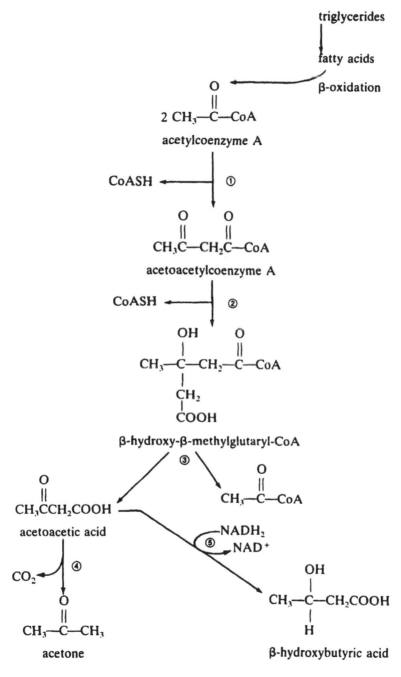

Figure 13.4 Synthesis of ketones from acetyl coenzyme A. 1. Condensation 2. β-Hydroxy-β-methylglutaryl-CoA synthetase 3. Cleavage 4. Acetoacetic decarboxylase 5. Acetoacetic reductase.

CHAPTER 14

Nucleic Acids, Genes, and Protein Synthesis

PURINES

The purines (adenine and guanine), components of the nucleic acids and hypoxanthine, are synthesized from three amino acids, carboxybiotin, and the N^{10}-formyl and N^5,N^{10}-methenyl derivatives of tetrahydrofolic acid (Figure 14.1). Six ATPs are consumed in the synthesis of the initial purine derivative, inosine monophosphate (IMP). The ATPs are expended in the incorporation of glycine, the nitrogens from aspartic acid and glutamine, and the activation of ribose-5-phosphate, forming 5-phosphoribosyl-1-pyrophosphate, which phosphorylates the mononucleotide, IMP (Figure 14.2). Figure 14.2 shows the pathway for the synthesis of adenosine monophosphate (AMP) and guanosine monophosphate (GMP) from IMP. Additional amounts of ATP are expended in synthesizing AMP and GMP. Two additional ATPs are consumed in converting each of the mononucleotides into trinucleotides with a total of 10 ATPs expended in the synthesis of one molecule of guanine triphosphate, GTP.

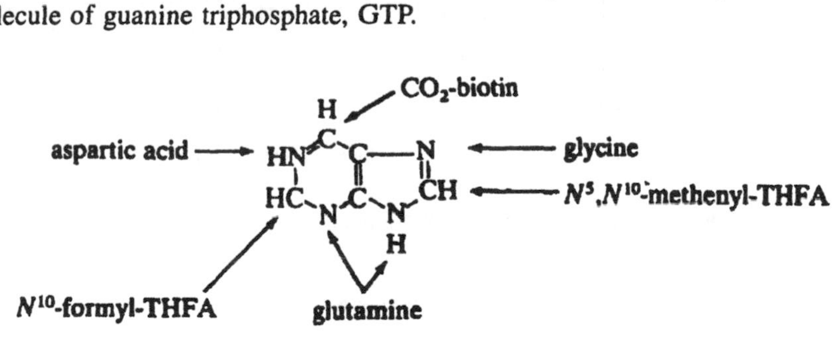

Figure 14.1 Synthesis of purines.

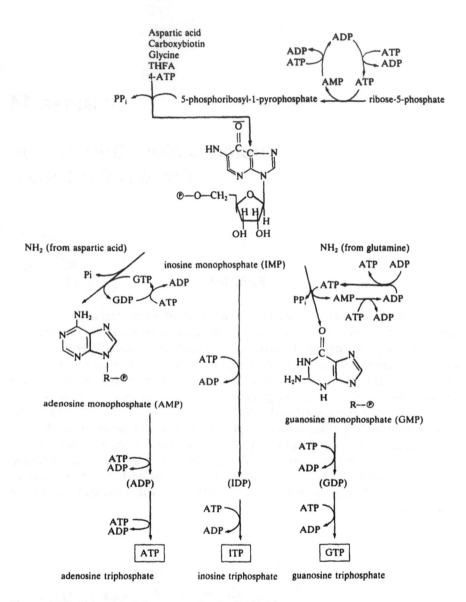

Figure 14.2 Abbreviated *de novo* synthesis of purines.

PYRIMIDINES

Pyrimidine (Figure 14.3) (cytosine, thymine, and uracil) components of the nucleic acids are synthesized from carbamoyl phosphate and aspartic acid (see urea cycle discussion in Chapter 12). Four ATPs are consumed in the synthesis of the initial pyrimidine derivative, uridine monophosphate (UMP). Two ATPs are consumed in the cytosolic synthesis of carbamoyl phosphate and two additional ATPs

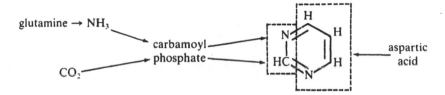

Figure 14.3 Synthesis of pyrimidines.

are consumed in the formation of the ribotide UMP (Figure 14.4). Cytidine triphosphate is derived from UTP with expenditure of an additional ATP for incorporating its amine being derived from glutamine. Thymidine triphosphate (TPP), through a series of metabolic steps, is derived from UMP and UTP, which yields pyrophosphate. N^5,N^{10}- methyltetrahydrofolic acid, probably in association with vitamin B_{12}, donates its methyl group in the synthesis of thymidine monophosphate (TMP) from UTP. TMP is then phosphorylated by two ATPs forming TTP. Nine ATPs are ultimately expended in the *de novo* synthesis of one molecule of thymidine triphosphate, TPP.

NUCLEOTIDES

Nucleotides (nucleic acids) are ubiquitous in animal and human diets, but they are not dietarily essential, as they are synthesized from rather simple components. The nucleic acids deoxyribonucleic acid (DNA) and ribonucleic acid (RNA) are carriers of cellular genetic information. The nucleic acid adenosine triphosphate (ATP) is the universal carrier of metabolic energy, and adenine is also found as a component of several coenzymes, including NAD^+ ($NADP^+$), FAD, CoA, and cyclic AMP. The building blocks of the nucleic acids are the nitrogenous heterocyclic bases, derivatives of purines or pyrimidines. Addition of the carbohydrates, ribose or deoxyribose, to a nitrogen base produces a nucleoside. Nucleosides with one phosphate moiety are called nucleotides. Adenosine mononucleotide, for example, is AMP. Additional phosphates yield the nucleotides adenosine diphosphate (ADP) and adenosine triphosphate (ATP). Names of purine and pyrimidine bases, and nucleosides and nucleotides, are given in Table 14.1.

DEOXYRIBONUCLEIC AND RIBONUCLEIC ACID

The previous sections of this chapter have shown how energy (ATP) is used in the *de novo* synthesis of the purine and pyrimidine trinucleotides. In this section we examine how the high-energy trinucleotides are used in the synthesis of deoxyribonucleic acid (DNA) and ribonucleic acid (RNA). DNA is a polymer assembled from the trinucleotides, dATP, dGTP, dCTP, and dTTP, in which the carbohydrate ribose has been reduced by $NADPH_2$, forming 2-deoxyribose (dADP) (Equation 14.1).

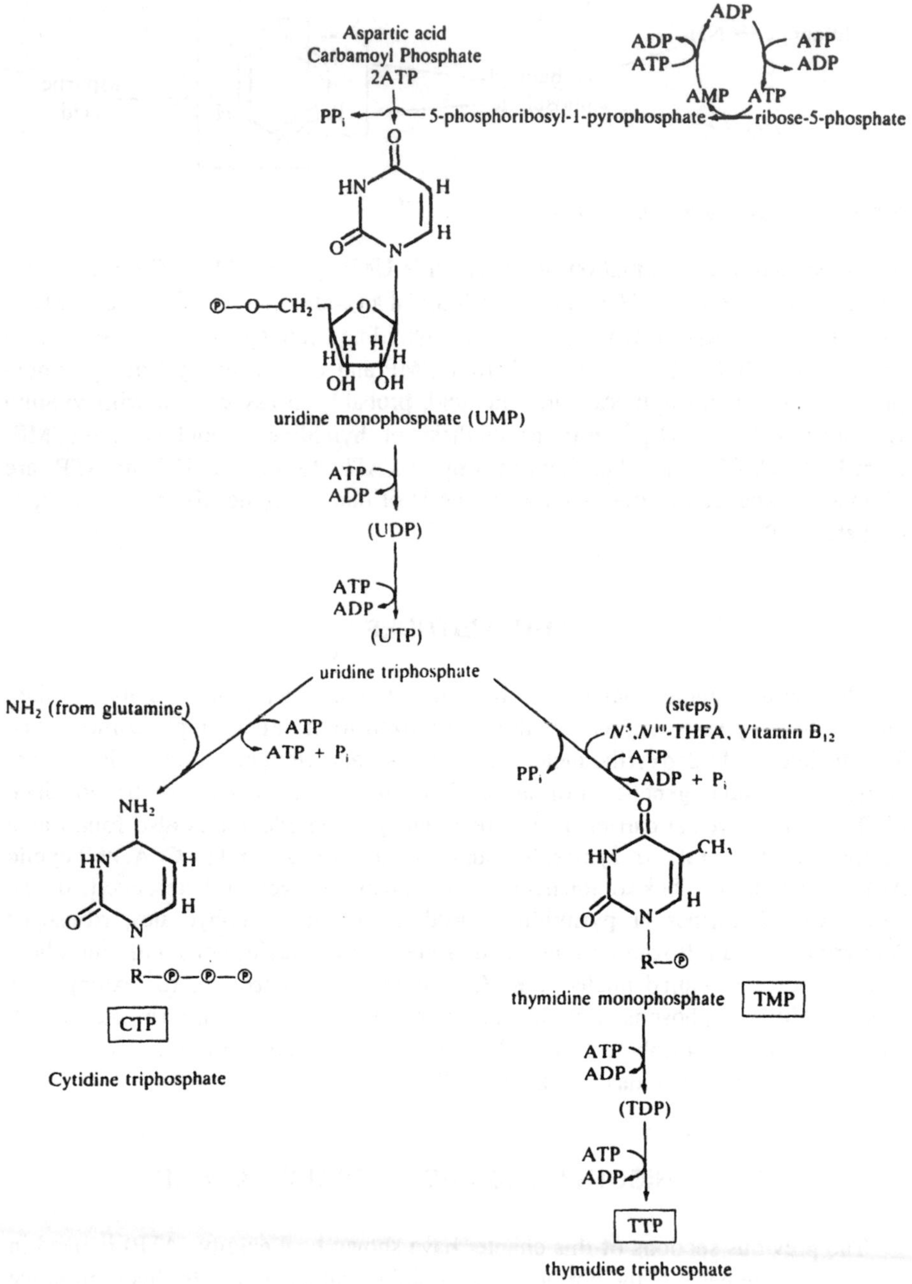

Aspartic acid
Carbamoyl Phosphate
2ATP

ADP
ADP — ATP
ATP — ADP
AMP ATP

PP_i ← 5-phosphoribosyl-1-pyrophosphate ← ribose-5-phosphate

O
HN — H
O — H
N

$\textcircled{P}$—O—CH$_2$ O
H H H H
OH OH

uridine monophosphate (UMP)

ATP
ADP
(UDP)

ATP
ADP
(UTP)

uridine triphosphate

NH$_2$ (from glutamine)

ATP
ATP + P$_i$

(steps)
N^5,N^{10}-THFA, Vitamin B$_{12}$
ATP
ADP + P$_i$

PP_i

NH$_2$
HN — H
O — H
N
R—$\textcircled{P}$—$\textcircled{P}$—$\textcircled{P}$

CTP

Cytidine triphosphate

O
HN CH$_3$
O — H
N
R—$\textcircled{P}$

thymidine monophosphate TMP

ATP
ADP
(TDP)

ATP
ADP
TTP

thymidine triphosphate

Figure 14.4 Abbreviated *de novo* synthesis of pyrimidines.

Table 14.1 Nomenclature of the Nucleic Acids

Heterocyclics	Nitrogen Bases	Nucleosides	Mononucleotides	Dinucleotides	Trinucleotides
Purine(s)	Adenine	Adenosine	Adenosine monophosphate (AMP)	(ADP)	(ATP)
	Guanine	Guanosine	Guanosine monophosphate (GMP)	(GDP)	(GTP)
	Hypoxanthine	Inosine	Inosine monophosphate (IMP)	(IDP)	(ITP)
Pyrimidine(s)	Cytosine	Cytidine	Cytidine monophosphate (CMP)	(CDP)	(CTP)
	Thymine	Thymidine	Thymidine monophosphate (TMP)	(TDP)	(TTP)
	Uracil	Uridine	Uridine monophosphate (UMP)	(UDP)	(UTP)

$$
\underset{\text{ribose (ADP)}}{
\begin{array}{c}
\text{adenine} \\
\textcircled{P}\text{—O—}\textcircled{P}\text{—O—}CH_2 \\
\end{array}
}
\xrightarrow[\text{NADPH, NADP}^+]{H_2O}
\underset{\text{2-deoxyribose (ADP)}}{
\begin{array}{c}
\text{adenine} \\
\textcircled{P}\text{—O—}\textcircled{P}\text{—}CH_2 \\
\end{array}
}
$$

Equation 14.1　Synthesis of 2-deoxyribose (dADP).

RNA is a polymer assembled from the trinucleotides ATP, GTP, CTP, and UTP. RNA differs from DNA in that the base thymidine is replaced by uracil and the carbohydrate ribose is utilized in place of 2-deoxyribose. The remaining structural differences between DNA and RNA are that DNA is predominantly double stranded, while RNA exists primarily in single-stranded form. Three forms of RNA have been distinguished in nature: messenger RNA (mRNA), transfer RNA (tRNA; sometimes referred to as soluble or sRNA), and ribosomal RNA (rRNA). Each form of RNA participates and functions differently in protein synthesis. RNA and DNA are structurally similar in that the phosphodiester linkage between ribose or 2-deoxyribose exists in 5′→3′ linkage. As DNA is predominantly double stranded, hydrogen bonding takes place between the complementary base pairs: adenine (A) and thymine (T), and guanine (G) and cytosine (C).

DNA is complementarily copied from a DNA template in a process called replication (Figure 14.5). In this process one strand of the double-stranded DNA serves as a template and the complementary base trinucleotides hydrogen bonds to its complement with the formation of the 5′→3′ phosphodiester bond being established. As the phosphodiester bond is formed, pyrophosphate (PP$_i$) is eliminated. DNA as well as RNA are therefore a polymer of mononucleotides. The energy used to synthesize the polymer exists within the trinucleotides prior to polymerization.

RNA is also complementarily copied from a DNA template. The difference between the DNA and the RNA is that the trinucleotides forming the RNA contain ribose and not 2-deoxyribose, and the pyrimidine uracil (as UTP) replaces thymine (as TTP) by the RNA polymerase. The process of complementarily copying DNA by RNA polymers and forming messenger RNA (mRNA) is called transcription. From DNA originates also the various transfer RNA (tRNA) molecules and ribosomal RNA (rRNA). Two molecules of ATP are therefore expended in adding one mononucleotide in establishing a 5′→3′ phosphodiester bond, extending either DNA or RNA by one nucleotide. This is demonstrated for cytosine monophosphate (CMP) and DNA in Equation 14.2.

GENES, CODONS, ANTICODONS, AND tRNAs

The sequence of nitrogen bases along the DNA molecule ultimately determines the amino acid sequence of a specific protein. This statement is the basis of the one gene–one protein theory of genetic regulation of protein synthesis of François Jacob

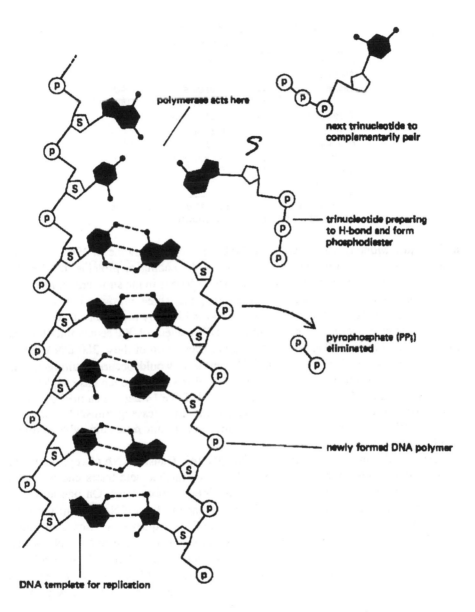

Figure 14.5 DNA replication.

$$dCMP + ATP \rightarrow dCDP + ADP$$

$$dCDP + ATP \rightarrow dCTP + ADP$$

$$dCTP(CTP) + DNA(RNA) \rightarrow DNA - dCMP \text{ or } RNA - CMP$$

$$5' \rightarrow 3' \text{ phosphodiester bond formed.}$$

Equation 14.2 Extension of nucleic acids (DNA and RNA) by one nucleotide.

Table 14.2 Codons of the Amino Acids Commonly Found in Proteins[a]

Glycine	GGU	Phenylalanine	UUU
Alanine	GCC	Proline	CCU
Valine	GUU	Histidine	CAU
Leucine	CUU	Aspartic acid	GAU
Threonine	ACU	Glutamic acid	GAA
Serine	UCU	Lysine	AAA
Methionine	AUG	Argine	AGA
Selenocysteine	UGA	Asparagine	AAU
Cysteine	UGU	Glutamine	GAA
Tyrosine	UGG		

[a] Some amino acids have more than one codon; for simplicity, only one codon is shown.

and Jacques Monod, who received the Nobel Prize in Medicine in 1965. The one gene–one protein theory provides not only for the coding of proteins, but for the control of protein synthesis. Our primary interest here is in the structural component of the (gene) DNA sequence. Within every gene, three nitrogen bases pair in sequence along the DNA code for one amino acid. Thus a protein of 100 amino acids would have a structural gene within a cell's nucleus of 300 sequential nitrogen bases coding for the 100 amino acids. During translation of these 300 DNA bases, complementary base pairing and mRNA synthesis would occur, resulting in the transfer of coded information to mRNA. Each of the 100 nitrogen base triplets is a codon that codes information for one amino acid. Table 14.2 gives an mRNA codon for each of the amino acids commonly found in protein. Messenger mRNA is directed from the cell's nucleus to the ribosomes of the endoplasmic reticulum, where protein synthesis occurs.

Derived also from DNA is transfer RNA (tRNA). Transfer RNA of approximately 80 mononucleotides may contain several unusual nucleic acid bases and is folded back upon itself in paper-clip fashion, with three or more arms. On one arm of a tRNA molecule is a complementary base sequence to the mRNA codon: the anti-codon. Attached to the tRNA through a terminal CCA sequence of bases is an amino acid. For each amino acid found in protein there is at least one specific tRNA which transfers that specified amino acid to the ribosome. The amino acids are activated by attachment to its specific tRNA, as shown in Equation 14.3. Two ATP equivalents are required to activate each amino acid, forming an amino-acyl-tRNA prior to peptide (protein) synthesis.

PROTEIN SYNTHESIS

Protein synthesis occurs in the rough endoplasmic reticulum (RER) of the cell's cytoplasm in association with ribosomes. Ribosomes, composed of rRNA and protein, are the focal point for the *de novo* synthesis of protein. It is at the ribosome that activated aminoacyl-tRNAs bearing their amino acids and mRNA come together to form a protein in the translation process. The ribosomes, moving along an mRNA,

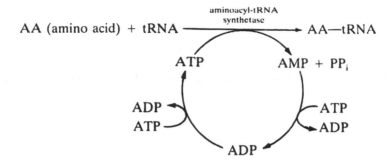

Equation 14.3 Amino acid activation.

keys in the anticodon of each tRNA to the complementary base pair with each codon along the mRNA. As the translational process occurs, peptide bonds are formed between amino acids in a growing polypeptide chain. The polypeptide is synthesized from the terminal free amine and as each amino acid is added to the growing polypeptide chain, the tRNA is cleaved from the amino acid which it had carried to the ribosome. Energy is required for the synthesis of each peptide bond in the new polypeptide chain and for the movement (translocation) of the ribosome along the mRNA. The energy for these events is provided by the aminoacyl- (activated) tRNA and two molecules of GTP. These reactions, summarized in Equation 14.4, take place within the ribosome. Two GTPs (two ATP equivalents) are expended in the elongation of a polypeptide chain by a single amino acid in the process of translation. Energy provided by the aminoacyl-tRNA, equivalent to two ATPs, is also expended in the synthesis of the new peptide bond, accounting for a total energy expenditure equivalent to four ATPs for the addition of each amino acid in polypeptide elongation.

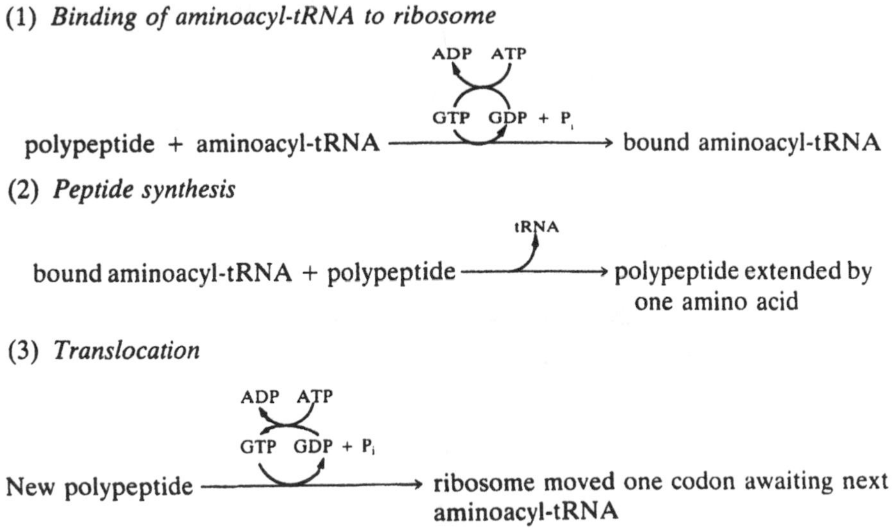

(1) *Binding of aminoacyl-tRNA to ribosome*

ADP ATP

GTP GDP + P$_i$

polypeptide + aminoacyl-tRNA ⟶ bound aminoacyl-tRNA

(2) *Peptide synthesis*

tRNA

bound aminoacyl-tRNA + polypeptide ⟶ polypeptide extended by
                                        one amino acid

(3) *Translocation*

ADP ATP

GTP GDP + P$_i$

New polypeptide ⟶ ribosome moved one codon awaiting next
                    aminoacyl-tRNA

Equation 14.4 Energy requirements for peptide synthesis and translocation.

$$\text{polypeptide} + \text{amino acid} + 4\text{ATP} \longrightarrow \text{polypeptide} + 1\,\text{amino acid} + 4\text{ADP} + 4P_i$$

Equation 14.5 Summary of energy requirement for peptide synthesis.

These reactions are summarized in Equation 14.5. Thus, it may be appreciated that much of the ATP formed in the catabolic pathways is used in the *de novo* synthesis of nitrogen bases and nucleic acids, in the activation of amino acids, and in the formation of the new proteins (Figure 14.6).

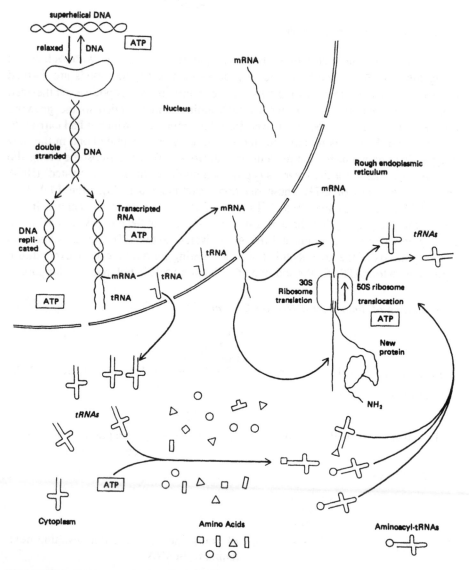

Figure 14.6 Energy use in protein synthesis.

Metabolic Aspects

CHAPTER 15

Free Radicals, Lipid Peroxidation, and the Antioxidants

TOXIC OXYGEN SPECIES

On earth, most life exists in a toxic atmosphere of oxygen. Oxygen is so toxic that an anaerobic organism can exist only in its absence. Aerobic organisms, including humans, require oxygen for cellular respiration and have concurrently evolved chemical and enzymatic systems to thwart the toxicity of oxygen and its reactive oxygen species.

Oxygen (really dioxygen) is an oxidant with an affinity for electrons and hydrogen. This fact is apparent in the mitochondrion, where oxygen accepts electrons and protons, forming metabolic water at the terminal end of the electron transport chain. This oxidative process is both desirable and normal. It is when dioxygen or one of its active reduced products uncontrollably and randomly oxidizes other biological molecules, such as lipid components of membranes, that biological damage is done. It is the oxidation of lipids, nucleic acids, proteins, and other molecules by oxygen and the reactive species of oxygen that is believed by many, but not all scientists, to be the molecular basis of aging. Such reactive oxygen species are initially produced by a single electron reduction of oxygen. From the approximately 250 grams of oxygen consumed each day by the average adult and reduced to metabolic water, an estimated 4% of the oxygen consumed forms superoxide (O_2^-) (Equation 15.1).

$$O_2^+ \xleftarrow{-e-} O_2 \xrightarrow{e-} O_2^- \xrightarrow{e-} O_2^{2-} + 2H^+ \longrightarrow H_2O_2 \xrightarrow[M^{2+}]{-e-} \begin{array}{c} \cdot OH \\ OH^- \end{array} \xrightarrow{RH} H_2O$$

$$O_2 \xrightarrow{h\nu} {}^1O_2$$

Equation 15.1 Pathway for the synthesis of superoxide and other reactive oxygen species.

Table 15.1 Reactive Oxygen Species

Oxygen Species	Name
O_2	Oxygen (dioxygen)
O_2^-	Superoxide
$^1O_2$	Singlet oxygen
H_2O_2	Hydrogen peroxide
$\cdot OH$	Hydroxyl radical
O_3	Ozone (environmental pollutant)
RO_2H	Organic peroxide
NO_2	Nitrogen dioxide

The most important species of reactive oxygen in biological systems are given in Table 15.1. Oxygen, superoxide anion, singlet oxygen, hydrogen peroxide, and the hydroxyl radical are all potentially reactive and capable of oxidizing organic molecules (RH), particularly unsaturated hydrocarbons. Peroxidation of mono- or polyunsaturated fatty acids (oxidation) is the cause of fats and oils becoming rancid, the cause of damage to cell membranes, and is perhaps a component of aging itself. Lipid peroxidation is caused by an initiator, an environmental component that induces formation of an organic free radical $(R\cdot)$, or one of the reactive species of oxygen (Table 15.1) which may react with an organic molecule, also initiating an organic free radical. The environmental initiators of lipid peroxidation *in vitro* include the presence of oxygen and trace metals, the absence of antioxidants, and moderate to high temperatures. Lipid peroxidation of cells *in vivo* is initiated by a variety of natural and environmental initiators. Since body temperature of most vertebrates is regulated, lipid peroxidation is initiated and occurs at a constant temperature. Table 15.2 lists some *in vitro* and *in vivo* initiators of lipid peroxidation.

Table 15.2 Initiators of Lipid Peroxidation

In Vitro (Fats and Oils)	*In Vivo* (Living Cells)
Oxygen	Oxygen
Metals	Ultraviolet radiation
High temperatures	X-irradiation
Ultraviolet light (?)	Metals: Fe, Cu; heavy metals: Pd, Cd, Hg, Ag
	Superoxide anion
	Singlet oxygen
	Hydrogen peroxide
	Hydroxyl radical
	Organic peroxide
	Ozone
	Nitrogen dioxide
	Alcohol
	Smoke (from cigarettes and other combustibles)
	Organic halogens
	Enzymes (e.g., glucose oxidase)
	Some drugs

Whereas lipid peroxidation is initiated by a number of species of oxygen derivatives, many endogenous metals and enzymes can either initiate directly, or be produced from organic substrates of these highly reactive and toxic oxygen derivatives, which cause lipid peroxidation. Many environmental factors, such as cigarette smoke, polluted air containing ozone, oxides of nitrogen, chlorinated hydrocarbons, and heavy metals (see Chapter 6) when inhaled, cause lipid peroxidation and damage living tissues. Either intensive or extensive exposure to ultraviolet light and x-irradiation can cause cellular peroxidation and when extreme, even cell death. Clearly, endogenous and environmental initiators of lipid peroxidation are diverse and extensive.

The result of lipid peroxidation by these initiators is membrane and genetic damage (i.e., aging), with the formation of degradative lipid products. The products of lipid peroxidation (Figure 15.1) are ethane, pentane, malondialdehyde, and lipofusion pigments. Ethane (C_2H_6) and pentane (C_5H_{12}) are gases formed as a result of lipid peroxidation and scission, and are exhaled.

CHAIN REACTIONS: ETHANE, PENTANE, MALONDIALDEHYDE, AND LIPOFUSION SYNTHESIS

Malondialdehyde is one of several aldehydes and ketones that may be synthesized from unsaturated fatty acids by scission of lipid hydroperoxides. Malondialdehyde is capable of acting as a cross-linking agent of protein and DNA, which contributes to cellular damage and the formation of lipofusion. Lipofusion pigments are fluorescent protein-derived molecules not found in young cells, but which accumulate in cells roughly proportionate with time. Such pigment formation and cellular deposition is thought to be associated with aging. Malondialdehyde, because it can cross-link protein to DNA, is at least mutagenic and may be carcinogenic.

In addition to lipid peroxidation, resulting in the formation of gases, malondialdehyde, and lipofusion, it may also result (if undetected) in the synthesis of other free radicals, as shown in Equation 15.2. Once lipid peroxidation is initiated, a single free radical can lead to the formation of many other free radicals and more ethane and pentane, more malondialdehyde, more lipofusion pigments, and so on. Such uncontrolled free-radical events are called chain reactions, and these reactions may continue until the reaction is quenched. Quenching is the elimination of the presence of a free radical. A chain reaction is given schematically in Equation 15.2.

Following initiation of lipid peroxidation, the formation of an organic peroxy free radical (ROO·) and an organic hydroperoxide (ROOH) can rapidly lead to a variety of new species of free radicals (R·, RO·, and ·OH) which in chain reactions result in the oxidation of still other molecules. These free-radical events are kept as low as possible by not allowing a lot of "free" oxygen to be available in tissues to promote uncontrolled oxidations. The diet provides a variety of antioxidants to cells which prevent free-radical reactions from being sustained. *In vivo*, additions to the dietary antioxidant armament are formed as cells synthesize molecules and enzymes which eliminate the cellular presence of most reactive oxygen species that initiate lipid peroxidation. These dietary factors and endogenous molecules and enzymes

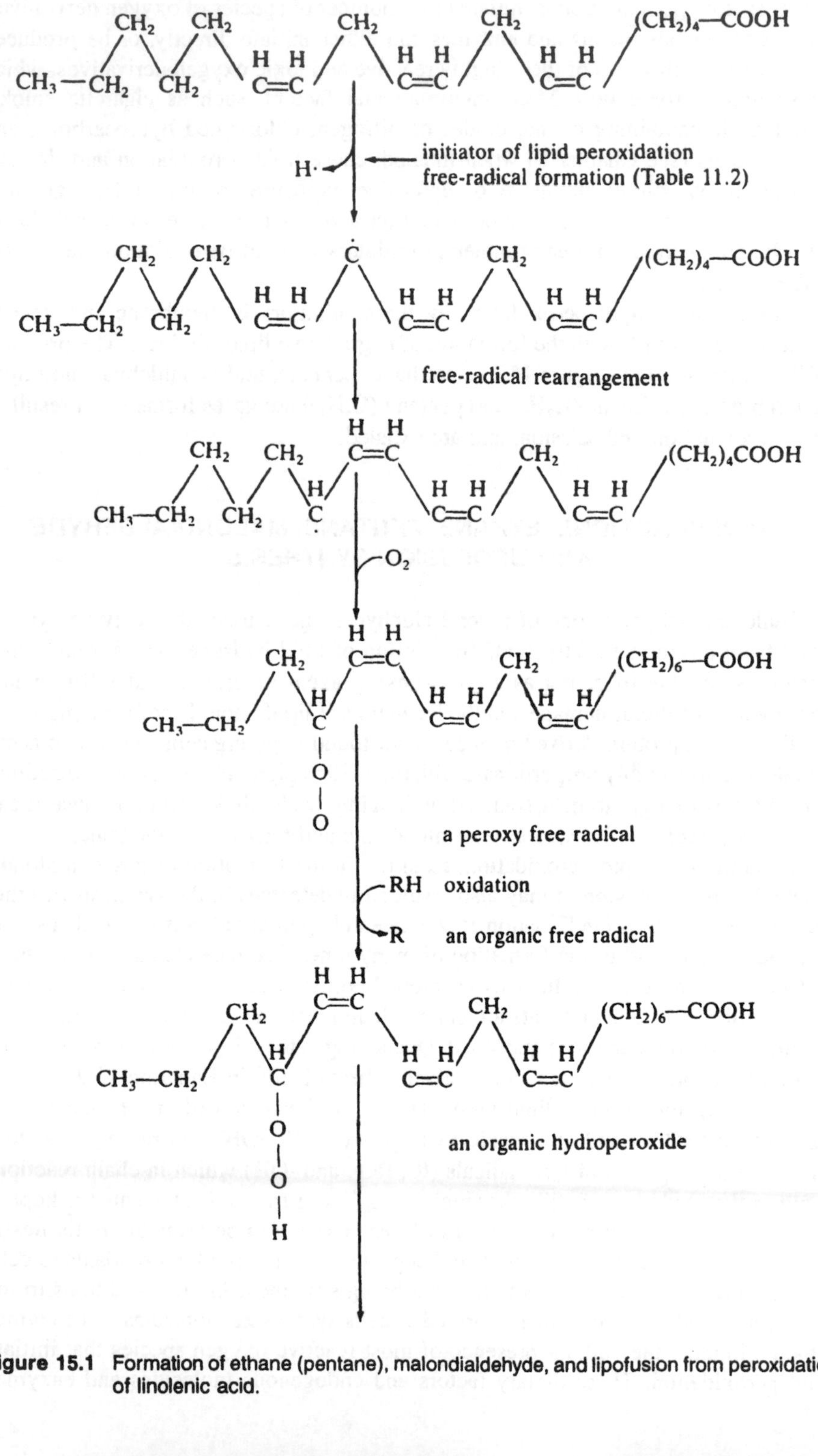

Figure 15.1 Formation of ethane (pentane), malondialdehyde, and lipofusion from peroxidation of linolenic acid.

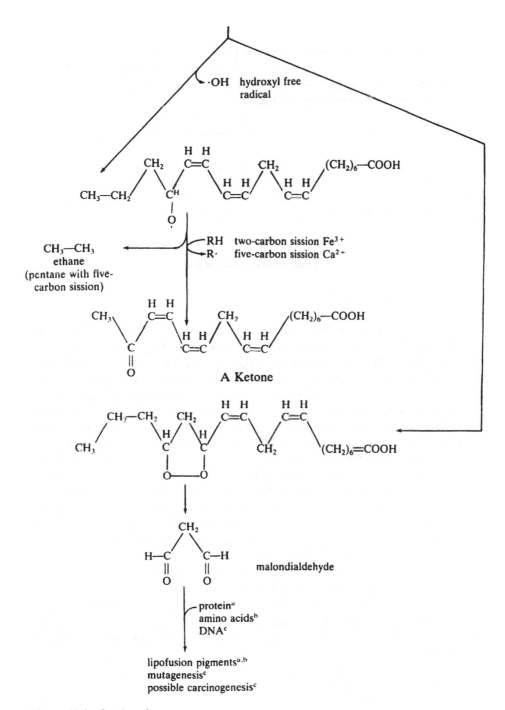

Figure 15.1 *Continued.*

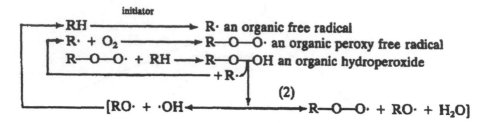

Equation 15.2 A chain reaction and lipid peroxidation.

are the cell's defenses against peroxidation and cell damage, which are collectively referred to as the antioxidant defense system of cells.

THE ANTIOXIDANTS

Antioxidants: Introduction

All cells contain endogenous initiators of lipid peroxidation and are also subject to a variety of environmental insults which, upon generating organic or inorganic free radicals, can lead to membrane damage and mutations that may contribute to aging and even produce cell death. These same cells contain antioxidants, a variety of molecules and macromolecules whose purpose is to prevent lipid peroxidation by either breaking free-radical chain reactions or preventing the cellular accumulation of the toxic molecular species of oxygen. The cellular antioxidant armamentarium can be divided into four classes of molecules. Group 1 molecules include the natural dietary antioxidants; group 2, the antioxidants found in foods as additives; group 3, the small-molecular-weight antioxidants synthesized by cells; and group 4, the antioxidant enzymes synthesized by cells. Table 15.3 lists these antioxidants.

Molecules found naturally in foods — vitamins A, C, E, β-carotene, and other carotenoids — are the cell's first line of defense against free-radical reactions, peroxidation, and cellular damage. These molecules protect the cell against peroxidation by becoming oxidized themselves, reacting with the toxic species of oxygen when they are found in the cell's cytoplasm, organelles, or membrane. They are free-radical traps that quench free-radical species such as superoxide ($O_2^{\cdot-}$) formed by a single electron reduction of oxygen. Each antioxidant vitamin generally protects a certain part of the cell and some antioxidants are found predominantly in certain types of cells. Vitamins A, E, β-carotene, and other carotenoids, because they are lipid-soluble, seem to protect cell membranes. They are the free-radical traps in membranes. Vitamin A and β-carotene are particularly effective in protecting ectodermal tissue: skin and the tissues lining the oral cavity and gastrointestinal tract. Vitamin C, being water-soluble, complements the lipid-soluble antioxidants by trapping free radicals in the aqueous portion of cells, the cytoplasm. Vitamin C is so easily oxidized that it may even help to protect vitamins A and E and even β-carotene from oxidation. The importance of vitamins C and E in protecting cell membranes and cytoplasmic components from oxidative damage is seen in the sparing effect of

Table 15.3 Antioxidants Found in Foods and Synthesized *De Novo* by Cells

Natural antioxidants in foods	Antioxidant food additives
Vitamin A	BHT (butylated hydroxytoluene)
β-Carotene, lycopene, and other	BHA (butylated hydroxyanisole)
carotenoids	Sodium benzoate
Vitamin C	Ethoxyquin
Vitamin E	Propyl galate
Minerals contributing to antioxidant enzymes	
Selenium	
Manganese	
Copper	
Zinc	
Iron	
Antioxidants synthesized by cells	Antioxidant enzymes synthesized by cells
Glutathione	Glutathione peroxidase
Cysteine	Phospholipidhydroperoxide glutathione
Uric acid	peroxidase
Hydroquinones	Glutathione-S-transferase
	Catalase
	CuZn-superoxide dismutase
	Mn-superoxide dismutase
	Fe-superoxide dismutase (bacterial)

both vitamins. It has been known for some time that vitamin C could replenish oxidized vitamin E, restoring membrane antioxidant protection. The reverse is also true in some tissues in that vitamin E at the membrane–cytoplasmic interface can restore oxidized vitamin C. Thus the functions of vitamin C in the cytoplasm and vitamin E in the membrane are not totally exclusive based upon solubility. These antioxidants are inclusive in protecting cells *in toto* from oxidative damage.

Figure 15.2 shows the proposed pathways for free-radical chain reactions following initiation, formation of hydrogen and lipid peroxides, and the points of prevention of cellular oxidation by the major antioxidants. The small dietary food additives and cellularly synthesized antioxidants are shown to block initiation and break closed-loop free-radical-chain reactions. The enzymes present in the cytoplasm and organelles of cells serve to protect the cells by catalytic elimination of superoxide by superoxide dismutase, hydrogen, and organic hydroperoxides by glutathione peroxidase, phospholipidhydroperoxide glutathione peroxidase, and catalase.

As an example of the action of antioxidants, free-radical trapping by vitamin E (α-tocopherol) is shown in Figure 15.3. One vitamin E molecule readily accepts two free radicals, either from superoxide or the organic peroxy radical. One electron oxidation of vitamin E results in the formation of an intermediate methyl-tocopheryl radical. This free radical is long lived relative to other free radicals and nonreactive. A complete two-electron reduction of vitamin E results in the formation of the tocophenyl quinone. The one-electron methyl-tocopheryl radical may be reduced by cellular glutathione, or as noted above, by vitamin C at the cytoplasmic–membrane interface. Vitamin E is normally present in cell membranes in a 1:1000 ratio with polyunsaturated fatty acids. Its absence from the diet leads to a decrease in vitamin C and an increase in the cellular production of ethane and pentane, malondialdehyde, and lipofusion pigments.

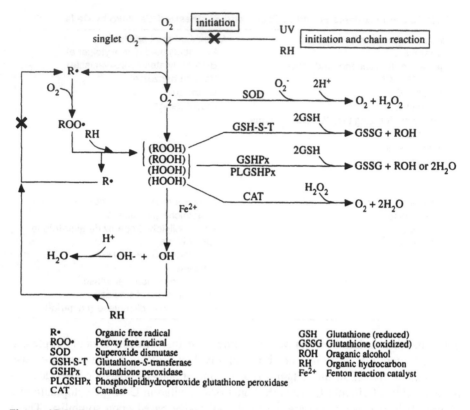

R•   Organic free radical   GSH   Glutathione (reduced)
ROO•   Peroxy free radical   GSSG   Glutathione (oxidized)
SOD   Superoxide dismutase   ROH   Oraganic alcohol
GSH-S-T   Glutathione-S-transferase   RH   Organic hydrocarbon
GSHPx   Glutathione peroxidase   Fe²⁺   Fenton reaction catalyst
PLGSHPx   Phospholipidhydroperoxide glutathione peroxidase
CAT   Catalase

Figure 15.2 Free-radical chain reactions and their prevention.

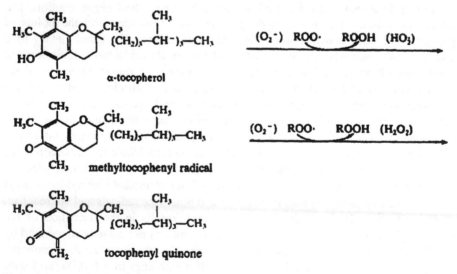

Figure 15.3 Antioxidant function of vitamin E. (Reproduced from *Nutrition of the Chicken*, with permission of M. Scott, Publisher, Ithaca, N.Y., 1977.)

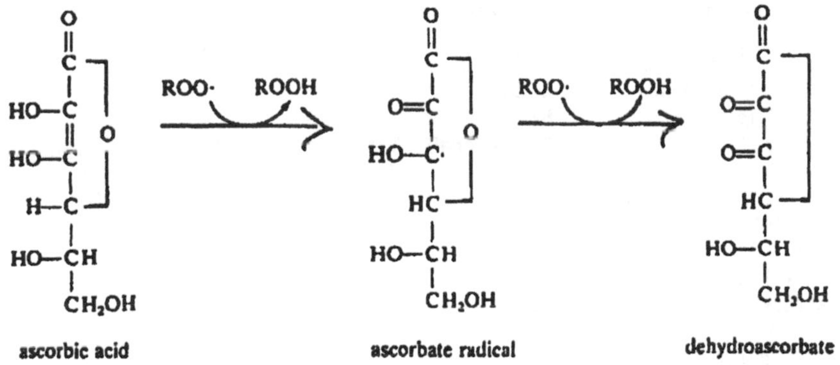

Figure 15.4 Antioxidant function of ascorbic acid.

Vitamin C, ascorbic acid, may be both an intracellular quencher of free radicals and an extracellular quencher of free radicals for the epithelial cellular lining of the lung. Intracellular ascorbate quenches the superoxide free radical, the organic peroxy free radical, and possibly the hydroxyl free radical. In the lung, ascorbate protects against free radicals generated from smoke, oxygen, and ozone. Ascorbate also protects organs from the peroxidative damage of drugs, chlorinated hydrocarbons, and peroxides.

Like vitamin E, ascorbic acid readily oxidizes and quenches free radicals in a two-electron process (Figure 15.4). Carotenoids and β-carotene in particular, like vitamins C and E, are effective quenchers of free-radical reactions *in vivo* in which (double) bonding electrons are oxidized. More importantly, β-carotene quenches induction of free radicals by ultraviolet light, a property not shared by any of the other antioxidants. β-carotene in skin blocks these free-radical chain reactions from occurring by quenching singlet oxygen. This reaction, unique to β-carotene, is shown in Figure 15.5. In this reaction, UV light interacting with oxygen produces excited singlet ($^1O_2$) oxygen. Singlet oxygen, instead of producing free radicals, interacts with β-carotene, transferring its energy to form "energized β-carotene." The UV energy present in β-carotene is dissipated from the molecule as heat.

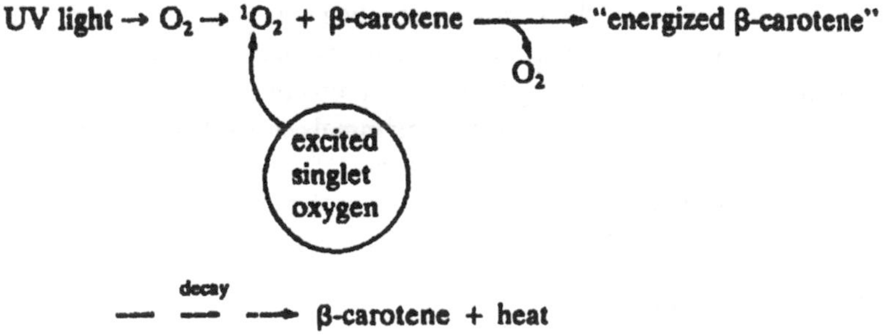

Figure 15.5 Quenching singlet oxygen by β-carotene.

Table 15.4 Antioxidant Enzymes Found in Aerobic Cells

Enzyme	Mineral	Reaction
Superoxide dismutase (EC 1.15.1.1) MW 32,500	CuZn Mn Fe (bacterial)	$2O_2^- + 2H^+ \rightarrow O_2 + H_2O_2$
Glutathione peroxidase	Se	$H_2O_2 + 2GSH \rightarrow GSSG + 2H_2O$
Phospholipidhydroperoxide glutathione peroxidase (EC 1.11.1.9) MW 84,000	Se Se	$ROOH + 2GSH \rightarrow GSSG + ROH + H_2O$
Catalase (EC 1.11.1.6) MW 250,000	Fe	$2H_2O_2 \rightarrow 2H_2O + O_2$
Glutathione-S-transferases (EC 2.5.1.18) MW various	—	$ROOH + 2GSH \rightarrow GSSG + ROH + H_2O$

Vitamin A, like β-carotene, vitamin C, and vitamin E, can also act as an anti-oxidant and quench free-radical reactions, but unlike β-carotene, it does not quench singlet-oxygen reactions. Other antioxidants added to foods such as butylated hydroxyanisole (BHA), or butylated hydroxytoluene (BHT), sodium benzoate, and so on, function similarly to the examples given for vitamins E and C in protecting cells from free-radical damage.

Antioxidant Enzymes

There exists in aerobic cells enzymes that act catalytically on free-radical sub-strates, and peroxides that generate free radicals, protecting cells from oxidative damage. These enzymes, which are present in the cytoplasm, are the superoxide dismutases and peroxidases. Four of these enzymes contain at least one mineral which participates in the dismutation of the superoxide anion or the reduction of peroxides. Table 15.4 provides data on each of these enzymes and shows the catalytic reaction in which it participates.

Superoxide Dismutase

Superoxide dismutase (SOD) catalyzes the dismutation of the superoxide anion into oxygen and hydrogen peroxide. This enzyme is ubiquitous in nature in aerobic cells in the mitochondria, providing them with protection from the superoxide free radical. Two SOD enzymes are known in mammals, a CuZn-SOD, blue-green in color, found in the cytoplasm of cells and a Mn-SOD, reddish in color, found in the mitochondrion. A pale yellow Fe-SOD has been isolated from *E. coli*. There are no aerobic organisms, including plants, that do not possess superoxide dismutases.

Glutathione Peroxidases

There are a number of members of different enzymes referred to as glutathione peroxidases. These enzymes are structurally similar but not identical. They all function to reduce hydrogen peroxide and organic hydroperoxides to water. Commonly all of the glutathione peroxidase enzymes contain a selenium amino acid residue, selenocysteine, at the active site. The first glutathione peroxidase (GSHPx) discovered was in the cytoplasm of red blood cells. It catalyzes the reduction of H_2O_2, which is produced by SOD via the dismutation of superoxide. The reduction of H_2O_2 and ROOH by all glutathione peroxidase enzymes requires the reduced tripeptide, glutathione (GSH), as a cofactor. In mammals, including humans, these enzymes are found in many tissues and are especially concentrated in muscle and liver, all being highly exposed to oxygen.

Catalase

Catalase (CAT) catalyzes the oxidation of hydrogen peroxide producing water without the need for a cofactor. The enzyme contains heme-iron and is widely distributed in nearly all aerobic cells. Catalase and glutathione peroxidases are complementary and are redundant enzymes for reducing hydrogen peroxide formed from superoxide and superoxide dismutase.

Glutathione-S-Transferases

The glutathione-S-transferases are a family of enzymes catalyzing conjugation of glutathione to xenobiotics, drugs, and non-nutritive dietary components (Chapter 16). In addition, some enzymes of this family catalyze the reduction of organic hydroperoxides (ROOH) to alcohols. The GSH-S-transferases help to protect cells from the damage that can occur from organic hydroperoxides. Cellular levels of these enzymes can be found elevated in some tissues when glutathione peroxidase is absent.

Digestive and Metabolic Interactions Between Medications and Nutrients/Foods

MEDICATION–NUTRIENT FOOD INTERACTIONS

It is well known that many drugs, particularly when used in chronic long-term drug therapy, can affect the nutritional status of individuals for certain nutrients. Effects on appetite, digestion of food, absorption, metabolism, and excretion of nutrients are consequences of some chronic drug therapies. Conversely, foods and the specific nutrient composition of certain foods can adversely affect the desired pharmacologic action of some drugs. Clinical practitioners of medicine and dietetics should be aware of both drug–nutrient and nutrient–drug interactions. Drug–nutrient interactions can be the consequence of chronic over-the-counter (OTC) or prescription drug therapy, particularly among the elderly, who are the principal consumers of drugs. Adverse nutrient–drug interactions can have short-term effects, usually reducing drug effectiveness without serious long-term nutritional consequences. Drugs and nutrients are both chemical entities and their interaction occurs because of (1) direct chemical reactivity, (2) competitive or noncompetitive inhibition of vitamins or coenzymes with enzymes, or (3) by alteration of membrane permeability or receptor sites.

Drugs are chemical substances used as medicines or as ingredients in medicines. They may or may not be toxic, and when they are toxic, toxicity is often dose related. Nutrients are chemical substances that are ingested to support growth, maintenance, and repair of tissues. When some nutrients are ingested in excess of 150% of the RDA for that nutrient, they may have a pharmacologic action or be toxic, and are considered drugs. In such cases when nutrients can have pharmacologic activity, nutrient–nutrient metabolic interactions are possible. Interest in drug–nutrient, nutrient–drug, and nutrient–nutrient interactions is the branch of science called pharmacology. Pharmacologists study, describe, and try to understand how chemicals (i.e., drugs) interact with living organisms. These goals are not much different from those of a nutritionist — only the molecules are different. The present status of understanding the many individual drug interactions with nutrients is often extensive, and such individual details exist well beyond the imposed limitations of this chapter. Table 16.1 lists many specific drug–nutrient interactions by chemical reactivity, interference with enzymatic activity, or alteration of membrane permeability or receptive sites. Three commonly used examples of drug–nutrient interactions are described for each category of pharmacologic effect.

DIRECT CHEMICAL REACTIVITY: CHELATION OF DIVALENT OR TRIVALENT CATIONS BY TETRACYCLINE

Several drugs and nutrients react directly with minerals by chelation, a process whereby organic molecules directly bind minerals usually through coordinate covalent bonding (see Chapter 6). The chelation of calcium (Ca^{2+}) and other divalent or trivalent cations (i.e., iron, magnesium, or aluminum) by the antibiotic tetracycline (Figure 16.1) in the gastrointestinal tract may reduce absorption of both the drug and the mineral by forming the chelate. Although short-term medicinal use of tetracycline would probably have little impact on the mineral status of an individual, the effect of minerals on reducing absorption of tetracycline would restrict the antibiotic's therapeutic effectiveness, so it is recommended that tetracycline not be taken at the same time as foods or supplements which are high in calcium, iron, magnesium, or aluminum.

Other drugs acting on minerals by chelation include penicillamine and EDTA (ethylenediaminetetraacetic acid) affecting calcium, copper, iron, and zinc absorption. In the treatment of some forms of arthritis, gold (gold-thioglucose) used in therapy may affect selenium metabolism.

COMPETITIVE INHIBITION OF DIHYDROFOLATE BY METHOTREXATE

Tetrahydrofolic acid (THFA) (Chapter 5) is an important coenzyme in the synthesis of purines and pyrimidines (Chapter 14) and in one-carbon metabolism. Reduction of dihydrofolic acid (DHFA) to the active form of folic acid, THFA, is inhibited by the anticancer drug methotrexate (aminopterin), resulting in a blockage of nucleic acid synthesis. This inhibition adversely affects replication and subsequently, cellular division. The reason that methotrexate blocks THFA synthesis is that it effectively competes with and blocks the binding site of DHFA on the enzyme dihydrofolate reductase because of its structural similarity to DHFA (Figure 16.2).

Methotrexate (Amethopterin, Folex, Rheumatrex) can induce folate deficiency, resulting in megaloblastic anemia, weight loss, weakness, diarrhea, and other adverse signs or symptoms. If methotrexate is being used as a chemotherapeutic agent against

Table 16.1 Some Medications Which Have Interactions with Foods and Nutrients

Medications*	Use	Possible Interactions
Acetylsalicylic acid	Analgesic Antipyretic	Loss of iron, folate, vitamin C, anticoagulant effect in patients with vitamin K deficiency
Aluminum hydroxide (Amphojel, Alternagel)	Antacid	Decreased absorption of phosphate, fluoride, iron, magnesium, vitamin A, and thiamin; aluminum toxicity is possible
Amitriptyline (Elavil)	Tricyclic Antidepressant	Interferes with riboflavin metabolism, riboflavin deficiency possible
Amphotericin B (Fungizone)	Fungicide	Decreased plasma potassium and magnesium
Barbiturates (Amytal, Nembutal, Seconal)	Sedative Anticonvulsant	Deficiency of folate, vitamin D, and vitamin C possible
Cephalosporin (Keflex)	Antibiotic	Risk of vitamin K deficiency
Chloramphenicol (Chloromycetin)	Antibiotic	Increased need for vitamin B_6, vitamin B_{12}, folate, and vitamin K
Cholestyramine (Questran)	Hypocholesterolemic	Decreased absorption of folate; vitamins A, D, K, E, B_{12}; carotenes; triglycerides; glucose, iron; and calcium
Cimetidine (Tagamet)	Antiulcer	Impaired vitamin B_{12} absorption, monitor vitamin K status
Clofibrate (Atromid-S)	Hypolipidemic	Decreased absorption of vitamin B_{12}, carotenes, glucose, medium-chain triglycerides, iron, and electrolytes
Colchicine (Colbenemid)	Antigout	Decreased absorption of vitamin B_{12}, fat, nitrogen, carotenes, sodium, potassium, and lactose
Colestipol (Colestid)	Hypercholesterolemic	Similar to cholestyramine
Contraceptives (oral)	Birth control	Increased hemoglobin, hematocrit, serum vitamins A and E, lipids, iron, and copper
Corticosteroids	Immune suppressor Anti-inflammatory	Decreased serum vitamin C, vitamin B_{12}, folate, vitamin B_6, riboflavin, magnesium, and zinc
Coumarin (Warfarin)	Anticoagulant Vitamin K antagonist	Vitamin K decreases its effect; vitamin E may increase its effect
Cycloserine (Seromycin)	Antibiotic (antitubercular)	Decreased serum vitamin B_6, folate, and vitamin B_{12}
Digitalis (Digoxin, Lanoxin)	Cardiac glycoside	Increased calcium, magnesium, zinc, and potassium excretion; toxicity increased with potassium or magnesium deficiency
Famotidine (Pepcid)	Antiulcer	Same as cimetidine

Table 16.1 Some Medications Which Have Interactions with Foods and Nutrients *(continued)*

Medications*	Use	Possible Interactions
Furosemide (Lasix)	Loop diuretic	Increased potassium, magnesium, calcium, and sodium excretion in the urine
Glutethimide (Doriden)	Sedative	Possible vitamin D deficiency
Hydralazine (Apresoline)	Antihypertensive	Vitamin B_6 deficiency possible; supplementation may be advisable
Imipramine (Tofranil)	Antidepressant	Decreased riboflavin status
Indomethacin (Indocin)	Anti-inflammatory	May cause fluid retention and hyperkalemia
Isoniazid (INH)	Antituberculosis	Induces vitamin B_6 deficiency, 25 to 50 mg pyridoxine HCl daily recommended prophylactically; avoid histamine
		Blocks conversion of tryptophan to niacin, risk of pellagra
		Vitamin B_{12} and vitamin D deficiencies possible
L-dopa (Levodopa)	Antiparkinson's	High intake of vitamin B_6 or protein may affect medication's effectiveness
Lithium carbonate (Carbonlith, Lithane)	Antidepressant Antimanic	Low fluid or sodium intake increases risk of toxicity
		Sodium intake may influence drug's effect
Methotrexate (Folex, Rheumatrex)	Anti-inflammatory Antineoplastic	Decreased active folate formation
Methyldopa (Aldomet)	Antihypertensive	Absorption reduced if taken with high-protein meal or iron supplements
Mineral oil (Agoral)	Laxative	Decreased absorption of vitamins, A, D, E, and K; carotenes, calcium, and phosphorus
Monoamine oxidase inhibitors (Marpan, Nardil, Parnate)	Antidepressant	Avoid high intake of tyramine and vasoactive amines
Neomycin, kanamycin (Mycifradin, Kantrex)	Antibiotic	Decreased absorption of fat; carbohydrate; protein; vitamins A, D, E, K, B_{12}; calcium; and iron
Nitrofurantoin (Macrodantin)	Antibiotic	Decreased serum folate
Penicillin	Antibiotic	Varies with type
		Increased excretion of potassium
		Decreased Vitamin K synthesis
		Folate and vitamin B_6 metabolism altered
		Decreased absorption of carotenes, vitamin B_{12}, calcium, and magnesium

Table 16.1 Some Medications Which Have Interactions with Foods and Nutrients *(continued)*

Medications*	Use	Possible Interactions
Penicillamine (Cuprimine, Depen)	Chelating agent	Increased excretion of copper, zinc, and vitamin B_6
Phenytoin (Dilantin)	Anticonvulsant	Tube feeding with standard non-whole food-based products may result in subtherapeutic levels of Dilantin at usual dosage levels
		Decreased serum vitamin D, K, B_{12}, and folate
		Supplement with less than 5 mg/day folate to avoid loss of seizure control
Potassium supplements	Potassium source	Decreased absorption of vitamin B_{12}
Primidone (Myidone)	Anticonvulsant	Decreased serum folate levels
Probenecid (Benemid)	Uriocosuric	Increased urinary excretion of calcium, magnesium, sodium, chloride, potassium, phosphate, and riboflavin
Pyrazinamide (PZA)	Antimalarial	Folic acid deficiency possible
Pyremethamine (Daraprim)	Antitubercular	Vitamin B_6 and niacin deficiency possible
Ranitidine (Zantac)	Antiulcer	Same as cimetidine
Sodium nitroprusside (Nitropress)	Antihypertensive	Increased vitamin B_{12} excretion
Spironolactone (Aldactone)	Potassium sparing diuretic	Risk of hyperkalemia and hyponatremia
Sucralfate (Carafate)	Antiulcer	Decreases vitamin E absorption and may increase requirement
Sulfasalazine (Azulfidine, Asacole, Dipentum)	Anti-inflammatory	Decreased serum folate
Sulfonamides: Sulfadoxine and pyrimethamine (Fansidar) Sulfamethoxazole (Gantanol)	Antibiotic	Decreased folate status
Tetracyclines (Decloycin, Minocin)	Antibiotic	*See text*
Theophylline, aminophylline (Theodur, Aerolate)	Anti-asthma Bronchodilator	Increased protein intake and intake of charbroiled meats causes excretion and decreased medication effect
		Caffeine and similar compounds may increase risk of toxicity
Thiazides (Diuril, Esidrix)	Diuretic	Increased urinary excretion of potassium, magnesium, zinc, and sodium; serum calcium elevation
Triamteren (Dyrenium)	Potassium sparing diuretic	Decreased serum folate, hyperkalemia, hyponatremia
Valproic acid (Depakene)	Anticonvulsant	Possible carnitine deficiency

* Generic name (trade name).

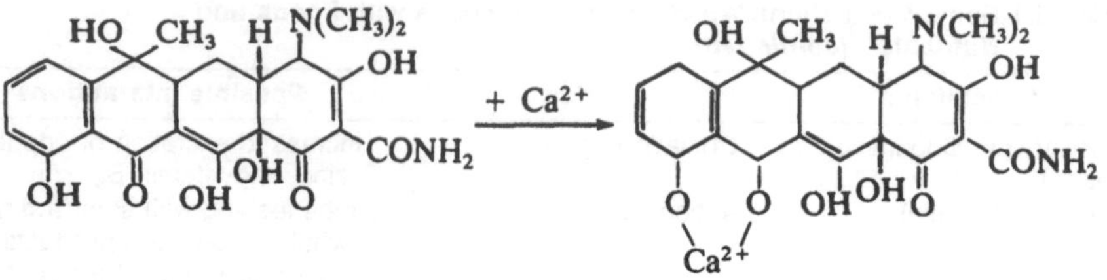

Figure 16.1 Chelation of calcium by tetracycline.

cancer, a high dietary intake of folate may decrease the anticarcinogenic action of the drug, and so a folate supplement should not be taken without the advice of a physician. When methotrexate is taken to treat rheumatoid arthritis or psoriasis, folate supplements may be used prophylactically to prevent a folate deficiency related to the side effects as drug efficacy has not been reported to be impaired when methotrexate is used to treat these conditions.

Many other drugs effectively compete to displace normal coenzymes and vitamins from their enzymes and block enzymatic catalysis because the drugs are structurally very similar to the coenzyme. This is particularly true of many of the vitamins for which there are known antimetabolites (i.e., drugs and poisons). Examples of drugs (poisons) that are competitive inhibitors of vitamins include isoniazid (vitamin B_6) used in the treatment of tuberculosis and dicumarol (and its derivatives, such as warfarin) which are antagonistic to vitamin K (see Chapter 5). Moderate supplements of vitamin B_6 generally do not decrease the antibiotic action of isoniazid. Large amounts of dietary supplements of vitamin K, however, will decrease the anticoagulant effect of dicumarol.

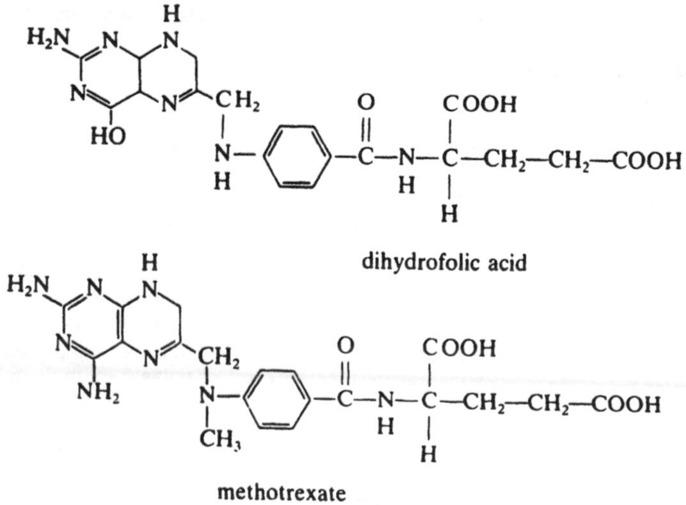

dihydrofolic acid

methotrexate

Figure 16.2 Structural similarity of dihydrofolic acid and methotrexate.

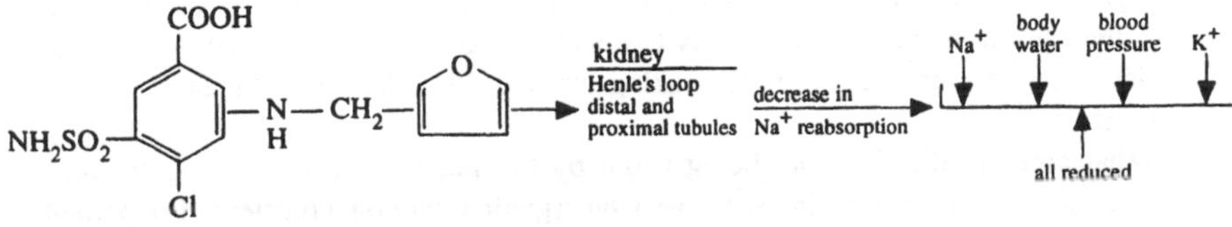

Figure 16.3 Alteration of Na+ reabsorption by furosemide.

DRUG ACTION ON MEMBRANE RECEPTOR SITES

Receptor sites on membranes are similar conceptually to the binding sites of coenzymes or substrates on enzymes. In the latter case, drugs may block catalysis. On membranes, blocking of receptor sites (which are proteins in most cases) may alter the membrane permeability, affecting molecular or ion transport. Furosemide is the generic name of a very commonly prescribed drug used as an antihypertensive to lower blood pressure or control edema. Furosemide pharmacologically is a diuretic drug which acts upon the receptor sites for Na+ in the proximal, distal, and Henle's loop of nephrotic tubules. The drug's action alters the ability of the tubules to reabsorb Na+ ions, facilitating excretion, which effectively reduces water retention and may lower blood pressure (Figure 16.3). The consequence of furosemide therapy for hypertension, in addition to loss of Na+, reduced blood pressure, and fluid retention, is the concomitant loss of potassium, K+. Potassium supplementation is therefore a frequent dietary recommendation for patients with normal renal function who are taking furosemide supplements to replace lost renal potassium. In some cases where body potassium levels are high or individuals are taking medications which promote potassium retention, the renal potassium loss promoted by furosemide may be a positive aspect of their treatment.

Many other drugs alter membrane permeability or affect membrane receptors. In addition, the diuretics and psychotropic drugs act on membranes and may affect utilization of nutrients. Phenytoin, an anticonvulsant used in the control of epilepsy, alters metabolism and may cause a decrease in nutritional status of folic acid and vitamins D and K.

Table 16.1 provides a list of some drugs and their interactions with nutrients and/or foods. The presence of a drug interaction with a nutrient does not always imply that nutrient supplementations need to be recommended. The following are factors that need to be considered before making a recommendation for medical nutritional therapy in the management of a food or nutrient–drug interaction.

1. Can the intake of the nutrient be increased without altering the efficacy of the medication in managing this patient's disorder? How severe are the consequences of the nutrient deficiency and what is the effect of lessening the medication's action on the patient's health by supplementing the nutrient? How long will the patient be on the medication and can nutritional status be restored after treatment? (*See Methotrexate* in Table 16.1.)
2. Assess the patient's risk of developing a deficiency in regard to factors such as dose, frequency, and length of treatment. For example, a patient taking two to three

aspirin a few times per year or taking one-half an aspirin tablet per day after having a myocardial infarction is not likely to develop a folic acid deficiency. Nutritional risk is much greater for a person taking ten aspirin tablets per day each day for arthritis.

3. What other medications are being taken by the patient and do the medications antagonize each other or do they have a synergistic effect on a nutrient? If a patient is taking a potassium-wasting diuretic such as furosemide (Lasix) in addition to a medication such as an angiotensin converting enzyme (ACE) inhibitor which promotes potassium retention, then this patient is not likely to need a potassium supplement.

4. What in the patient's medical or dietary history would increase the risk of a drug–nutrient interaction?
   • Poor intake of a nutrient
   • Nutrient deficiency
   • High intake or supplement use
   • Protein energy malnutrition
   • Alcohol consumption
   • History of poor drug compliance
   • Mental status
   • Age
   • Diseases
   • Idiosyncratic factors

5. Seek input from the pharmacist, nurse, or physician. A health care team working in cooperation is best in assessing and managing potential drug–nutrient interactions.

Table 16.1 is not an all-inclusive list of all drug–nutrient interactions and some interactions are controversial. Medications may also have additional effects which are not included in Table 16.1. Many medications can cause appetite depression, diarrhea, or other side effects.

In addition to direct drug–nutrient interactions, foods and fiber in the diet often affect drug absorption by altering gastrointestinal pH, diluting medications, and causing nonspecific binding. These effects may alter the efficacy of medication by reducing drug absorption. Thus, the timing of medications with or without food is important as foods may decrease drug effectiveness or the drug(s) may effect nutrient absorption and metabolism. In addition, for many medications avoidance of alcoholic beverages is highly recommended during therapy.

DRUG METABOLISM: EFFECT OF NUTRITIONAL STATUS

In addition to consuming drugs, we also consume food dyes, agricultural chemicals, and other unnatural compounds. Such manufactured compounds that adulterate foods are called xenobiotics, from the Greek word, *xenor*, meaning "strange," "foreign," or "extraneous." We also consume naturally, in many foods, chemical compounds which are not nutrients, which if homogeneously isolated and consumed in sufficient quantity would possibly be mutagenic, carcinogenic, or at the least, toxic.

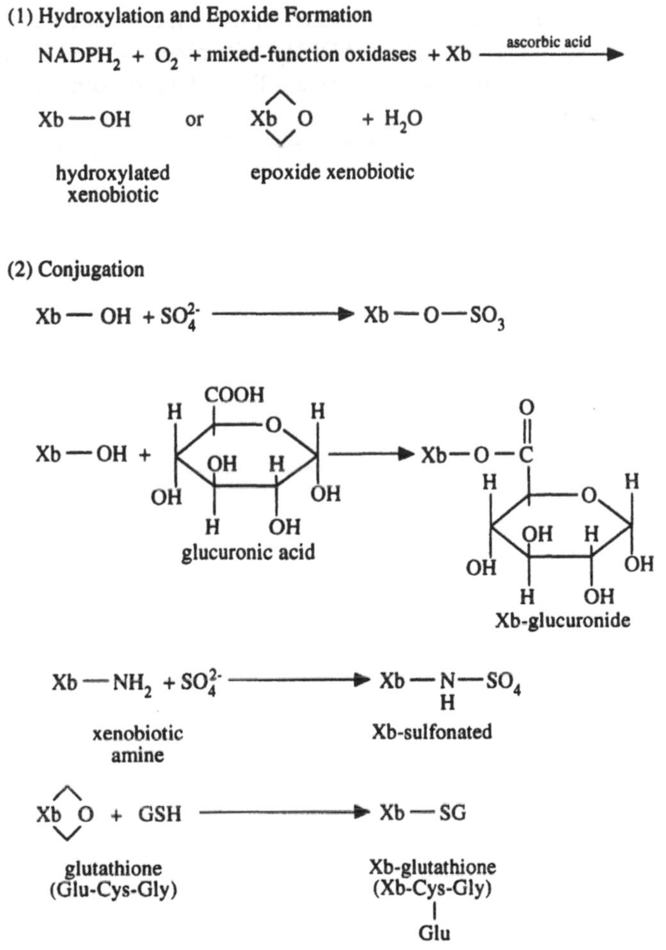

(1) Hydroxylation and Epoxide Formation

$$NADPH_2 + O_2 + \text{mixed-function oxidases} + Xb \xrightarrow{\text{ascorbic acid}}$$

$$Xb-OH \quad \text{or} \quad Xb\overset{\triangle}{\underset{\triangledown}{O}} \quad + H_2O$$

hydroxylated   epoxide xenobiotic
xenobiotic

(2) Conjugation

$$Xb-OH + SO_4^{2-} \longrightarrow Xb-O-SO_3$$

$$Xb-NH_2 + SO_4^{2-} \longrightarrow Xb-\underset{H}{N}-SO_4$$

xenobiotic   Xb-sulfonated
amine

$$Xb\overset{\triangle}{\underset{\triangledown}{O}} + GSH \longrightarrow Xb-SG$$

glutathione   Xb-glutathione
(Glu-Cys-Gly)   (Xb-Cys-Gly)
                                 |
                                Glu

Figure 16.4 Two-step metabolism and conjugation of xenobiotics (Xb) and nonnutritive food chemicals.

All such molecules absorbed from the diet have to be metabolized, conjugated, and excreted.

A good nutritional status influences the metabolisms of xenobiotics and natural toxins. Most of these molecules are metabolized by the liver in a two-step process (Figure 16.4). In the first step, (1) mixed-function oxidases (MFOs) make nonpolar hydrocarbons more polar, usually by inserting a hydroxyl moiety or epoxide. Two cytochrome enzymes in the endoplasmic reticulum complete the polarization process. NADPH$_2$ and O$_2$ are then enzymatically combined for either the hydroxylation or epoxide reactions. These reactions in the liver make the compounds more water soluble. In a second set of reactions, (2) a conjugating enzyme adds to a xenobiotic phenol, alcohol, or amine, either sulfate, glucuronic acid, or glutathione to the hydroxyl amine, or epoxide moiety. The apolar conjugated hydrocarbon is now made more water soluble to be excreted in the urine. Adequate protein intake (for methionine), vitamins (niacin for $NADPH_2$), vitamins A, C, and E (antioxidants), and minerals are all important for the metabolism of food-borne xenobiotics and nonnutritive food chemicals.

CHAPTER 17

Nutrient Metabolism and Dietary Recommendations

Throughout this book nutrition has been discussed almost completely at the nutrient level. Humans get the vast majority of their nutrients from food. Some individuals may get some of their nutrients from various types of dietary supplements.

Dietary recommendations and guidelines for the consumption of a diet that meets an individual's requirements for nutrients as well as promotes health and reduces the risks of chronic diseases are available. Information regarding dietary recommendations and guidelines developed by the committees/subcommittees of the National Academy of Sciences, United States Department of Agriculture, and United States Department of Health and Human Services will be briefly described. The reader is referred to the original publications if additional information is desired. Other organizations and individuals have also issued dietary recommendations and guidelines.

RECOMMENDED DIETARY ALLOWANCES

The nutrient standards used in the United States are developed by a committee/subcommittee of the Food and Nutrition Board of the National Academy of Sciences. According to the 1989 edition (or 10th edition), the Recommended Dietary Allowances (RDAs) are "the levels of intake of essential nutrients that, on the basis of scientific knowledge, are judged by the Food and Nutrition Board to be adequate to meet the known nutrient needs of practically all healthy persons." The 1989 Recommended Dietary Allowances dealt with the minimal amounts plus safety margins of nutrients needed to protect against possible nutrient deficiency. Currently, the Recommended Dietary Allowances are being updated and expanded. According to V. Young the recommended intakes will be levels believed to help people "achieve measurable physical indicators of good health." To date, revised dietary recommendations are available for calcium and related nutrients (phosphorus, magnesium, vitamin D, and fluoride) and for B-vitamins (thiamin, riboflavin, niacin, vitamin B_6, folate, vitamin B_{12}, pantothenic acid, and biotin) and choline. Until revised dietary recommendations are released for other essential nutrients, the 1989 Recommended Dietary Allowances will remain in use.

The 1989 Recommended Dietary Allowances as presently being used are listed in Table 17.1. The 1989 RDA revision also included the category Estimated Safe and Adequate Daily Dietary Intakes (ESADDIs). Estimated Safe and Adequate Daily Dietary Intakes for essential nutrients are used when data were deemed to be sufficient for estimating a range of requirements, but not a Recommended Dietary Allowance. The 1989 Estimated Safe and Adequate Daily Dietary Intakes are listed in Table 17.2. The 1989 revision also included Estimated Minimum Requirements for three electrolytes. These Estimated Minimum Requirements are given in Table 17.3.

In the 1989 RDAs, the recommended energy allowances are reflective of the mean requirement of each category:age group. These allowances are for reference adults with light to moderate physical activity. These recommended energy intakes were discussed in Chapter 10 (Table 10.5). Safety margins were not added to these allowances as was done with those for the nutrients. This is because doing so could lead to obesity in most individuals.

DIETARY REFERENCE INTAKES

The new recommended intakes are known as Dietary Reference Intakes (DRIs). There are four types of Dietary Reference Intakes — Estimated Average Requirements (EARs), Recommended Dietary Allowances (RDAs), Adequate Intakes (AIs), and Tolerable Upper Intake Levels (ULs). Together these four categories constitute a complete set of reference values. Definitions and intended uses of these Dietary Reference Intake values are given in Table 17.4. The Recommended Dietary Allowance is the value intended for use in "guiding individuals to achieve adequate nutrient intake." Having a set of Dietary Reference Intakes should permit health professionals to utilize the appropriate reference value designed for the intended usage.

The Dietary Reference Intakes for calcium, phosphorus, magnesium, vitamin D, and fluoride released in 1997 are given in Tables 17.5 through 17.9. Tolerable Upper Intake Levels for these five nutrients are listed in Table 17.10. Dietary Reference Intakes were released in April 1998 for thiamin, riboflavin, niacin, vitamin B_6, folate, vitamin B_{12}, pantothenic acid, biotin, and choline. The Estimated Average Requirements (EARs) and reported dietary intakes of six of the B-complex vitamins are given in Table 17.11. The Recommended Levels for Individual Intakes of the B-vitamins and choline are given in Table 17.12. These recommended levels are given as Recommended Dietary Allowances or as Adequate Intakes. Tolerable Upper Intake Levels for niacin, vitamin B_6, synthetic folic acid, and choline are listed in Table 17.13. Dietary Reference Intakes will be released in the next couple or years or so for the following nutrient groups: energy and macronutrients (tentative); antioxidants, carotenoids, vitamin E, vitamin C, and selenium; trace elements; electrolytes; and other food components (tentative).

Table 17.1 Recommended Dietary Allowances,[a] Revised 1989 (*Designed for the maintenance of good nutrition of practically all healthy people in the United States*)

Category	Age (years) or Condition	Weight (kg)	Weight (lb)	Height (cm)	Height (in)	Protein (g)	Fat-Soluble Vitamins Vitamin A (µg RE)[c]	Vitamin E (mg α-TE)[d]	Vitamin K (µg)	Iron (mg)	Minerals Zinc (mg)	Iodine (µg)	Selenium (µg)	Vitamin C (mg)
Infants	0.0–0.5	6	13	60	24	13	375	3	5	6	5	40	10	30
	0.5–1.0	9	20	71	28	14	375	4	10	10	5	50	15	35
Children	1–3	13	29	90	35	16	400	6	15	10	10	70	20	40
	4–6	20	44	112	44	24	500	7	20	10	10	90	20	45
	7–10	28	62	132	52	28	700	7	30	10	10	120	30	45
Males	11–14	45	99	157	62	45	1,000	10	45	12	15	150	40	50
	15–18	66	145	176	69	59	1,000	10	65	12	15	150	50	60
	19–24	72	160	177	70	58	1,000	10	70	10	15	150	70	60
	25–50	79	174	176	70	63	1,000	10	80	10	15	150	70	60
	51+	77	170	173	68	63	1,000	10	80	10	15	150	70	60
Females	11–14	46	101	157	62	46	800	8	45	15	12	150	45	50
	15–18	55	120	163	64	44	800	8	55	15	12	150	50	60
	19–24	58	128	164	65	46	800	8	60	15	12	150	55	60
	25–50	63	138	163	64	50	800	8	65	15	12	150	55	60
	51+	65	143	160	63	50	800	8	65	10	12	150	55	60
Pregnant						60	800	10	65	30	15	135	65	70
Lactating	1st 6 mo					65	1,300	12	65	15	19	200	75	95
	2nd 6 mo					62	1,200	11	65	15	16	200	75	90

[a] The allowances, expressed as average daily intakes over time, are intended to provide for individual variations among most normal persons as they live in the United States under usual environmental stresses. Diets should be based on a variety of common foods in order to provide other nutrients for which human requirements have been less well defined.

[b] Weights and heights of Reference Adults are actual medians for the U.S. population of the designated age, as reported by NHANES II. The median weights and heights of those under 19 years of age were taken from Hamill et al. (1979). The use of these figures does not imply that the height-to-weight ratios are ideal.

[c] Retinol equivalents. 1 retinol equivalent = 1 µg retinol or 6 µg β-carotene.

[d] α-Tocopherol equivalents. 1 mg d-α-tocopherol = 1 α-TE.

Note: The 1989 Recommended Dietary Allowances for Vitamin D, Calcium, Phosphorus, and Magnesium were replaced by Dietary Reference Intakes in 1997. The 1989 Recommended Dietary Allowances for Thiamin, Riboflavin, Niacin, Vitamin B$_6$, Folate, and Vitamin B$_{12}$ were replaced by Dietary Reference Intake in 1998.

From *Recommended Dietary Allowances.* © 1989 National Academy of Sciences. Courtesy of National Academy Press, Washington, DC. Table has been updated to reflect only recommendations not replaced in 1997 and 1998 by *Dietary Reference Intakes.*

Table 17.2 Estimated Safe and Adequate Daily Dietary Intakes of Trace Elements[a,b,c,d]

Category	Age (y)	Copper (mg)	Trace Elements Manganese (mg)	Chromium (µg)	Molybdenum (µg)
Infants	0–0.5	0.4–0.6	0.3–0.6	10–40	15–30
	0.5–1	0.6–0.7	0.6–1.0	20–60	20–40
Children & Adolescents	1–3	0.7–1.0	1.0–1.5	20–80	25–50
	4–6	1.0–1.5	1.5–2.0	30–120	30–75
	7–10	1.0–2.0	2.0–3.0	50–200	50–150
	11+	1.5–2.5	2.0–5.0	50–200	75–250
Adults		1.5–3.0	2.0–5.0	50–200	75–250

[a] Because there is less information on which to base allowances, these figures are not given in the main table of RDA and are provided here in the form of ranges of recommended intakes.

[b] The Estimated Safe and Adequate Daily Dietary Intakes of Fluoride were replaced by Dietary Reference Intakes in 1997.

[c] The Estimated Safe and Adequate Daily Dietary Intakes of Biotin and Pantothenic Acid were replaced by the Dietary Reference Intakes in 1998.

[d] Since the toxic levels for many trace elements may be only several times usual intakes, the upper levels for the trace elements given in this table should not be habitually exceeded.

From *Recommended Dietary Allowances.* © 1989 National Academy of Sciences. Courtesy of National Academy Press, Washington, DC. Table has been updated to reflect only recommendations not replaced in 1997 and 1998 by *Dietary Reference Intakes.*

Table 17.3 Estimated Sodium, Chloride, and Potassium Minimum Requirements of Healthy Persons[a]

Age	Weight (kg)[a]	Sodium (mg)[a,b]	Chloride (mg)[a,b]	Potassium (mg)[c]
Months				
0–5	4.5	120	180	500
6–11	8.9	200	300	700
Years				
1	11.0	225	350	1000
2–5	16.0	300	500	1400
6–9	25.0	400	600	1600
10–18	50.0	500	750	2000
>18[d]	70.0	500	750	2000

[a] No allowance has been included for large, prolonged losses from the skin through sweat.
[b] There is no evidence that higher intakes confer any health benefit.
[c] Desirable intakes of potassium may considerably exceed these values (~3500 mg for adults).
[d] No allowance included for growth.

From *Recommended Dietary Allowances*. ©1989 National Academy of Sciences. Courtesy of National Academy Press, Washington, DC.

Table 17.4 Dietary Reference Intakes and Their Intended Usage[a]

Estimated Average Requirements (EAR) — the intake that meets the estimated nutrient need of 50% of the individuals in a specific life-stage group. This reference value is to be used as the basis for developing the Recommended Dietary Allowances and is to be used by policy-makers in the evaluation of the adequacy of nutrient intakes of the group and for planning how much the group should consume.

Recommended Dietary Allowance (RDA) — the intake that meets the nutrient need of almost all (97 to 98%) individuals in a specific life-stage group. This reference value should be used in guiding individuals to achieve nutrient intake aimed at decreasing the risk of chronic disease. It is based on estimating an average requirement plus an increase to account for the variation within a particular group.

Adequate Intake (AI) — average observed or experimentally derived intake by a defined population or subgroup that appears to sustain a defined nutritional state, such as normal circulating nutrient values, growth, or other functional indicators of health. Adequate Intakes have been set when sufficient scientific evidence is not available to estimate an average requirement. Individuals should use the Adequate Intake as a goal for intake where no Recommended Dietary Allowances exist.

Tolerable Upper Intake Level (UL) — the maximum intake by an individual that is unlikely to pose risks of adverse health effects in almost all (97 to 98%) individuals in a specified life-stage group. This figure is not intended to be a recommended level of intake, and there is no established benefit for individuals to consume nutrients at levels above the Recommended Dietary Allowances or Adequate Intakes. For most nutrients, this figure refers to total intakes from food, fortified food, and nutrient supplements.

[a] Refers to daily intakes averaged over time.

From *Uses of Dietary Reference Intakes and New Report Recast Dietary Requirements for Calcium and Related Nutrients*. ©1997 National Academy of Sciences. Courtesy of National Academy Press, Washington, DC.

Table 17.5 Criteria and Dietary Reference Intake Values for Calcium by Life-Stage Group

Life-Stage Group[a]	Criterion	AI (mg/day)
0 to 6 months	Human milk content	210
6 to 12 months	Human milk + solid food	270
1 through 3 years	Extrapolation of maximal calcium retention from 4 through 8 years	500
4 through 8 years	Maximal calcium retention	800
9 through 13 years	Maximal calcium retention	1,300
14 through 18 years	Maximal calcium retention	1,300
19 through 30 years	Maximal calcium retention	1,000
31 through 50 years	Calcium balance	1,000
51 through 70 years	Maximal calcium retention	1,200
>70 years	Extrapolation of maximal calcium retention from 51 through 70 years	1,200
Pregnancy		
<19 years	Bone mineral mass	1,300
19 through 50 years	Bone mineral mass	1,000
Lactation		
<19 years	Bone mineral mass	1,300
19 through 50 years	Bone mineral mass	1,000

[a] All groups except Pregnant and Lactation are males and females.

From *Dietary Reference Intakes Series.* ©1997 National Academy of Sciences. Courtesy of National Academy Press, Washington, DC.

Table 17.6 Criteria and Dietary Reference Intake Values for Phosphorus by Life-Stage Group

Life-Stage Group[a]	Criterion	EAR (mg/day)	RDA (mg/day)	AI (mg/day)
0 to 6 months	Human milk content	—	—	100
6 to 12 months	Human milk + solid food	—	—	275
1 through 3 years	Factorial approach	380	460	—
4 through 8 years	Factorial approach	405	500	—
9 through 13 years	Factorial approach	1,055	1,250	—
14 through 18 years	Factorial approach	1,055	1,250	—
19 through 30 years	Serum P_i	580	700	—
31 through 50 years	Serum P_i	580	700	—
51 through 70 years	Extrapolation of serum P_i from 19 through 50 years	580	700	—
>70 years	Extrapolation of serum P_i from 19 through 50 years	580	700	—
Pregnancy				
<19 years	Factorial approach	1,055	1,250	—
19 through 50 years	Serum P_i	580	700	—
Lactation				
<19 years	Factorial approach	1,055	1,250	—
19 through 50 years	Serum P_i	580	700	—

[a] All groups except Pregnancy and Lactation are males and females. P_i = Serum inorganic phosphate concentration.

From *Dietary Reference Intakes Series.* ©1997 National Academy of Sciences. Courtesy of National Academy Press, Washington, DC.

Table 17.7 Criteria and Dietary Reference Intake Values for Magnesium by Life-Stage Group

Life-Stage Group[a]	Criterion	EAR (mg/day) Male/Female	RDA (mg/day) Male/Female	AI (mg/day) Male/Female
0 to 6 months	Human milk content	—/—	—/—	30/30
6 to 12 months	Human milk + solid food	—/—	—/—	75/75
1 through 3 years	Extrapolation of balance from older children	65/65	80/80	
4 through 8 years	Extrapolation of balance from older children	110/110	130/130	
9 through 13 years	Balance studies	200/200	240/240	
14 through 18 years	Balance studies	340/300	410/360	
19 through 30 years	Balance studies	330/255	400/310	
31 through 50 years	Balance studies	350/265	420/320	
51 through 70 years	Balance studies	350/265	420/320	
>70 years	Intracellular studies; decreases in absorption	350/265	420/320	
Pregnancy				
<19 years	Gain in lean mass	—/335	—/400	
19 through 30 years	Gain in lean mass	—/290	—/350	
31 through 50 years	Gain in lean mass	—/300	—/360	
Lactation				
<19 years	Balance studies	—/300	—/360	
19 through 30 years	Balance studies	—/255	—/310	
31 through 50 years	Balance studies	—/265	—/320	

[a] All groups except Pregnancy and Lactation are males and females.

From *Dietary Reference Intakes Series*. ©1997 National Academy of Sciences. Courtesy of National Academy Press, Washington, DC.

Table 17.8 Criteria and Dietary Reference Intake Values for Vitamin D by Life-Stage Group

Life-Stage Group[a]	Criterion	AI (micrograms/day)[b,c]
0 to 6 months	Serum 25(OH)D	5
6 to 12 months	Serum 25(OH)D	5
1 through 3 years	Serum 25(OH)D	5
4 through 8 years	Serum 25(OH)D	5
9 through 13 years	Serum 25(OH)D	5
14 through 18 years	Serum 25(OH)D	5
19 through 30 years	Serum 25(OH)D	5
31 through 50 years	Serum 25(OH)D	5
51 through 70 years	Serum 25(OH)D	10
>70 years	Serum 25(OH)D	15
Pregnancy		
<19 years	Serum 25(OH)D	5
19 through 50 years	Serum 25(OH)D	
Lactation		
<19 years	Serum 25(OH)D	5
19 through 50 years	Serum 25(OH)D	

[a] All groups except Pregnancy and Lactation are males and females.
[b] As cholecalciferol. 1 μg cholecalciferol = 40 IU vitamin D.
[c] In the absence of adequate exposure to sunlight.

From *Dietary Reference Intakes Series*. ©1997 National Academy of Sciences. Courtesy of National Academy Press, Washington, DC.

294   NUTRITION: CHEMISTRY AND BIOLOGY

Table 17.9   Criteria and Dietary Reference Intake Values for Fluoride by Life-Stage Group

Life-Stage Group[a]	Criterion	AI (mg/day) Male/Female
0 to 6 months	Human milk content	0.01/0.01
6 to 12 months	Caries prevention	0.5/0.5
1 through 3 years	Caries prevention	0.7/0.7
4 through 8 years	Caries prevention	1.1/1.1
9 through 13 years	Caries prevention	2.0/2.0
14 through 18 years	Caries prevention	3.2/2.9
19 through 30 years	Caries prevention	3.8/3.1
31 through 50 years	Caries prevention	3.8/3.1
41 through 70 years	Caries prevention	3.8/3.1
>70 years	Caries prevention	3.8/3.1
Pregnancy		
<19 years	Caries prevention	—/2.9
19 through 50 years	Caries prevention	—/3.1
Lactation		
<19 years	Caries prevention	—/2.9
19 through 50 years	Caries prevention	—/3.1

[a] All groups except Pregnancy and Lactation are males and females.

From *Dietary Reference Intakes Series.* ©1997 National Academy of Sciences. Courtesy of National Academy Press, Washington, DC.

Table 17.10   Tolerable Upper Intake Levels (UL) of Calcium, Phosphorus, Magnesium, Vitamin D, and Fluoride by Life-Stage Group

Life-Stage Group[a]	Calcium (g/day)	Phosphorus (g/day)	Magnesium[b] (mg/day)	Vitamin D (µg/day)[c]	Fluoride (mg/day)
0 to 6 months	ND[d]	ND	ND	25	0.7
6 to 12 months	ND	ND	ND	25	0.9
1 through 3 years	2.5	3	65	50	1.3
4 through 8 years	2.5	3	110	50	2.2
9 through 18 years	2.5	4	350	50	10
19 through 70 years	2.5	4	350	50	10
>70 years	2.5	3	350	50	10
Pregnancy					
<19 years	2.5	3.5	350	50	10
19 through 50 years	2.5	3.5	350	50	10
Lactation					
< 19 years	2.5	4	350	50	10
19 through 50 years	2.5	4	350	50	10

[a] All groups except Pregnancy and Lactation are males and females.
[b] The UL for magnesium represents intake from a pharmacological agent only and does not include intake from food and water.
[c] As cholecalciferol, 1 µg cholecalciferol = 40 IU vitamin D.
[d] ND. Not determinable due to lack of data of adverse effects in this age group and concern with regard to lack of ability to handle excess amounts. Source of intake should be from food only in order to prevent high levels of intake.

Based on *Dietary Reference Intakes Series.* ©1997 National Academy of Sciences. Courtesy of National Academy Press, Washington, DC.

Table 17.11 Estimated Average Requirements and Reported Dietary Intakes of Six B-Complex Vitamins by Gender for Young and Elderly Adults

Life-Stage Group	Thiamin (mg/d)	Riboflavin (mg/d)	Niacin (mg/d)	B$_6$ (mg/d)	Folate (µg/d)[a]	B$_{12}$ (µg/d)
Males						
19–30 yr						
EAR[b]	1.0	1.1	12	1.1	320	2.0
CSFII Median Dietary Intake,[c]	1.95,	2.33,	30.5,	2.31,	297,	5.60,
Range (5th–95th percentiles)	1.16–3.14	1.32–4.00	17.60–50.60	1.25–4.01	148–584	2.90–13.10
NHANES-III Median Dietary Intake,[d]	1.78,	2.09,	25.30,	2.02,	277,	5.22
Range (5th–95th percentiles)	1.07–3.41	1.18–3.90	15.00–45.60	1.16–3.91	163–564	4.42–7.56
>70 years						
EAR	1.0	1.1	12	1.4	320	2.0
CSFII Median Dietary Intake,[c]	1.64,	1.97,	21.7,	1.89,	276,	5.10,
Range (5th–95th percentiles)	0.97–2.62	1.09–3.30	12.60–35.30	1.01–3.29	137–527	2.40–10.30
NHANES-III Median Dietary Intake,[d]	1.56,	1.84,	20.8,	1.72,	269,	4.99,
Range (5th–95th percentiles)	1.03–2.68	1.13–3.28	13.84–35.67	1.02–3.22	163–542	4.45–6.81
Females						
19–30 yr						
EAR	0.9	0.9	11	1.1	320	2.0
CSFII Median Dietary Intake,[c]	1.22,	1.49,	17.5,	1.38,	200,	3.45,
Range (5th–95th percentiles)	0.80–1.99	0.80–2.55	9.50–29.10	0.76–2.31	100–374	1.67–6.47
NHANES-III Median Dietary Intake,[d]	1.45,	1.63,	19.69	1.54,	223,	4.77,
Range (5th–95th percentiles)	0.94–2.49	0.99–2.85	13.23–33.56	0.93–2.77	145–497	4.27–6.23
>70 yr						
EAR	0.9	0.9	11	1.3	320	2.0
CSFII Median Dietary Intake,[c]	1.18,	1.40,	16.8,	1.41,	212,	3.32
Range (5th–95th percentiles)	0.68–1.86	0.83–2.34	9.70–26.60	0.76–2.35	105–383	1.49–11.63
NHANES-III Median Dietary Intake,[d]	1.38,	1.60,	18.78,	1.53,	252,	4.74
Range (5th–95th percentiles)	0.94–2.21	1.01–2.71	12.74–30.30	0.92–2.76	152–474	4.37–5.99

Note: The Estimated Average Requirement (EAR) can be used to assess the adequacy of nutrient intakes by groups. To do this, one determines the percentage of individuals whose usual intakes are less than the EAR. From this table it can be seen that less than 5 percent of young men have thiamin intakes less than the EAR, but more than half of young women have reported folate intakes less than the EAR. Appendixes C and D allow more accurate estimates of percentages for all age groups than does this excerpted table.

[a] As dietary folate equivalents for the Estimated Average Requirement but not for reported dietary intakes. Reported intakes are likely to underestimate true intakes because of limitations of the methods used to analyze the folate content of food (see Chapter 8) and because adjustment has not been made for the higher bioavailability of the folic acid consumed in fortified foods and supplements: 1 dietary folate equivalent = 1 µg food folate = 0.6 µg of folic acid (from fortified food or supplement) consumed with food = 0.5 µg of synthetic (supplemental) folic acid taken on an empty stomach.

[b] EAR = Estimated Average Requirement.

[c] SOURCE: CSFII data on B vitamin intake from food, A. Carriquiry, Iowa State University, unpublished, 1997.

[d] SOURCE: NHANES-III, 1988–1994, unpublished data on B vitamin intake from food, C. Johnson, National Center for Health Statistics, 1997.

From *Dietary Reference Intakes Series*. © 1998 National Academy of Sciences. Courtesy of National Academy Press. Washington, DC.

Table 17.12 Recommended Levels for Individual Intakes of the B-Vitamins and Choline

Life-Stage Group	Thiamin (mg/d)	Riboflavin (mg/d)	Niacin (mg/d)[a]	B_6 (mg/d)	Folate (µg/d)[b]	B_{12} (µg/d)	Pantothenic Acid (mg/d)	Biotin (µg/d)	Choline[c] (mg/d)
Infants									
0.5– mo	0.2*	0.3*	2*	0.1*	65*	0.4*	1.7*	5*	125*
6–11	0.3*	0.4*	3*	0.3*	80*	0.5*	1.8*	6*	150*
Children									
1–3 yr	0.5	0.5	6	0.5*	150	0.9	2*	8*	200*
4–8 yr	0.6	0.6	8	0.6	200	1.2	3*	12*	250*
Males									
9–13 yr	0.9	0.9	12	1.0	300	1.8	4*	20*	375*
14–18 yr	1.2	1.3	16	1.3	400	2.4	5*	25*	550*
19–30 yr	1.2	1.3	16	1.3	400	2.4	5*	30*	550*
31–50 yr	1.2	1.3	16	1.3	400	2.4	5*	30*	550*
51–70 yr	1.2	1.3	16	1.7	400	2.4[d]	5*	30*	550*
>70 yr	1.2	1.3	16	1.7	400	2.4[d]	5*	30*	550*
Females									
9–13 yr	0.9	0.9	12	1.0	300	1.8	4*	20*	375*
14–18 yr	1.0	1.0	14	1.2	400*	2.4	5*	25*	400*
19–30 yr	1.1	1.1	14	1.3	400*	2.4	5*	30*	425*
31–50 yr	1.1	1.1	14	1.3	400*	2.4	5*	30*	425*
51–70 yr	1.1	1.1	14	1.5	400*	2.4[d]	5*	30*	425*
>70 yr	1.1	1.1	14	1.5	400	2.4[d]	5*	30*	425*
Pregnancy (all ages)	1.4	1.4	18	1.9	600[f]	2.6	6*	30*	450*
Lactation (all ages)	1.5	1.6	17	2.0	500	2.8	7*	35*	550*

Note: This table presents Recommended Dietary Allowances (RDAs) in bold type and Adequate Intakes (AIs) in ordinary type followed by an asterisk (*). RDAs and AIs may both be used as goals for individual intake. RDAs are set to meet the needs of almost all (97 to 98 percent) individuals in a group. For healthy breast-fed infants, the AI is the mean intake. The AI for other life stage groups is believed to cover their needs, but lack of data or uncertainty in the data prevent clear specification of this coverage.

[a] As niacin equivalents. 1 mg of niacin = 60 mg of tryptophan.

[b] As dietary folate equivalents (DFE). 1 DFE = 1 µg food folate = 0.6 µg of folic acid (from fortified food or supplement) consumed with food = 0.5 µg of synthetic (supplemental) folic acid taken on an empty stomach.

[c] Although AIs have been set for choline, there are few data to assess whether a dietary supply of choline is needed at all stages of the life cycle, and it may be that the choline requirement can be met by endogenous synthesis at some of these stages.

[d] Since 10 to 30 percent of older people may malabsorb food-bound B_{12}, it is advisable for those older than 50 years to meet their RDA mainly by taking foods fortified with B_{12} or a B_{12}-containing supplement.

[e] In view of evidence linking folate intake with neural tube defects in the fetus, it is recommended that all women capable of becoming pregnant consume 400 µg of synthetic folic acid from fortified foods and/or supplements in addition to intake of food folate from a varied diet.

[f] It is assumed that women will continue taking 400 µg of folic acid until their pregnancy is confirmed and they enter prenatal care, which ordinarily occurs after the end of the periconceptional period — the critical time for formation of the neural tube.

From Dietary Reference Intakes Series. © 1998 National Academy of Sciences. Courtesy of National Academy Press. Washington, DC.

Table 17.13 Tolerable Upper Intake Levels for Niacin, Vitamin B₆, Synthetic Folic Acid, and Choline

Life-Stage Group (y)	Niacin (mg/d)	Vitamin B₆ (mg/d)	Synthetic Folic Acid (µg/d)	Choline (µg/d)
1–3	10	30	300	1.0
4–8	15	40	400	1.0
9–13	20	60	600	2.0
14–18	30	80	800	3.0
≥19	35	100	1,000	3.5
Pregnant	35	100	1,000	3.5
Lactating	35	100	1,000	3.5

Based on *Dietary Reference Intakes Series*. © 1998 National Academy of Sciences. Courtesy of National Academy Press. Washington, DC.

DIETARY GUIDELINES FOR AMERICANS

These guidelines are designed to be used in advising healthy Americans 2 years of age and older about "food choices that promote health and prevent disease." The Dietary Guidelines for Americans, in its 4th edition in 1995, was prepared jointly by the United States Departments of Agriculture and of Health and Human Services. The 1995 Dietary Guidelines for Americans are given in Figure 17.1. The Dietary Guidelines for Americans are meant to apply to diets eaten over several days not just a 24-hour period.

FOOD GUIDE PYRAMID

The Food Guide Pyramid is a food guidance system developed by the United States Department of Agriculture and supported by the United States Department of Health and Human Services. It was first published in 1992. The Food Guide Pyramid provides information for putting the Dietary Guidelines for Americans into action. The Food Guide Pyramid recommends "what and how much to eat from each food group to get the nutrients you need and not too many calories, or too much fat, saturated fat, cholesterol, sugar, sodium, or alcohol." The Food Guide Pyramid helps individuals design a healthful diet that is appropriate for them. The Food Guide Pyramid focuses on fat because many individuals in the United States consume diets high in fat. The consumption of diets low in fat has been associated with decreased incidence of chronic diseases. The Food Guide Pyramid is given in Figure 17.2.

In using the Food Guide Pyramid in dietary planning, one needs to know what counts as a serving (Table 17.14). These serving sizes are general guidelines. If you consumed a sandwich, you would be consuming foods from several of the food groups. A typical sandwich might contain 2 servings of the bread group, half a serving of the meat group, half a serving of the milk group, and perhaps a partial serving of the vegetable group. Table 17.15 lists daily sample diets at three different

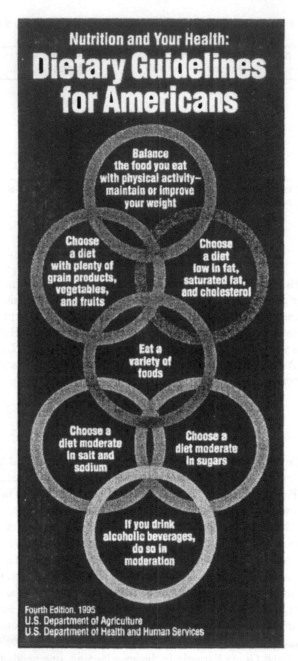

Figure 17.1 Dietary Guidelines for Americans.

Food Guide Pyramid
A Guide to Daily Food Choices

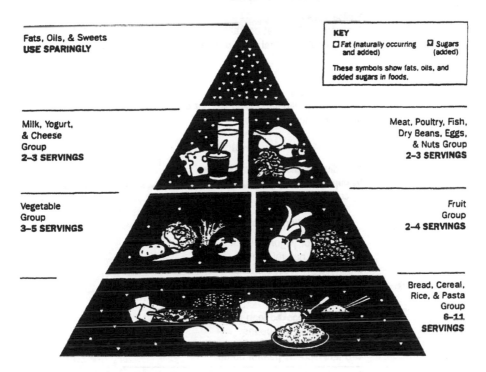

Fats, Oils, & Sweets
USE SPARINGLY

KEY
☐ Fat (naturally occurring ▨ Sugars
   and added)   (added)

These symbols show fats, oils, and
added sugars in foods.

Milk, Yogurt,
& Cheese
Group
2–3 SERVINGS

Meat, Poultry, Fish,
Dry Beans, Eggs,
& Nuts Group
2–3 SERVINGS

Vegetable
Group
3–5 SERVINGS

Fruit
Group
2–4 SERVINGS

Bread, Cereal,
Rice, & Pasta
Group
6–11
SERVINGS

Figure 17.2 Food Guide Pyramid.

calorie levels. The amount of fat in the daily diet can be estimated using information given in Table 17.16. The total fat consumed can be compared to the number of calories listed in Table 17.15 for your caloric intake or you may calculate how many grams of fat represents <30% of your caloric intake.

NUTRITIONAL LABELING

The Nutrition Labeling and Education Act of 1990 directed that all processed foods must have food labels. The United States Department of Agriculture is responsible for the regulation of meat and poultry products and eggs, while the United States Food and Drug Administration regulates all other foods, nutrient supplements, and drugs.

Information provided on food products as Nutrition Facts may be used by the consumer in planning and consuming healthful diets. An example of a Nutrition Facts label is shown in Figure 17.3. The label provides information as to the serving size of the product and the calories and percentage of the Daily Value (DV) of

**Table 17.14 What Counts as a Serving of Each
of the Food Groups**

Bread, Cereal, Rice, and Pasta

1 slice bread
1 ounce ready-to-eat cereal
$^1/_2$ cup cooked cereal, rice, or pasta

Vegetable

1 cup raw leafy vegetables
$^1/_2$ cup other vegetables, cooked or chopped raw
$^3/_4$ cup of vegetable juice

Fruit

1 medium apple, banana, orange
$^1/_2$ cup chopped, cooked, or canned fruit
$^3/_4$ cup fruit juice

Milk, Yogurt, and Cheese

1 cup milk or yogurt
$1^1/_2$ ounces natural cheese
2 ounces processed cheese

Meat, Poultry, Fish, Dry Beans, Eggs, and Nuts

2–3 ounces cooked lean meat, poultry, or fish
$^1/_2$ cup cooked dry beans
1 egg
4–6 tablespoons peanut butter

Taken from USDA's Home and Garden Bulletin No.
252.

Table 17.15 Sample Diets for a Day at 3 Calorie Levels

	Lower ~1,600	Moderate ~2,200	Higher ~2,800
Bread Group Servings	6	9	11
Vegetable Group Servings	3	4	5
Fruit Group Servings	2	3	4
Milk Group Servings	2–3[a]	2–3[a]	2–3[a]
Meat Group[b] (ounces)	5	6	7
Total Fat (grams)	53	73	93
Total Added Sugars (teaspoons)	6	12	18

[a] Women who are pregnant or breast-feeding, teenagers, and young
adults to age 24 need 3 servings.
[b] See Table 17.14 as to what constitutes a serving.

Taken from USDA's Home and Garden Bulletin No. 252.

Table 17.16 Counting Grams of Fat

	Servings	Grams Fat		Servings	Grams Fat		Servings	Grams Fat
Bread, Cereal, Rice, & Pasta Group			**Fruit Group**			**Meat, Poultry, Fish, Dry Beans, Eggs, & Nuts Group**		
Bread, 1 slice	1	1	Whole fruit: medium apple, orange, banana	1	trace	Lean meat, poultry, fish, cooked	3 oz.	6
Hamburger roll, bagel, english muffin	2	2	Fruit, raw or canned, 1/2 cup	1	trace	Ground beef, lean, cooked	3 oz.	16
Tortilla, 1	1	3	Fruit juice, unsweetened, 3/4 cup	1	trace	Chicken, with skin, fried	3 oz.	13
Rice or pasta, cooked, 1/2 cup	1	trace	Avocado, 1/4 whole	1	9	Bologna, 2 slices	1 oz.	16
Plain crackers, small, 3–4	1	3				Egg, 1	1 oz.	5
Breakfast cereal, 1 oz.	1	*	**Milk, Yogurt, & Cheese Group**			Dry beans and peas, cooked, 1/2 cup	1 oz.	trace
Pancakes, 4" diameter, 2	2	3	Skim milk, 1 cup	1	trace	Peanut butter, 2 tbsp.	1 oz.	16
Croissant, 1 large, 2 oz.	2	12	Nonfat yogurt, plain, 8 oz.	1	trace	Nuts, 1/3 cup	1 oz.	22
Doughnut, 1 medium, 2 oz.	2	11	Lowfat milk, 2%, 1 cup	1	5	* Ounces of lean meat these items count as		
Danish, 1 medium (2 oz.)	2	13	Whole milk, 1 cup	1	8			
Cake, frosted, 1/16 average	1	13	Chocolate milk, 2%, 1 cup	1	8	**Fats, Oils & Sweets**		
Cookies, 2 medium	1	4	Lowfat yogurt, plain, 8 oz.	1	5	Butter, margarine, 1 tsp	—	4
Pie, fruit, 2-crust, 1/6 8" pie	2	19	Lowfat yogurt, fruit, 8 oz.	1	4	Mayonnaise, 1 tbsp.	—	11
* Check product label			Natural cheddar cheese, 1 1/2 oz.	1	14	Salad dressing, 1 tbsp.	—	7
			Processed cheese, 2 oz.	1	18	Reduced calorie salad dressing, 1 tbsp.	—	*
Vegetable Group			Mozzarella, part skim, 1 1/2 oz.	1	7	Sour cream, 2 tbsp.	—	6
Vegetables, cooked, 1/2 cup	1	trace	Ricotta, part skim, 1/2 cup	1/4	10	Cream cheese, 1 oz.	—	10
Vegetables, leafy, raw, 1 cup	1	trace	Cottage cheese, 4% fat, 1/2 cup	1/3	5	Sugar, jam, jelly, 1 tsp.	—	0
Vegetables, nonleafy, raw, chopped, 1/2 cup	1	trace	Ice cream, 1/2 cup	1/3	7	Cola, 12 fl. oz.	—	0
Potatoes, scalloped, 1/2 cup	1	4	Ice milk, 1/2 cup	1/3	3	Fruit drink, ade, 12 fl. oz.	—	0
Potato salad, 1/2 cup	1	8	Frozen yogurt, 1/2 cup	1/2	2	Chocolate bar, 1 oz.	—	9
French fries, 10	1	8				Sherbet, 1/2 cup	—	2
						Fruit sorbet, 1/2 cup	—	0
						Gelatin dessert, 1/2 cup	—	0
						* Check product label		

Taken from USDA's Home and Garden Bulletin No. 252.

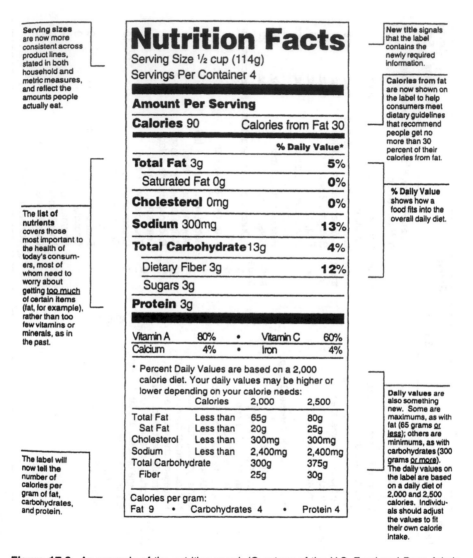

Figure 17.3 An example of the nutrition panel. (Courtesy of the U.S. Food and Drug Administration.)

selected nutrients per serving. These Daily Values are meant to be used as a rough guide to ensure that daily nutrient needs are met. The United States Food and Drug Administration has regulations in which serving sizes are defined.

Standardized descriptors for nutrient content to be used on food labels were set by the Food and Drug Administration as a result of the Nutrition Labeling and Education Act of 1990. These terms are given in Table 17.17. The food industry also is allowed only to make scientifically verified appropriate health claims. These approved health claims are listed in Table 17.18.

The dietary recommendations and guidelines are useful in advising individuals regarding the consumption of nutritionally adequate diets. By appropriate planning,

Table 17.17 Nutrient Content Descriptors that May be Used on Food Labels

Descriptor	Definition
Free	A serving contains no or a physiologically inconsequential amount: <5 calories; <5 mg sodium; <5 g fat; <0.5 g saturated fat; <2 mg cholesterol; or <0.5 g sugar.
Low	A serving (and 50 g food if the serving size is small) contains no more than 40 calories; 140 mg sodium; 3 g fat; 1 g saturated fat and 15% of calories from saturated fat; or 20 mg cholesterol; not defined for sugar; for "very low sodium," no more than 35 mg sodium.
Lean	A serving (and 100 g) of meat, poultry, seafood, and game meats contains <10 g fat, <4 g saturated fat, and <95 mg cholesterol.
Extra lean	A serving (and 100 g) of meat, poultry, seafood, and game meats contains <5 g fat, <2 g saturated fat, and <95 mg cholesterol.
High	A serving contains 20% or more of the Daily Value (DV) for a particular nutrient. Also referred to as "major source of" and "rich in."
Good source	A serving contains 10–19% of the DV for the nutrient. Also referred to as "source of" and "important source of."
Reduced	A nutritionally altered product contains 25% less of a nutrient or 25% fewer calories than a reference food; cannot be used if the reference food already meets the requirement for a "low" claim.
Less	A food contains 25% or less of a nutrient or 25% fewer calories than a reference food.
Light	An altered product contains 1/3 fewer calories or 50% of the fat in a reference food; if 50% or more of the calories come from fat, the reduction must be 50% of the fat; or
	The sodium content of a low-calorie, low-fat food has been reduced by 50% (the claim "light in sodium" may be used); or
	The term describes such properties as texture and color, as long as the label explains the intent (examples, "light brown sugar" and "light and fluffy").
More	A serving contains at least 10% of the Daily Value (DV) of a nutrient more than a reference food. Also applies to fortified, enriched, and added claims for altered foods.
% Fat-Free	A product must be low-fat or fat-free, and the percentage must accurately reflect the amount of fat in 100 g of food. Thus, 2.5 g of fat in 50 g of food results in a "95% fat-free" claim.
Fresh	A food is raw, has never been frozen or heated, and contains no preservatives (irradiation at low levels is allowed), or
	The term accurately describes the product (examples, "fresh milk" and "freshly baked bread").
Fresh frozen	The food has been quickly frozen while still fresh; blanching is allowed before freezing to prevent nutrient breakdown.

Table 17.18 Approved Health Claims

Claims for the following relationships between diet and disease are allowed on appropriate food products:
- Calcium and osteoporosis
- Fat and cancer
- Saturated fat and cholesterol and coronary heart disease
- Fruits, vegetables, and grain products and cancer
- Fruits, vegetables, and grain products and coronary heart disease
- Fruits and vegetables and cancer
- Sodium and hypertension
- Folic acid during pregnancy and neural tube defects

The claim must use "may" or "might" in describing the relationship and must add that other factors play a role in that disease.

healthy individuals may obtain all the nutrients needed by the body from foods. Every day individuals make food choices that affect their health for better or worse. The making of beneficial choices may decrease the risk of chronic diseases. Good nutrition is important to good health.

Appendices and Index

Review of Chemistry and Biology Concepts of Importance in Nutrition

THE PERIODIC TABLE

The periodic table, first established by the Russian chemist Dmitri Mendeleev (1834–1907) in 1869, and independently by the German chemist Julius Meyer (1830–1895) in 1870, now contains more than 110 elements (atoms), of which 90 occur naturally. The periodic table is given in Figure A.1. Beginning with the smallest element, hydrogen (element 1), and progressing through the periodic table, the elements become increasingly larger by the addition of protons, neutrons, and electrons. As the elements get physically larger, they increase in mass correspondingly. For the experimental nutritionist, the periodic table contains and retains fascinating information. On the practical side, the periodic table provides information on atomic numbers and atomic weights. As discussed in Chapter 1, life's elements have been selected, often in groups and clusters, with great specificity. On the basis of physical and chemical properties alone, the elements of the periodic table have been grouped into light metals, transition metals, heavy metals, and nonmetals.

MOLECULAR WEIGHTS

Weights of the elements are obtained from the periodic table and are standardized against the atomic weight of the element carbon (C) equal to 12. The atomic weight of the smallest element, hydrogen, is 1. The heaviest element is the man-made element ununuium, of atomic weight 110. All other elements have atomic weights between hydrogen and ununuium. In determining the molecular weights of molecules of two or more atoms, the sum of the atomic weights of the atoms equals its molecular weight. Thus, the molecular weight of oxygen (O_2) is 32; water (H_2O),

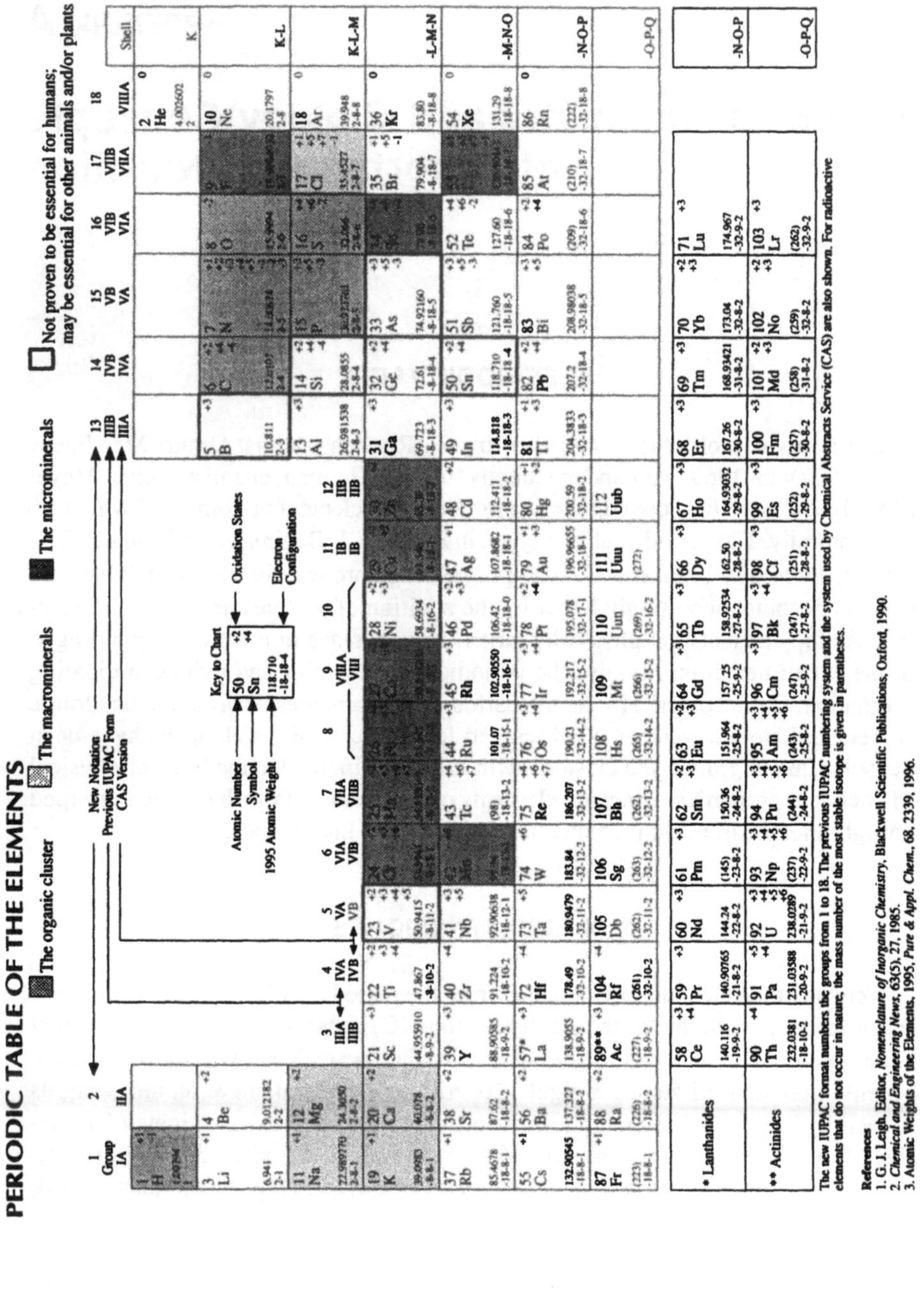

Figure A.1 Periodic Table of the Elements.

18; and ethane (C_2H_6), 30. The molecular weight of any molecule, regardless of size, can be calculated by addition of the atomic weights of the constituent atoms.

BONDING

In the biological world, as in the more inanimate chemical world, few elements exist entirely by themselves. Almost all elements are found in association with other elements as molecules. Elements are composed of neutrons and protons which comprise the nucleus. Surrounding the nucleus of each element are ordered layers of orbiting electrons. It is electrons (e^-), small, negatively charged particles orbiting the nucleus with its positively charged protons (p^+) and uncharged neutrons (n^0), which permit the bonding of elements into molecules. There are many possible combinations of elements that make up molecules, and there are then additional interactions between molecules involving bonding forces related to orbiting electrons.

THE COVALENT BOND

The most important bond in the biological world is the covalent bond. In the simplest case, two atoms of hydrogen share their single orbiting electron to form a single covalent bond (Figure A.2). Most biological molecules exist by sharing a pair of outer orbital electrons which comprise the covalent bond, designated by —. Whereas the covalent bond of hydrogen (H_2) is relatively simple, more complex and important covalent bonds exist in the bioorganic molecules, including the carbon–carbon bond (—C—C—), the carbon–hydrogen bond (—C—H), and the carbon–oxygen double bond (—C=0) as well as other carbon bonds. Every covalent bond of every molecule represents a small amount of stored energy.

THE IONIC BOND

The ionic bond is commonly found in inorganic compounds, such as salts. Examples of this class of compounds include NaCl, KI, and $FeSO_4$. Like the covalent bond, outer orbiting electrons of atoms enter into ionic bonds that also exist in pairs. Unlike the covalent bond, in which each atom donates and shares an electron pair, in the ionic bond electrons in the shared pair of electrons are donated by only one of the paired atoms. For this reason, NaCl can also be written $Na^+ + Cl^-$. In this

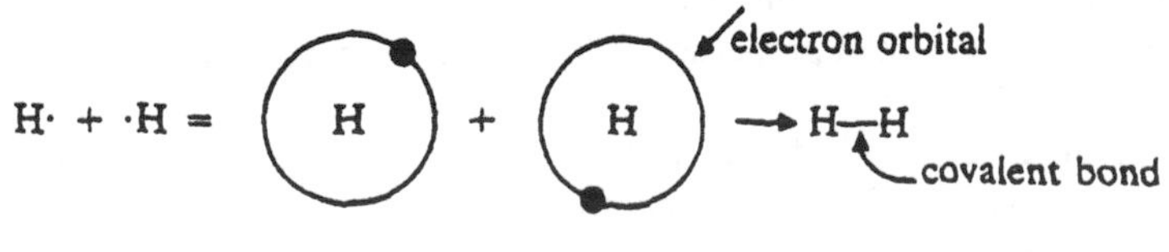

Figure A.2   Covalent bond of hydrogen.

$$NaCl \rightarrow Na^+ + Cl^-$$

Equation A.1

example of an ionic bond, the sodium (Na^+) cation's outermost electron shell is deficient by one electron. In contrast, the chloride (Cl^-) anion has an extra electron (e^-) in its outer electron shell. In NaCl the sodium atom accepts a single electron from the chloride atom forming the ionic bond. When dissolved in water, many salts undergo either partial or total dissociation. Dissociated salts in solution separate, with the electrons that formed the ionic bond being retained by the donor atom. For example, NaCl in solution is fully dissociated, producing the sodium cation (Na^+) and the chloride anion (Cl^-). In Equation A.1, Na^+ has lost its electron, forming anionic Cl^-. The ionic bond and principles of dissociation are of more importance to the inorganic chemist and biochemist than to the nutritionist.

THE COORDINATE COVALENT BOND

The coordinate covalent bond possesses properties of both the covalent bond and the ionic bond. In the coordinate covalent bond, two electrons are donated from one atom to another atom, forming the bond. In many instances, coordinate covalent bonds are formed between nitrogen (N) atoms and metal ions. Molecules called chelates (meaning "claw") form coordinate covalent bonds between two or more nitrogens and a metal ($\ddot{N} \rightarrow Fe^{2+}$). Molecules derived from pyrroles form tetrapyrroles, which form coordinate covalent bonds with iron (Fe), cobalt (Co), and magnesium (Mg). These molecules are of particular interest, for they form the biologically important molecules hemoglobin, myoglobin, cytochromes, vitamin B_{12}, and the chlorophyll family of molecules.

OTHER BONDING

The covalent, ionic, and coordinate covalent bonds are forms of intramolecular associations of atoms in the assembly of molecules. There are other forms of intramolecular and intermolecular bonding which are probably of less interest but are no less important in biological systems. These bonding associations include hydrophobic bonding, hydrogen bonding, electrostatic bonding, and van der Waals forces. An appreciation of hydrophobic interactions (bonding) and hydrogen bonding is essential, for such interactions are important in lipids (hydrophobic bonds) and contribute to water's special properties (hydrogen bonding). The hydrogen bond and its hydrogen oxide dipole moment are unique properties of the most important nutrient, water. Electrostatic forces and van der Waals forces occur as a result of charged separation in molecules (bond dipoles) and may exist as either intermolecular or intramolecular partitioning of polar molecular species.

Table A.1 Functional Organic Groups in Nutrients

Functional group name	Formula	Found in these nutrients
Hydroxyl	R—OH (primary)	Carbohydrates, proteins, lipids, vitamins
Amino	R—NH$_2$ (primary)	Proteins
Carboxylic acid	R—COOH	Proteins, lipids
Ester	R—O—C(=O)—R	Lipids
Ether	R—O—R	Carbohydrates
Amide	R—N(H)—C(=O)—R	Proteins, vitamins
Phosphate esters	R—O—P(=O)(OH)—O—R	Lipids, vitamins
Methylene	R—CH$_2$—R	Proteins, lipids, vitamins
Alkyl	R—CH$_2$—CH$_2$—CH$_3$	Lipids, proteins
α-Keto acid	R—C(=O)—COOH	Important metabolic intermediates
Imine	R—NH (secondary)	Proteins, heterocyclics
Methyl	R—CH$_3$	Lipids, vitamins, proteins
Aldehyde	R—CHO	Carbohydrates, vitamins
Keto	R$_2$C=O	Carbohydrates, proteins
Thiol	R—SH	Proteins
Selenol	R—SeH	
Aryl	R—C$_6$H$_5$	Proteins
Phosphate	R—O—P(OH)(=O)—OH	Energy intermediates, phospholipids
Halide	R—I	Thyroid hormones (minerals)

FUNCTIONAL ORGANIC GROUPS OF NUTRITIONALLY IMPORTANT COMPOUNDS

While the study of the chemistry of carbon and its compounds is the purview of organic chemistry, it is useful to review and again become familiar with those functional organic groups that are important in the nutrients and their metabolic intermediates. Table A.1 lists the names of these functionally important groups.

THERMODYNAMICS

Thermodynamics is often viewed as being an esoteric concept of the chemist, biochemist, or physicist. Not so! General thermodynamic principles are easily understandable and should be familiar to all advanced students who study nutrition. Understanding nutrition — why animals and people eat — as well as understanding photosynthesis, energy flow, and food chains, is to have an understanding of thermodynamics. The principles of thermodynamics are embodied in the three laws of thermodynamics.

1. The first law of thermodynamics is a statement of the conservation of matter and energy: matter and energy can be neither created nor destroyed, but their form can be changed. In nutritional terminology, matter consists of carbohydrates, lipids, and protein, which is converted into physical movement (work) and heat or is stored as body fat. The first law of thermodynamics is embodied in Einstein's equation, $E = mc^2$ (E = energy, m = mass, c = speed of light). Both obesity and starvation are realities of the first law.
2. The second law of thermodynamics is only slightly more esoteric than the first law but is no less important to the understanding of the biological world. The second law is embodied in the idea of a semblance of order within any system: molecule, machine, man, or universe. The law states that the entropy (S) of the universe tends toward maximum disorder. In different words, the second law says that all order of the universe generally progresses in a unilateral direction toward ever-increasing disorder. Entropy, then, is a quantitative measure of how much order exists in the universe or in any other defined system at any given time.
3. The third law of thermodynamics states that the entropy (S) of a perfect crystal, like a perfect diamond with perfect order, is equal to zero [at absolute temperature (0°K)]. In a state of perfect order, $S = 0$. Combining the second and third laws of thermodynamics provides the limits for entropy where S exists within theoretical values of $S = 0$ (perfect order) to $S = \infty$ (maximum or infinite disorder). In the real world, S never equals zero or infinity in any system, but possesses intermediate values. The amount of entropy of any system can be either increased or decreased, but any decrease in entropy of one system is always at the expense of increased entropy within another system. This is what happens when people eat. Decreasing body entropy is accomplished at the expense of an increase in entropy of food and the environment.

ENZYMOLOGY

The study and understanding of enzymes, enzymology, and their functions are described by biochemical specialists called enzymologists. General concepts of enzymology are important aspects of an understanding of the biological world. It is within the study of enzymes that we discover the nutritional needs and functions of

(1) sucrose $\xrightarrow{\text{sucrase}}$ fructose + glucose

(2) fructose + glucose $\xrightarrow[\text{synthetase}]{\text{sucrose}}$ sucrose

Equation A.2 Enzyme–substrate terminology.

the vitamins and many minerals. Here, a general presentation is made of the action of enzymes, simple enzyme kinetics, and the thermodynamic concepts of "free" or biologically useful energy, G. (G stands for J.W. Gibbs, who was the first person to describe useful biological energy.)

Structurally, enzymes are proteins of varied molecular weights and differing amino acid composition. Functionally, enzymes are organic catalysts often possessing extraordinary specificity. Enzymes exist because the reactions in which they participate normally would not proceed at the human body temperature or at the subzero temperatures often encountered by cold-water fish. As catalysts, enzymes enter into reactions that would not ordinarily occur by lowering the "energy of activation," which results in a reaction proceeding at a faster (sometimes very fast) rate without itself being consumed in the reaction.

In the simplest case, an enzyme acts on a substrate or substrates to produce one or more products. The enzyme is often named for the function it performs, and/or for the substrate upon which it acts, by adding the suffix *ase*. Examples are shown in Equation A.2. In example (1), sucrose, the substrate, is hydrolyzed to yield the products fructose and glucose by the enzyme sucrase. In example (2), fructose and glucose, the substrates for the reaction, are combined by the enzyme, a synthetase, to yield the product, sucrose. The substrate in reaction (1) becomes the product in reaction (2). In the reactions above, the enzymes are shown to react without the requirement for cofactors or coenzymes. Many enzymatic reactions require organic coenzymes or vitamins to complete the structural requirements of the active site of an enzyme.

Enzymes acting on substrates have physical and chemical limits to their catalytic activity. This notion is demonstrated in Figure A.3. In this example, the rate of the enzymatic reaction or velocity is seen to increase with increasing substrate concentration until further increases in substrate concentration beyond the maximum substrate concentration (MSC) result in no increase in reaction velocity. At [S] equal to the (MSC), the enzyme is said to be saturated and it is operating at V_{max}, maximum

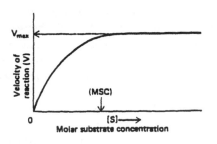
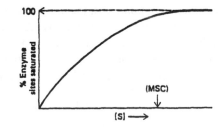

Figure A.3 Enzyme–substrate kinetics.

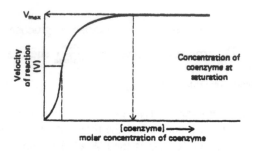

Figure A.4   Enzyme–coenzyme–substrate kinetics.

velocity. V_{max} is also a measure of how fast an enzyme is able to convert substrate(s) to products, and V_{max} is different for each enzyme.

Enzymes acting on substrates in cooperation with coenzymes or vitamins often exhibit different kinetics. The kinetics exhibited with the cooperative binding of coenzymes in completing the active site is sigmoidal, as shown in Figure A.4. In this example of enzyme kinetics, the concentration of coenzyme in the presence of excess substrate [S] is the limiting factor in attaining maximum enzyme catalytic activity (V_{max}) when the concentration of enzyme is held constant. Each enzyme molecule in this situation is not able to function catalytically until there is enough coenzyme present to fulfill the binding requirements to structurally complete all the active sites on the enzymes for substrate attachment. Such limiting conditions of coenzyme saturation are paramount to the induction of a vitamin deficiency, and if the deficiency is severe enough, the onset of disease.

ENERGY REQUIREMENTS OF ENZYMATIC REACTIONS

Many enzymatic reactions proceed with either a requirement for energy or the liberation of energy. When enzyme reactions proceed without any energy require-ment, they often, but not always, liberate internal energy contained within the substrate. The difference in internal energy — the difference in energy contained within the substrate and the energy contained within the products — is called the "free energy" of the enzymatic reaction and is designated (G), Gibbs' free energy, G, or more appropriately ΔG, the change in free energy, a thermodynamic property of the reaction. In addition to the change in the thermodynamic property of the enzymatic reaction (ΔG), there will be an associated change in the overall state of order of the reaction: the entropy (ΔS) of the reaction. The relationship between the free energy of the enzymatic reaction and the change in the entropy, the internal order of the reaction, is shown in Equation A.3. In example (1), the enzyme reaction proceeds spontaneously and may be exothermic, releasing energy, $-\Delta G$. The net result within the reaction at completion is an increase in the entropy of the substrate and a decrease in the total energy of the reaction. In example (2), the enzyme reaction cannot proceed without an input of energy, $+\Delta G$, and is therefore a reaction that will not proceed spontaneously. If this reaction is completed to yield a product, energy, often supplied to the enzymatic reaction as adenosine triphosphate (ATP),

		$\Delta G^{\circ\prime}$	ΔS	E_{total}
(1) substrate $\xrightarrow{\text{enzyme}}$ product(s)		reaction $(-)$ exothermic and spontaneous	increased $(+)$ disorder	$(-)$ declines
(2) substrate(s) $\xrightarrow{\text{enzyme}}$ product(s)		reaction $(+)$ endothermic and nonspontaneous	increased $(-)$ order	$(+)$ increases

Equation A.3 Free energy, entropy, and total energy within enzyme reactions.

will be consumed during catalysis. Entropy in this reaction will decline; there will be increased order within the reaction products and the total energy, E_{total}, within the product will increase. The relationships in enzyme reaction (2) between ΔG, ΔS, and E_{total} is an example of the thermodynamic state of nutrition, which relates free energy, entropy, and total energy to growth, food (energy source), maintenance, and aging.

OXIDATION–REDUCTION REACTIONS

Oxidation–reduction reactions, redox reactions, are important in nutrition because the release of "energy" from food is a basic oxidative process. Reduction reactions are also important, as these processes are paramount in the synthesis of carbohydrates by plants, the synthesis of fatty acids and the subsequent storage of body fat, and the synthesis of other essential organic compounds by animals and humans. No oxidation reaction will take place without a concurrent reduction reaction taking place. Conversely, no reduction reaction will take place without an oxidation reaction also taking place. Therefore, oxidation and reduction reactions occur simultaneously in close contact and are referred to as redox reactions. Redox reactions are most easily understood by example and the application of three rules.

1. No oxidation reaction takes place without something being reduced, and no reduction reaction takes place without something being oxidized.
2. In inorganic chemistry, oxidation is the loss of electrons (e^-), and in organic chemistry oxidation is the loss of hydrogen (H).
3. In inorganic chemistry, reduction is the gain of electrons (e^-), and in organic chemistry reduction is the gain of hydrogen (H).

These rules are almost absolute and should be retained as a guide to recognizing redox reactions. In Equation A.4 a simple redox reaction is shown for iron (Fe). This reaction can be viewed as an example of an inorganic redox reaction. *In vivo*, such reactions are carried out biologically by a group of iron-containing proteins, the cytochromes.

In biological systems, instead of transferring electrons (e^-), redox reactions more often transfer hydrogen (H), as shown in Equation A.5. In this reaction, flavin adenine dinucleotide (FAD) is a coenzyme in which the vitamin riboflavin participates in the redox reaction.

(reduced) Fe^{2+} $\underset{-\ e^-}{\overset{+\ e^-}{\rightleftharpoons}}$ Fe^{3+} (oxidized)

Iron(II)	Iron(III)
Ferrous ion	Ferric ion
[Fe(II) has been	[Fe(III) has been
oxidized to produce	reduced to produce
Fe(III)]	Fe(II)]

Equation A.4 Inorganic redox reaction.

$$FAD \underset{-\ 2H}{\overset{+\ 2H}{\rightleftharpoons}} FADH_2$$
$$\text{(oxidized form)} \qquad\qquad \text{(reduced form)}$$

Equation A.5 Organic redox reaction.

Examples of several vitamin redox reactions are presented in Chapter 5. Additional redox reactions of vitamin-containing and nonvitamin coenzymes and minerals will also be encountered in metabolism.

ENERGY, WORK, AND ATP

As defined by physics, energy is the capacity for doing work and overcoming resistance. Work, for example, physical movement, is movement through a measured distance. There are, in the biological world, several types of work and various forms of energy. The various types of work that require energy include mechanical work, chemical work, and osmotic and electrical work. All are different types of biological work. In animals and humans, the energy that sustains the various forms of biological work is derived from the carbohydrates, lipids, and proteins of the diet. Animals and humans, which derive their energy from a variety of food sources, are called heterochemotropes. Plants, on the other hand, derive their primary energy from photosynthesis (see Appendix B) from the sun and are called phototropes. In an indirect way, mediated by plants, people are solar powered.

All forms of energy may be described as consisting of either potential or kinetic energy. Gasoline (hydrocarbons) in the tank of an automobile is potential energy. A gasoline engine transforms the fuel into the kinetic energy of a flywheel or momentum for work to be accomplished. For people, food is a source of potential energy. A second source of potential energy for people is represented by the body's own store of its carbohydrates, lipids, and proteins, which can be called upon in the absence of an intake of food to provide the body with energy.

Whereas potential energy sources — the sun, food, and plant and body stores of carbohydrates, lipids, and proteins — are rather extensive for biological processes, most chemical, mechanical, osmotic, and electrical work (kinetic energy) is mediated by a single energy-bearing molecule, adenosine triphosphate (ATP). When energy-requiring processes of the body do not use ATP directly, they are mediated by ATP in a preexisting or subsequent step in metabolism. Energy flows through great

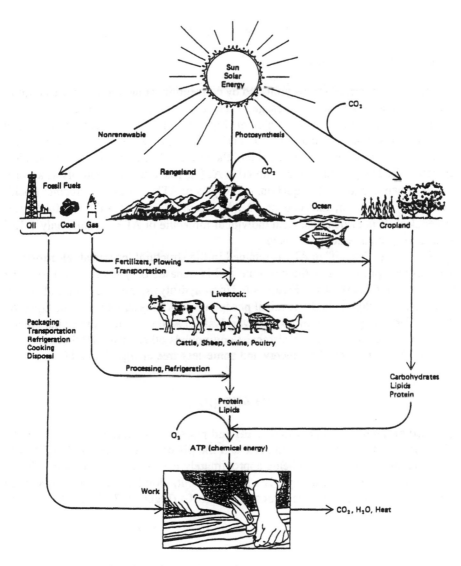

Figure A.5 Energy flow from the sun to people.

biological systems from the sun to people in food chains. This energy transfer is shown in Figure A.5.

Energy flow and energy requirements are measured in calories, kilocalories, or joules. By definition, the energy content of 1 calorie (cal) is the amount of heat needed to raise the temperature of 1 gram (g) of water 1°C. The amount of heat needed to raise the temperature of 1 kilogram (1000 g) of water 1°C is the kilocalorie (kcal). Thus 1000 calories equals 1 kcal. A normal human diet containing 2000 kcal contains 2,000,000 calories. It is technically correct to define energy units as either calories (actually kcal) or joules (1 J = 0.239 kcal). Whereas the use of the joule

$$\text{ATP} \xrightarrow[\text{H2O}]{\text{ATPase}} \text{ADP} + \text{P}_i + (\Delta G^{\circ\prime} = -7.3 \text{ kcal/mol})$$

Equation A.6 Hydrolysis of ATP.

for quantitating energy is now preferred by convention. However, there is a continuing widespread acceptance and usage of the calorie as a measure of energy.

The caloric values of the major energy-yielding nutrients are: proteins and carbohydrates, 4 kcal/g, and lipids, 9 kcal/g. Through the metabolic processes, the potential energy of food is converted into the universal carrier of potential chemical energy, ATP. The potential energy stored in ATP is released upon hydrolysis according to Equation A.6. In the equation, hydrolysis of ATP is shown to liberate (yield) free energy, $\Delta G^{\circ\prime}$, in the amount -7.3 kcal/mol (1 mol of ATP = 6.02×10^{23} molecules). It is evident that each individual molecule of ATP contains only $6/10^{23}$ kcal, a very small amount of energy.

The energy "stored" in ATP is retained in the structural, chemical, electrostatic, and resonant properties of the molecule and is released only upon hydrolysis. The structure of ATP is shown in Figure A.6. Upon hydrolysis, the -7.3 kcal/mol energy that has been "stored" in the terminal phosphate of ATP is summarized in Equation A.7. Under biological conditions, the hydrolysis of ATP may yield somewhat greater amounts of free energy. There also exist compounds other than ATP that can yield free energy, some more free energy and some less free energy than ATP.

pH AND pOH

Also of importance in nutrition is pH and pOH. It is important to recall that the pH of the stomach may approach pH 1 and the pH of the duodenum, 7 to 10, with the remaining small intestine being approximately neutral, pH 7. The letter p in pH stands for "–the log of"; thus pH is a measurement, $-\log [\text{H}^+]$, the molar hydrogen ion concentration. The pH scale runs from 0 to 14 (Figure A.7). The pH value and

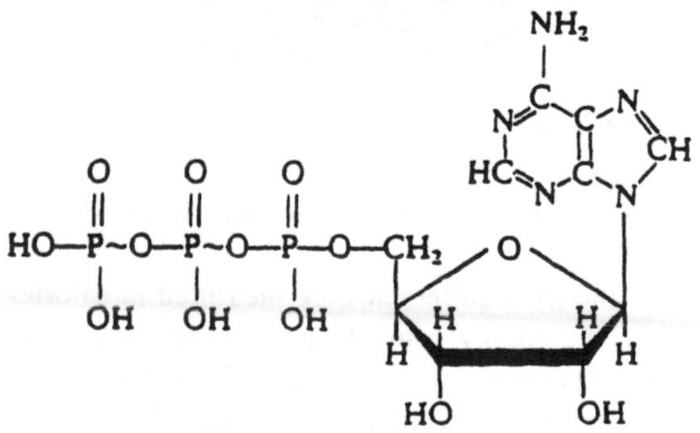

Adenosine triphosphate (ATP)

Figure A.6 Chemical structure of ATP.

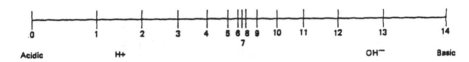

	kcal/mol
Energy contribution from hydrolysis of the terminal phosphate	$\Delta G^{o\prime} = -3.0$
Energy contribution from phosphoric acid electrostatic repulsion	$\Delta G^{o\prime} = -2.0$
Energy from change in resonance structure of π electrons	$\Delta G^{o\prime} = -2.3$
Summary: $ATP \rightarrow ADP + P_i$	$\Delta G^{o\prime} = -7.3$

Equation A.7 Energy stored within ATP.

```
 |——+———+——+——+——+——+—|||+——+——+——+——+——|
 .0      1      2     3    4  5 6 8 9  10   11    12    13          14
                               7
Acidic         H+                                        OH⁻        Basic
```

Figure A.7 pH scale (not to proper log scale).

the pOH (–log of the [OH⁻], the molar hydroxyl ion concentration) value, are always equal to 14.

Pure water is only weakly dissociated; $HOH \rightleftharpoons H^+ + OH^-$, with a concentration of $[H^+] =$ to $10^{-7}\ M$ and $[OH^-] = 10^{-7}\ M$. This condition is commonly referred to as neutral pH, pH 7. Values (pH) below 7 are acidic, while pH values greater than 7 are basic or alkaline. The [pH-pOH] scale is shown in Figure A.7. The pH scale is logarithmic, so that the difference between pH 7 and 8 is a factor of 10 in the [H⁺], whereas between 7 and 9 the [H⁺] is decreased by a factor of 100, and so on.

POLARITY AND SOLUBILITY

Wherever life exists as we know it, water is necessary as the primary sustenance of that life. The property of water that allows it to sustain life is its fluidity and versatility as a solvent. Water's most unique property in these respects is its polarity. Water possesses a dipole moment (Figure A.8) that is considerably larger than that of other liquid solvents. This property, the large dipole moment, permits solvation of inorganic salts; solvation of carbohydrates and proteins; and in the presence of certain amphipathic molecules, such as soaps and detergents, the solubilization of lipids that are hydrophobic. Most organic solvents are generally poor biological solvents because of their smaller dipole moment (Table A.2).

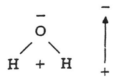

Figure A.8 Dipole moment of water.

Table A.2 Dielectric Constants

Solvent		Dielectric constant (measure of polarity, Debye units)	
Water	HOH	80	
Methanol	CH_3OH	33	
Ethanol	CH_3CH_2OH	24	
Butanol	$CH_3CH_2CH_2OH$	18	
Acetone	CH_3—C—CH_3 ‖ O	21	increasing polarity
Benzene	⬡ or ⬡	2.3	
N-Hexane	$CH_3CH_2CH_2CH_2CH_2CH_3$	1.9	

WEIGHTS AND MEASURES

Commonly used weights and measures are listed in Table A.3.

Table A.3 Commonly Used Weights and Measures

(m) 1 meter	= 3.2808 feet
(cm) 1 centimeter	= 0.3937 inch
(g) 1 gram	= 0.035274 ounce
(kg) 1 kilogram	= 2.2046 pounds
1 liter	= 1.05671 quarts
1 mm	= 10^7 Å
100 mm	= 1 centimeter
100 cm	= 1 meter
1000 ng	= 1 μg
1000 μg	= 1 mg
1000 mg	= 1 g
1000 g	= 1 kg
1000 μl	= 1 ml
1000 ml	= 1 L
1 dl	= 100 ml
1000 ppb	= 1 ppm
1 ppm	= 1 μg/mg = 1 mg/kg
1 ppm	= 1 μg/ml = 1 mg/L
1000 calories	= 1 Calorie (1 kilocalorie)
1 mole	= 1 gram-molecular weight
temperature: °C	= $\frac{5}{9}$ (°F − 32)
212°F	= 100°C
32°F	= °C
1 Cal (1 kcal)	= 4.184 kilojoules (kJ)

Photosynthesis and Energy Transfer

Located just 93×10^6 miles (150×10^6 km) from Earth (next door by astronomical distances) is a middle-aged star, our sun. Driven by hydrogen fusion ($1H^4 \rightarrow {}_2He^4 + 2e^-$), the sun's surface temperature is raised to about 10,800°F (6000°C). From its surface is emitted a continuous flow of thermal, ultraviolet, and visible energy in discrete energy packets called quanta. Calculations estimate that the emission of all forms of solar energy is equivalent to 7.2×10^{31} cal per day. Each day Earth receives about $5 \times 10^{-13}\%$ of the total emitted solar energy. The land area of Earth receives approximately 30% of each day's allocation of solar energy, equivalent to 1.1×10^{21} cal. More than 99.9% of all this solar energy received on Earth is either absorbed as heat, reflected back into space, or is used to drive our weather systems, consisting of evaporation, precipitation, and the convection currents of air and oceans. Of the remaining 0.1% of solar energy, 0.00005% is captured, stored, and utilized by algae and higher plants in a metabolic process called photosynthesis. All biologically useful energy enters and begins its journey through food chains by the photosynthetic process. With the exception of direct energy solar power conversion, nuclear power, wind power, tidal power, hydroelectromechanical power, and gravitational attraction, all other energy is supplied from the fossil fuels: oil, natural gas, and coal. These hydrocarbon energy sources are the remnants of the photosynthetic plants and animals existing millions of years ago. Energy derived from these fossil fuels is irreplaceable; once used, it is gone forever. In contrast, energy sources derived from photosynthesis — foods, nonfossil fuels, and fiber — are forever renewable on a seasonal or annual basis. Energy trapped by algae and higher plants by photosynthesis may enter a complex food web of nature or an agricultural food chain devised by humans. Energy transfer through a food chain from algae and crop plants to humans is shown in Figure B.1. In this hypothetical food chain, energy stored by photosynthesis by algae and cereal grains would be 100% transferable if eaten by humans. Energy transferred between levels of a food chain, between the primary energy producers (plants) and humans, may result in a 60% loss of the energy stored in each preceding level of organization. Such organization of food chains makes it

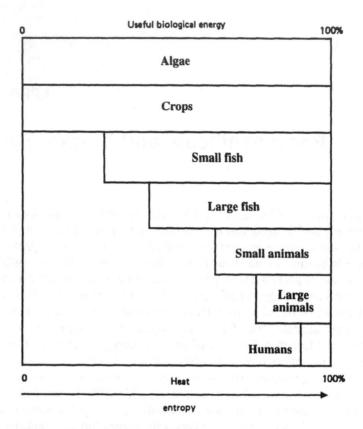

Figure B.1 Energy transfer within a food chain.

clear that a large agricultural base must be sustained and remain productive to supply energy to an ever-growing human population.

PHOTOSYNTHESIS

Plants, in the presence of sunlight, with adequate carbon dioxide and water, initially photosynthesize carbohydrates and can then use this carbohydrate energy to synthesize proteins and lipids. Photosynthesis is generally expressed by Equation B.1. In this equation the organic product is glucose and the oxygen gas evolved is derived from water. Nearly all atmospheric oxygen is produced by plants from water by photosynthesis. The carbon dioxide is provided to the plants by the atmosphere from oxidations and animal and human respiration. Water is absorbed in higher

$$6CO_2 + 6H_2O \xrightarrow{hv} C_6H_{12}O_6 + 6O_2 \uparrow$$

Equation B.1 Equation of photosynthesis.

plants from the soil by roots. Light (hv) energy is provided by the sun in quanta, discrete units of light energy sufficient to excite electrons. Photosynthesis is a dynamic process of plants which is affected by light intensity, temperature, and availability of carbon dioxide. For descriptive purposes the photosynthetic process is often divided into two major sets of chemical equations: (1) the light reactions and (2) the dark reactions. In plants, both light and dark reactions are operative in the presence of light, but in the absence of sufficient light only the dark reactions are operative.

LIGHT REACTIONS

The light reactions are the "photo" half of photosynthesis in plants and are shown in Figure B.2. Light energy (hv) falling on a plant's cellular surface is absorbed by the plant and converted to chemical (ATP) energy. The selective absorption of light energy of the wavelengths 400 to 525 nm and 600 to 680 nm are accomplished by the primary photosensitive pigments, chlorophylls a and b, and accessory pigments, the carotenoids (β-carotene) and the xanthophylls (Figure B.2). Absorbed light energy is transferred within the plant's thylakoid and chloroplast (Figure B.3) at photoreactive center I to an electron (e^-). The light energy transferred causes it to be excited, and it is raised to a higher energy level and a primary electron acceptor, PEA. This process is equivalent to using a large rubber mallet at the county fair (light) to raise the ringer (e^-) to the bell (PEA). With the potential energy raised, the e^- travels through a series of electron carriers, cytochromes, to which is coupled the enzymatic capacity for the synthesis of ATP from ADP and P_i. As a result of this process, called cyclic phosphorylation, some of the light energy transferred to the e^- is captured, stored, and retained by the chloroplast as molecules of ATP. To the extent that it occurs within the thylakoids in plants, cyclic phosphorylation requires only photocenter I and its accompaniment of enzymes and electron carriers.

Synthesis of ATP by noncyclic phosphorylation requires the integration of both photoreactive centers I and II (Figure B.2). In noncyclic phosphorylation, photoreactive center II, found in the intergranal lamella, absorbs light, and an excited electron (e^-) is raised to a higher potential energy level. This e^- cascades through a portion of the same electron carrier system as that responsible for the synthesis of ATP by cyclic phosphorylation, terminating in an electron void left by the excitation of an e^- from photoreactive center I. In this process ATP is synthesized from ADP and P_i and chemical energy is now transferable. Electrons from photoreactive center I have an alternative chemical pathway from the primary electron acceptor for cyclic (ATP) phosphorylation. These electrons may alternatively reduce $NADP^+$ formed from the oxidation of $NADPH_2$ during the synthesis of glucose (see next section, "Dark Reactions"). In this reaction $NADP^+$ is reduced by a flavoprotein. The protons of hydrogen (H^+) and electrons needed to form $NADPH_2$ for further biosynthesis of glucose are provided to $NADP^+$ by the splitting (oxidation) of water by the plant. Assisted by Mn^{2+}, the water split by the plant provides for

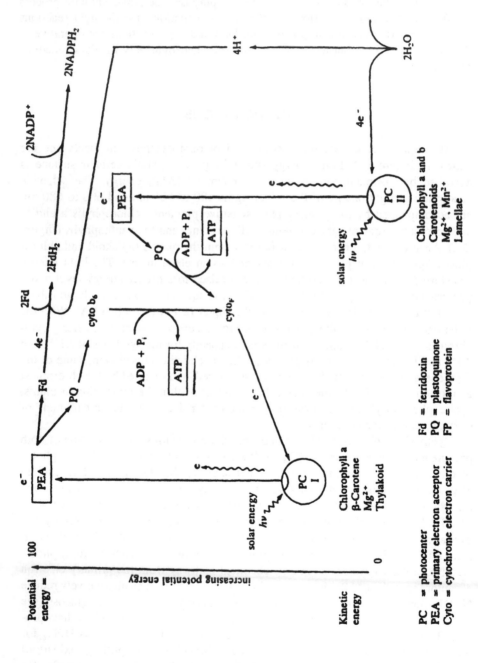

Figure B.2 Light reactions of photosynthesis (schematically simplified).

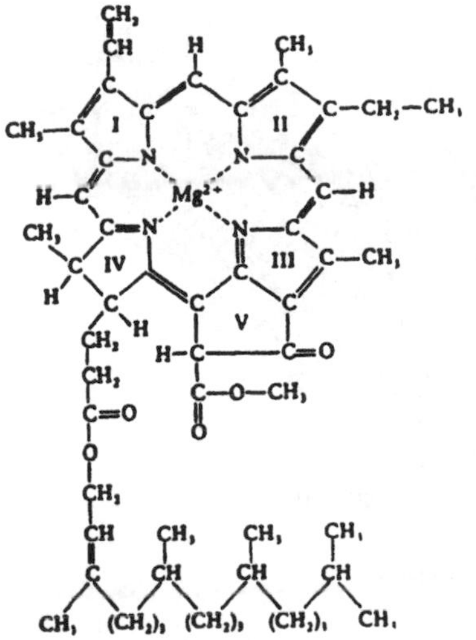

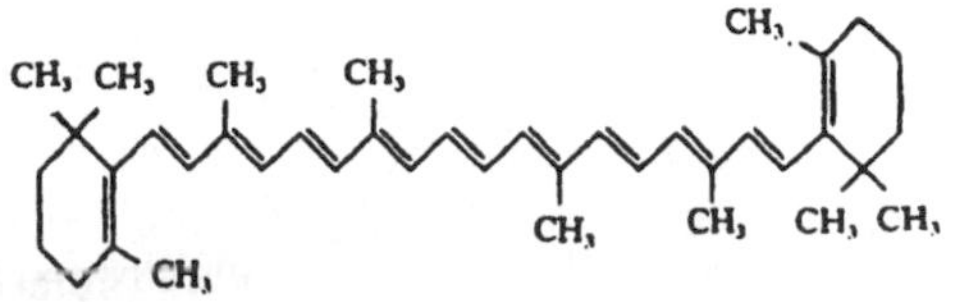

β-Carotene

Responsible for autumn folage color and precursor to vitamin A. β-Carotene, a carotenoid, absorbs light energy with transference to chlorophyll.

Chlorophyll a

Chlorophyll a is the major photoreceptive pigment in plants and is responsible for our green world. Replacement of —CH₃ in ring II by —CHO produces chlorophyll b. The chlorophylls are a major source of dietary magnesium.

Note: The extensive use of isoprene, a five-carbon monomeric unit is demonstrated here in the side chain of chlorophyll, β-carotene, and spirilloxanthin.

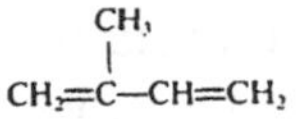

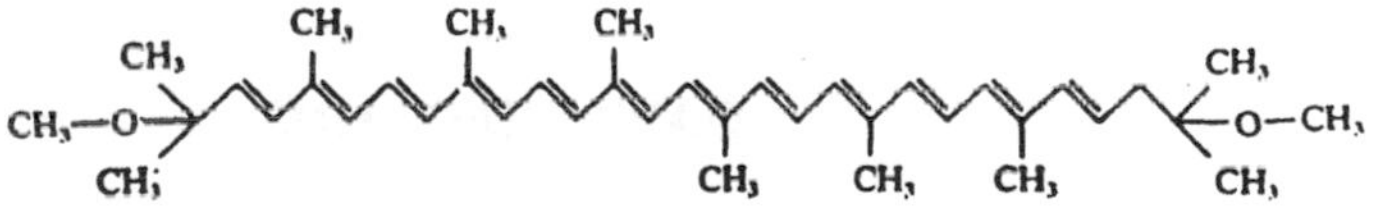

Xanthophylls contain oxygen but are otherwise similar to the carotenoids. This xanthophyll is spirilloxanthin.

Figure B.3 Chlorophyll and the secondary light-absorbing pigments.

the evolution of oxygen (O_2) gas, electrons for photocenter II for noncyclic phosphorylation, and electrons and hydrogen (protons) for reduction of $NADP^+$ to $NADPH^+ + H^+$. This entire process is energetically driven by sunlight, from which it derives its name, the light reactions. A chemical summation of noncyclic phosphorylation events and $NADP^+$ reduction is given in Equation B.2. The electrons and hydrogen for $NADPH + H^+$ in Equation B.2 are derived from the first two water molecules. The second water molecule is derived from the condensation of ADP and P_i in the synthesis of ATP.

$$2H_2O + ADP + P_i + 2NADP^+ \rightarrow ATP + 2NADPH + 2H^+ + O_2\uparrow + H_2O$$

Equation B.2 Equation of noncyclic phosphorylation.

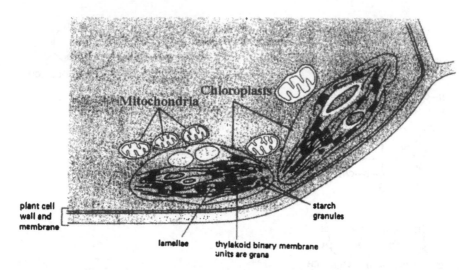

Figure B.4   Plant chloroplasts. Drawn from an electron micrograph of a soybean plant cell.
(Courtesy of Dr. John Burke, Plant Stress and Water Conservation Laboratory,
U.S. Department of Agriculture.)

The important products of the light reactions are the synthesis of ATP and
NADPH + H+, for both are used in the dark reactions of photosynthesis. The oxygen
produced during the light reactions by higher plants is important to animals, humans,
and even for plant life.

DARK REACTIONS

The dark reactions are the "synthetic" half of photosynthesis. In the chloroplast,
ATP and NADPH+ + H+ synthesized in the light reactions are consumed in the
reduction and conversion of CO_2 to glucose and other carbohydrates. The chemical
details of the reduction of CO_2 to glucose became possible when the radioisotope,
$^{14}CO_2$, was made available toward the end of World War II. M. Calvin and his
associates at the University of California at Berkeley are responsible for providing
much of the information on how CO_2 is incorporated into glucose. For this work,
Calvin received the Nobel Prize in Chemistry in 1961 and the chemical cycle for
the photosynthetic reduction of CO_2 bears his name, the Calvin cycle (Figure B.5).

THE CALVIN CYCLE

The Calvin cycle (Figure B.5) is thermodynamically driven by the ATP and
NADPH + H+ synthesized by the light reactions. No light or other external energy
is needed beyond the ATP requirement; thus CO_2 reduction may occur in the presence
or absence of light. The first two reactions of the Calvin cycle are the most important,
as they use the ATP and NADPH + H+ produced by the light reactions for CO_2

fixation. The first reaction (Equation B.3) is the carboxylation of ribulose-1,5-diphosphate (a five-carbon sugar), forming two molecules of a three-carbon carbohydrate, 3-phosphoglycerate (six carbons total).

The ATP and NADPH + H$^+$ produced in the light reactions are used in the second chemical reaction of the cycle (Equation B.4). Equation B.5 is the reverse of the glycolysis reaction (see Chapter 12), in which 3-phosphoglyceraldehyde is converted to 3-phosphoglycerate with the accompanying synthesis of ATP and NADH + H$^+$. Equation B.5 is thermodynamically very much "uphill," requiring the expenditure of two molecules of ATP to ensure the reaction's completion.

In the remaining reactions of the Calvin cycle (see Figure B.5), isomerization of one of the molecules of glyceraldehyde-3-phosphate to dihydroxyacetone phosphate and its condensation with another molecule of 3-phosphoglyceraldehyde yields the hexose, fructose-1,6-diphosphate. Fructose-1,6-diphosphate loses P$_i$, yielding 6-phosphofructose-6-phosphate, which can isomerize to glucose-6-phosphate. Glucose (six carbons) may then polymerize, becoming cellulose [β-(1→4) glycosides] or starch [α-(1→4)glycosides], or dimerize with fructose to become sucrose. To this point the cycle has added only the one carbon atom from CO_2. To complete the cycle, ribulose-1,5-diphosphate must be regenerated. This is accomplished by the condensation of fructose-6-phosphate with glyceraldehyde-3-phosphate (nine carbons) in lieu of glucose synthesis, which yields a four-carbon carbohydrate, erythrose-4-phosphate, and a five-carbon carbohydrate, xylulose-5-phosphate. Ribulose-1-5-diphosphate is then regenerated in two possible ways. Xylulose-5-phosphate is epimerized to ribulose-5-phosphate, which is phosphorylated by ATP to ribulose-1,5-diphosphate or sedhepulose-7-phosphate (seven carbons). Sedhepulose-7-phosphate combines with glycerate-3-phosphate (three carbons) to yield two molecules of ribulose-5-phosphate, which are phosphorylated with two ATP molecules (one ATP each), completing the cycle. One complete turn of the Calvin cycle for each added CO_2 can be summarized as shown in Equation B.5. To complete the synthesis of one completely new glucose molecule, six turns of the cycle are necessary. Three molecules of ATP are used in reducing one molecule of CO_2 and 18 molecules of ATP are expended in the synthesis of one molecule of glucose. With this information and knowing the $\Delta G^{o\prime}$ energy value for ATP and the caloric value of glucose, an estimate of the efficiency for the Calvin cycle can be made (Figure B.6).

The calculated value of efficiency for the Calvin cycle, 81%, demonstrates the metabolic conservation of energy for this single pathway. Overall, thermodynamic efficiency of plants, however, is much, much lower. Taking into consideration the needed quantum light energy capable of synthesizing sufficient ATP to make a mole of glucose, plant thermodynamic efficiency drops to about 35%. When thermodynamic calculations consider the entire solar energy falling on the surface of a plant's leaf, conservation of solar energy for cultivated crops is around 1%, and much less than 1% of total solar energy is stored by plants for use as food, fuels, and fiber. Every year, however, 106 metric tons of CO_2 are converted by plants into organic matter by photosynthesis, dwarfing any other single annual human effort. Table B.1 provides estimates of annual grain production and compares the photosynthetic event to annual meat production.

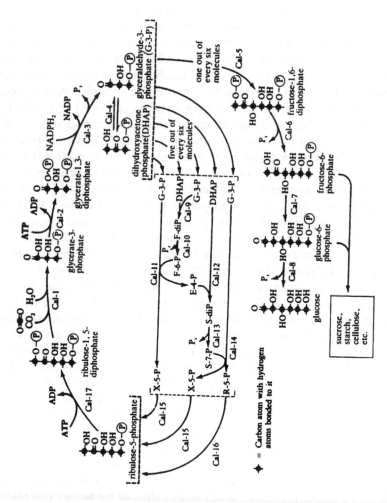

Figure B.5 The Calvin cycle.

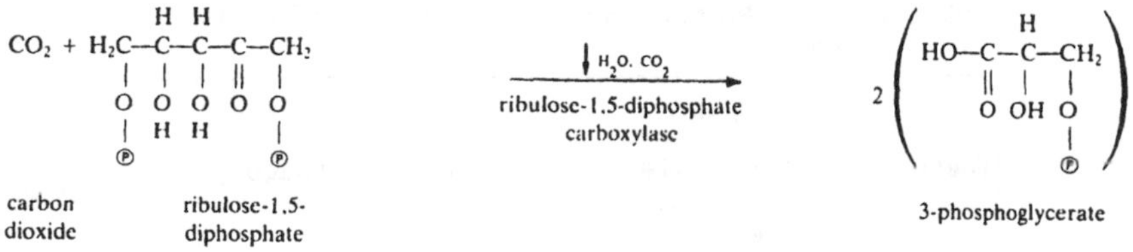

$$CO_2 + H_2C-C-C-C-CH_2$$

carbon
dioxide

ribulose-1,5-
diphosphate

$$\xrightarrow[\text{carboxylase}]{\text{ribulose-1,5-diphosphate}} \quad H_2O, CO_2$$

$$2\left(HO-C-C-CH_2\right)$$

3-phosphoglycerate

Equation B.3 Carbon dioxide formation by plants.

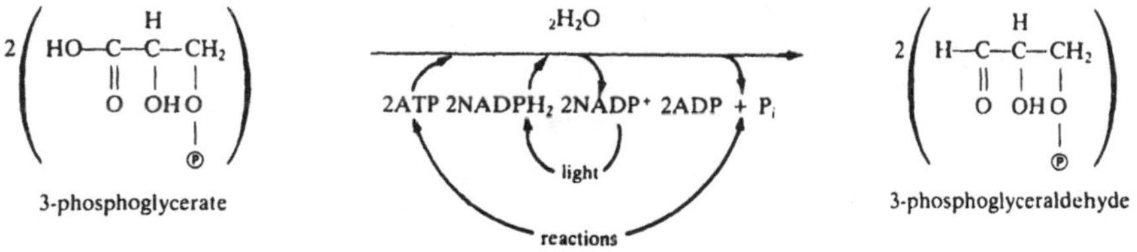

$$2\left(HO-C-C-CH_2\right)$$

3-phosphoglycerate

$$\xrightarrow{2H_2O}$$

2ATP 2NADPH$_2$ 2NADP$^+$ 2ADP + P$_i$

light

reactions

$$2\left(H-C-C-CH_2\right)$$

3-phosphoglyceraldehyde

Equation B.4 Reduction of 3-phosphoglycerate.

$$\text{ribulose-1,5-diphosphate} + CO_2 + 3ATP + 2NADPH + 2H^+ + 2H_2O \xrightarrow{\text{one turn}}$$

$$\text{ribulose-1,5-diphosphate (regenerated)} + \tfrac{1}{6}(C_6H_{12}O_6) + 3P_i + 3ADP + 2NADP^+$$

Equation B.5 Chemical summary of the Calvin cycle.

$\Delta G^{\circ\prime}$ of hydrolysis for ATP $\quad = -7.3$ kcal/mol

Glucose (caloric value) $\quad = 686$ kcal/mol

ATP consumed $(-7.3 \text{ kcal} \times 18) = 131$ kcal

$$\frac{131 \text{ kcal}}{686 \text{ kcal}} \times 100 = 19\%$$

$100\% - 19\% = 81\%$ efficiency for the conversion of "ATP energy" into "glucose energy"

Figure B.6 Energy efficiency of the Calvin cycle.

Table B.1   Annual Production of Grains and Meats (10^6 Metric Tons)

Grains				<15
Wheat	360	Millet	45	Cabbage
Rice	320	Banana	35	Onions
Corn	300	Tomato	35	Beans
Potato	300	Sugarbeet	30	Peas
Barley	170	Rye	30	Sunflower seeds
Sweet potato	130	Oranges	30	Mango
Cassava	100	Coconut	30	
Grapes	60	Cottonseed oil	25	
Soybeans	60	Apples	20	
Oats	50	Yams	20	
Sorghum	50	Peanuts	20	
Sugarcane	50	Watermelon	20	

Meats	
Pork	43
Beef	42
Poultry	21
Lamb	5
Goat	1.5
Buffalo	1
Horse	0.7

Source: Jack R. Harlan, The plants and animals that nourish man, in Human Nutrition, Chapter 6, Scientific American Press, New York (1978).

PLANT RESPIRATION

As described above, plants produced ATP and $NADPH_2$ in the light reactions for the fixation and reduction of CO_2 in the dark reactions. Plants continue to undergo metabolism and growth in the absence of light and without the synthesis of ATP and $NADPH_2$ by noncyclic phosphorylation. Continuation of plant metabolism in the dark is possible because of respiration. Like animals (Chapter 12), plants metabolize their own carbohydrates from photosynthesis, producing $NADPH_2$ by the hexose monophosphate shunt, and plants possess mitochondria, which synthesize ATP by oxidative phosphorylation. During respiration, plants, like animals, produce CO_2 and consume O_2.

APPENDIX C

REFERENCES

Books

Berdanier, C.D. *Advanced Nutrition: Macronutrients*. Boca Raton, FL: CRC Press, 1995.

Berdanier. C.D. *Advanced Nutrition: Micronutrients*. Boca Raton, FL: CRC Press, 1998.

Bezkorovainy, A. and Rafelson, M.E., Jr. *Concise Biochemistry*. New York: Marcel Dekker, Inc., 1996.

Deglin, J.H., and Vallerand A.H. *Davis's Drug Guide for Nurses*, 5th ed. Philadelphia, PA: F.A. Davis Co., 1997.

Federation of American Societies for Experimental Biology. *ThirdReport on Nutrition Monitoring in the United States*, Vol. 1 and 2. Washington, D.C.: U.S. Government Printing Office, 1995.

Gibson, R.S. *Principles of Nutritional Assessment*. New York: Oxford University Press, 1990.

Grant, A. and DeHoog, S. *Nutritional Assessment and Support*, 4th ed. Seattle, WA: Anne Grant and Susan DeHoog Publ., 1991.

Harper, L.J., Deaton, B.J., and Driskell, J.A. *Food, Nutrition, and Agriculture: Textbook*. Rome: FAO, 1984.

Machlin, L.J., Ed. *Handbook of Vitamins*, 2nd ed. New York: Marcel Dekker, Inc., 1991.

Murray, R.K., Granner, D.K., Mayes, P.A., and Rodwell, V.W. *Harper's Biochemistry*, 23rd ed. Norwalk, CN: Appleton & Lange, 1993.

National Research Council, National Academy of Sciences. *Diet and Health: Implications for Reducing Chronic Disease Risk*. Washington, DC: National Academy Press, 1989.

National Research Council, National Academy of Sciences. *Dietary Reference Intakes: Calcium, Phosphorus, Magnesium, Vitamin D, and Fluoride*, Prepublication copy. Washington, DC: National Academy Press, 1997.

National Research Council, National Academy of Sciences. *Dietary Reference Intakes: Thiamin, Riboflavin, Niacin, Vitamin B_6, Folate, Vitamin B_{12}, Pantothenic Acid, Biotin, and Choline*, Prepublication copy. Washington, DC: National Academy Press, 1998.

National Research Council, National Academy of Sciences. *Recommended Dietary Allowances*, 10th ed. Washington, DC: National Academy Press, 1989.

Physician's Desk Reference. Montvale, NJ: Medical Economics Data Production Co., 1998.

Sizer, F., and Whitney, E. *Nutrition Concepts and Controversies*, 7th ed. Belmont, CA: West/Wadsworth, 1997.

Shils, M.E., Olson, J.A., and Shike, M. *Modern Nutrition in Health and Disease*, Vol. 1 and 2, 8th ed. Malvern, PA: Lea & Febiger, 1994.

Ziegler, E.E., and Filer, L.J., Jr., Eds. *Present Knowledge in Nutrition*, 7th ed. Washington, DC: International Life Sciences Institute Press, 1996.

Journal Articles

Ames, B.N. Dietary carcinogens and anticarcinogens. *Science*, 1983; 221:1256-1264.

Arthur, J.R., Nicol, F., and Beckett, G.J. Selenium deficiency, thyroid hormone metabolism and thyroid hormone deiodinases. *Am. J. Clin. Nutr.*, 1993;57:236S-239S.

Bock A., Forchhammer, K., Heider, J., Leinfelder, W., Sawers, G., Veprek, B., and Zinoni, F. Selenocysteine: The 21st amino acid. *Mol. Microbiol.* 1991; 5:515-520.

Buettner, G.R. The pecking order of free radicals and antioxidants: Lipid peroxidation, - tocopherol and ascorbate. *Arch. Biochem. Biophys.*, 1993; 300:535-543.

Burk, R.F. Recent developments in trace element metabolism and function: Newer roles of selenium in nutrition. *J. Nutr.*, 1989; 119:1051-1054.

Chung, A., Suttie, J.W., and Bernatowicz, M. Vitamin K-dependent carboxylase: Structural requirements for propeptide activation. *Biochem. Biophys. Acta*, 1990; 1039:90-93.

Frieden, E. New perspectives on the essential trace elements. *J. Chem. Educ.*, 1985; 62:917-923.

Hudnall, M.V., Connor, S.L., and Connor, W.E. Position of The American Dietetic Association: Fat replacement. *J. Am. Diet.Assoc.*, 1991; 91:1285-1288.

Hahn, N.E. Replacing fat with food technology. *J. Am. Diet. Assoc.*, 1997; 97:15-16.

Mermelstein, N.H. A new era in food labeling. *Food Tech.*, 1993; 47(2):81-92.

Olson, J.A. Hypervitaminosis A: Contemporary scientific issues. *J. Nutr.*, 1994; 124:1461S-1466S.

Prasad, A.S. Discovery and importance of zinc in human nutrition. *Fed. Proc.*, 1984; 43:2829-2834.

Spallholz, J.E. On the nature of selenium toxicity and carcinostatic activity. *Free Rad. Biol. and Med.*, 1994; 17:45-64.

Suttie, J.W. Synthesis of vitamin K dependent proteins. *FASEB J.*, 1993; 7:445-452.

Vidal-Cros, A., Gaudry, M., and Andree, M. Vitamin K-dependent carboxylation. *Biochem. J.*, 1990; 266:749-755.

Pamphlets

Hassel, C. *Olean Briefing*. Cincinnati, OH: Proctor and Gamble Co., 1997.

United States Department of Agriculture and of Health and Human Services. *Nutrition and Your Health: Dietary Guidelines for Americans*, 4th ed. Washington, DC: U.S. Government Printing Office, 1995 [Home and Garden Bulletin No. 232].

United States Department of Agriculture. *The Food Guide Pyramid*. Hyattsville, MD: U.S. Department of Agriculture, Human Nutrition Information Service, 1992 [Home and Garden Bulletin No. 252].

Federal Register

Food and Drug Administration. Food Labeling: Mandatory Status of Nutrition Labeling and Nutrient Content Revision, Format for Nutrition Label. *Federal Register*, 1992; 58:2079-2205.

Food and Drug Administration. Food Labeling: Nutrient Content Claims, General Principles, Petitions, Definition of Terms; Definitions of Nutrient Content Claims for the Fat, Fatty Acid, and Cholesterol Content of Food. *Federal Register*, 1992; 58:2302-2426.

Food and Drug Administration. Food Labeling: Reference Daily Intakes and Daily Reference Values. *Federal Register*, 1992; 58:2206-2228.

Food and Drug Administration. Food Labeling: Serving Sizes. *Federal Register*, 1992; 58:2229- 2300.

Internet

National Research Council, National Academy of Sciences. New Report Recasts Dietary Requirement for Calcium and Related Nutrients. *Internet release* of August 13, 1997.

Index

A

Abetalipoproteinemia, 72
Abortions, spontaneous, 65
ACE, *see* Angiotensin converting enzyme
Acetic, acid, 25
Acetylkinase, 132
Acetylphosphate, 229
Acetylsalicylic acid, 279
Activity factor, 206
Adenosine
  diphosphate (ADP), 201
  monophosphate (AMP), 253
  triphosphate (ATP), 201, 316
    energy, 316
    release of, 318
    synthesis, 227
    work, 316
Adipose tissue, 167
ADP, *see* Adenosine diphosphate
Adrenocorticotropins, 24
Alanine, 49, 260
Aldehyde oxidase, 141
Algae, 321
Algal polysaccharides, 18
Alkalosis, 135
Aluminum hydroxide, 279
Amino acid(s), 188
  classification, 41
  essential, 49
  metabolism, 235
  secondary, 45
γ-Amino butyric acid, 43
Amitriptyline, 279
Ammonia, elimination of, 235
AMP, *see* Adenosine monophosphate
Amphotericin, 279

Amylose, 12
Anabolic pathways, 241–251
  cholesterol and steroid biosynthesis,
    247–251
  fatty acid synthesis, 244–247
  fatty acid and triglyceride synthesis, 244
  gluconeogenesis, 241–243
  glycogenic amino acids and glycerol, 244
Anabolic reactions, 228
Androgens, 24
Anemia, 72
Angiotensin converting enzyme (ACE), 284
Anorexia, 91
Anticarcinogen, 22
Antidiuretic hormone, 169
Antihemorrhagic Factor, 57
Antimetabolites, 282
Antioxidants, 58, 78, 270
Appendicitis, 20
Arachidonic acid, 39, 71
Arginine, 49
Ariboflavinosis, 57
Ascorbic acid, 45, 273
  lack of dietary, 77
  major functions of, 78
Asparagine, 49, 260
Aspartame, 43
Aspartic acid, 49, 260
Ataxia, 149
Atherosclerosis, 72, 81
ATP, *see* Adenosine triphosphate
Autism, 95

B

Bacteria, elements required by, 6
Barbiturates, 279

Basal metabolic rate (BMR), 152
Behenic acid, 25, 191
Beriberi, 57
BHA, *see* Butylated hydroxyanisole
BHT, *see* Butylated hydroxytoluene
Bile
  acids, 24, 30, 42, 192
  salts, 192
  secretion, 177
Biotin, 56, 104, 181
Birth defects, 65
Blood coagulation, 74
BMR, *see* Basal metabolic rate
Body energy, 201–207
  aerobic and anaerobic energy release,
    201
  anaerobic and aerobic energy from foods,
    202
  basal and resting metabolism, 203–204
  body calorimetry, 203
  calories, 202–203
  components of energy expenditure, 203
  energy reservoir, 201–202
  estimating energy expenditure, 204–207
  thermic effect of exercise, 204
  thermic effect of food, 204
Bomb calorimeter, 202
Bonding, 309
Bone(s)
  abnormalities, 65
  porous, 126
Buccal cavity, 174
Butylated hydroxyanisole (BHA), 274
Butylated hydroxytoluene (BHT), 274
Butyric acid, 22, 25

C

Calcitonin, 127
Calcium, 125
  absorption, 126
  dietary reference intake values for, 292
Calmodulin, 127
Caloric density, of selected foods, 239
Calvin cycle, 327
Cancer, 20, 72
Caprenin, 191
Caproic acid, 25
Caprylic acid, 25

Carbohydrates, 9–22
  catabolism of, 222
  chemistry of dietary fiber, 16–18
    cellulose, 16
    gums, mucilages, and algal
      polysaccharides, 18
    hemicellulose, 16
    lignin, 18
    pectins, 16–18
  dietary fiber, 15–16
  disaccharides, 10–12
    lactose, 11
    maltose, 12
    sucrose, 10–11
  fermentation, 19
  fiber and cholesterol, 20–21
  fiber and colon cancer, 21–22
  hydration, 19
  importance of fiber as nutrient, 20
  loss of, 234
  metal binding, 19–20
  monosaccharides, 9–10
    fructose and galactose, 9–10
    glucose, 9
  nutritional properties of dietary fiber, 19
  polysaccharides, 12–15
    cellulose, 13–14
    dietary fiber, 14–15
    glycogen, 13
    starch, 12–13
Caries prevention, 294
Carnitine, 111, 114
Carotenoids, 65, 273
Carpal tunnel syndrome, 95
Catabolic pathways, 219–240
  of carbohydrates, 219–230
    citric acid cycle, 223–225
    electron transport system and oxidative
      phosphorylation, 225–227
    glycolysis, 219–222
    thermodynamics of ATP and ATP
      synthesis, 227–230
  of lipids, 230–233
  of proteins, 234–240
    caloric density of foods, 239–240
    elimination of ammonia, 235–236
    energy, ATP, and catabolic pathways,
      236–239
Catalase, 141, 275

Cataracts, 10, 72
Cells, components of, 209–216
    animal and plant metabolism, 212–215
    mammalian cells, 209–211
    metabolic maps, 216
    plant cells, 211–212
Cellulose, 13, 16
Ceramide, 32
Cereal grains, 321
Cerebroside, 32, 35
Ceruloplasmin, 154
Cheilosis, 86
Chinese disease, 151
Chlorine, 134
Chloroplasts, 211, 212
Cholesterol, 24, 180
    esters, in plasma, 29
    serum, 178
    synthesis, 247
Cholestyramine, 178, 279
Choline, synthetic, 297
Chromium, 157
    dietary, 158
    picolinate, 158
Chromoproteins, 48
Cimetidine, 279
Citric acid, 202, 222
Clofibrate, 279
Coast disease, 162
Cobalamin, 100
Cobalt, 161
Coenzyme A, 223
Colchicine, 279
Collagen, 45
Colloid, 177
Colon cancer, 21
Constipation, 20
Convulsion, 169
Copper, 153
Coronary heart disease, 58, 78
Coumarins, 73, 279
Covalent bond, 309
Creatine
    kinase, 131
    phosphate, 229
Creatinine, 51
Cyanocobalamin, 196
Cycloserine, 279
Cysteine, 49, 260, 271

Cytochrome C, 141, 154
Cytosine, 254

D

Dehydration, 169
Deoxyribonucleic acid (DNA), 1, 211, 255
Dermatitis, 57
Dextrans, 190
DFEs, see Dietary folate equivalents
Diabetic neuropathy, 95
Diet, American, 219
Dietary fiber, 15, 120
Dietary folate equivalents (DFEs), 98
Dietary reference intakes (DRIs), 288, 291
Digestive enzymes, 18
Digitalis, 279
Diglycerides, 24
Dihydroxyacetonephosphate, 244, 247
Dipeptides, 188
Dipole moment, 319
Disaccharides, 10
Diverticulosis, 20
DNA, see Deoxyribonucleic acid
L-Dopa, 280
Dopamine, 93
Down's syndrome, 95
DRIs, see Dietary reference intakes
Drug therapy, prescription, 277

E

EDTA, see Ethylenediaminetetraacetate
Eicosapentaenoic acid, 38, 39
Eicosatetraenoic acid, 37
Eicosatrienoic acid, 37
Electrocardiographic abnormalities, 107
Electrolytes, 170
Electron micrograph, of a soybean plant, 325
Electron transport chain (ETC), 225
Elements, naturally occurring, 118
Endocrine diseases, 20
Energy
    expenditure, 204
    intake, recommended, 207
    potential, 316
    sources, 321
Enolase, 131
Enterokinase, 179, 181

Enteropeptidases, 179
Enzyme activity, regulator of, 130
Enzymology, 312
Ergosterol, 66
Erythrocuprein, 154
Esterases, 179
Estrogens, 24
ETC, see Electron transport chain
Ethylenediaminetetraacetate (EDTA), 122
Exercise, thermic effect of, 204

F

FAD, see Flavin adenine dinucleotide
Famotidine, 279
Fat
    counting grams of, 301
    -soluble vitamins, 23
Fatty acid(s), 24, 185
    catabolism of, 222
    short-chain, 22
    synthesis, 245
Feces formation, 183
Fermentation reactions, 18
Ferridoxins, 141
Ferritin, 141
FFAs, see Free fatty acids
Fiber, of vegetable origin, 19
Fish liver oils, 68
Flavin adenine dinucleotide (FAD), 84, 85
Flavin mononucleotide (FMN), 84, 85
Flavoprotein, 231
Fluoride, dietary, 144
FMN, see Flavin mononucleotide
Folate, 96
    antagonists, 99
    deficiency, 282
    precipitation, 100
    status, 99
Folic acid
    absorption, 196
    rich sources of 98
    synthetic, 297
Follicle-stimulating hormone (FSH), 46
Food
    chains, 317
    chemicals, nonnutritive, 286
    groups, 300
    labels, 303
    thermic effect of, 204

Free fatty acids (FFAs), 230
Free radicals, lipid peroxidation, and
        antioxidants, 265–275
    antioxidants, 270–275
        antioxidant enzymes, 274
        antioxidants, 270–274
        catalase, 275
        glutathione peroxidases, 274–275
        glutathione-S-transferase, 275
        superoxide dismutase, 274
    chain reactions, 267–270
    toxic oxygen species, 265–267
Fructokinase, 131
Fructose, 9
FSH, see Follicle-stimulating hormone
Fungicide, 279
Furosemide, 280

G

GABA, see γ-Amino butyric acid
Galactose, 9, 14
Gallbladder, 167
Ganglioside, 32, 36
Gastric juice, 136
Gastrin, 183
Gestational diabetes, 95
Gibbs' free energy, 314
Gluconeogenesis, 243
Glucose, 14, 170
Glutamic acid, 49, 260
Glutamine, 49, 236, 260
Glutamylglycine, 237
Glutathione reductase activity, 88
Glycine, 42, 49, 260
Glycogen
    storage disease (GSD), 13
    structure of, 13
Glycogenolysis, 183
Glycolipids, 24
Glycolysis, 220
Glycoproteins, 48
GSD, see Glycogen storage disease

H

HDL cholesterol, 21
Health claims, approved, 303
Heart, irreversible calcification of, 69
Heat stroke, 169

Heme iron, 48
Hemicellulose, 15, 16, 187
Hemocyanin, 154
Hemoglobin, 141
Hemolytic anemia, 76
Hemorrhoids, 20
Hemosiderin, 140, 141
Hemovanadin, 163
Hepatic lipogenesis, 21
Heptanoic acid, 25
Herbivores, 219
Hexosemonophosphate (HMP), 210
Histamine, 93
Histidine, 49, 260
HMP, see Hexosemonophosphate
Humans, elements required by, 6
Hydralazine, 280
Hydrochloric acid, 136
Hydroquinones, 271
Hydroxyapatite, 128
Hydroxyproline, 41, 49
Hyperbilirubinemia, 76
Hypercholesterolemia, 107
Hyperoxaluria, 95
Hyponatremia, 134

I

IF, see Intrinsic factor
Imipramine, 280
Immune function, optimal, 80
IMP, see Inosine monophosphate
Index nutrient, 83
Indomethacin, 280
Inosine monophosphate (IMP), 253
Inositol metabolism, 116
Insomnia, 91
Insulin secretion, 65, 68
Insulin, 47
International Union of Pure and Applied
    Chemists, (IUPAC), 26
Intestinal microflora, 112
Intestines, bacterial synthesis in, 74
Intrinsic factor (IF), 175
Ionic bond, 309
Iron
    homeostasis, 140
    sources of, 142
    toxicity, 142
Isoleucine, 42, 49

Isoniazid, 280
IUPAC, see International Union of Pure and
    Applied Chemists

K

Kanamycin, 280
Kernicterus, 76
Keshan's disease, 121
Ketone formation, 250
Kidney(s)
    disorders, 52
    irreversible calcification of, 69
Krebs cycle, 82
Kwashiorkor, 51

L

Lactase, 181
Lactic acid bacteria, 96
Lactoflavin, 85
Lactose intolerance, 11
Lauric acid, 25
Laxative, 280
Leucine, 49, 260
    aminopeptidase, 146
    metabolism of, 42
Leukopenia, 103
Leukotrienes, 39
Life, elements of, 1–6
    distribution of elements in universe, on
        earth, and in human body, 3–4
    elemental requirements of
        microorganisms, plants, animals, and
        humans, 5
Lignin, 15, 19, 187
Lignoceric acid, 25
Linoleic acid, 36, 93
Lipids, 23–40, 311
    cholesterol and derivatives, 29–30
    classification, 23–24
    essential fatty acids, 35–36
    fatty acids, 24–27
    mono-, di-, and triglycerides, 27–29
    phosphatidic acid and derivatives, 30–35
    prostanoic acid and prostaglandins, 38–40
    synthesis of eicosatrienoic,
        eicosatetraenoic, and
        eicosapentaenoic acids, 36–38
    eicosatrienoic acid, 37

  eicosatetraenoic acid, 37–38
  eicosapentaenoic acid, 38
Lipoproteins, 24, 48
Liver
  alcohol dehydrogenase, 146
  cell, human, 209
  cirrhosis of, 10
  damage, 76
Loop diuretic, 280
Lungs, irreversible calcification of, 69
Lycopene, 192
Lymph system, 185
Lysine, 49, 260
Lysyl oxidase, 154

M

Macrominerals, 121
Magnesium, 293
Malondialdehyde, 267
Maltose, 12, 181
Malt sugar, 10
Manadione, 73
Maple syrup urine disease (MSUD), 42
Marasmus, symptoms of, 52
Margaric acid, 25
Margarine, 27
Maximum substrate concentration (MSC),
    313
Medications, digestive and metabolic
    interactions between nutrients/foods
    and, 277–286
  competitive inhibition of dihydrofolate,
    278–282
  direct chemical reactivity, 278
  drug action on membrane receptor sites,
    283–284
  drug metabolism, 284–286
  medication–nutrient food interactions,
    277–278
Megaloblastic anemia, 57, 103
Melanin, 43
Mental retardation, 10
Metabolic maps, 216
Metabolic water, 168
Metabolism, resting, 203
Metalloenzymes, 119
Metalloproteins, 48
Methionine, 49, 137, 260
Methotrexate, 280, 282

Methylcobalamin, 100
Methyldopa, 280
Methylene, 311
MFOs, see Mixed-function oxidases
Micelles, formation of, 177
Microminerals, 117
Milk fat, 29
Minerals, 117–163
  absorption and metabolism of, 123–125
  calcium, 125–128
  chlorine, 134–136
  chromium, 157–158
  cobalt, 161–162
  coordination and chelation of, 122–123
  copper, 153–155
  essentiality and bioavailability of, 121
  fluorine, 142–144
  iodine, 150–153
  iron, 139–142
  magnesium, 130–133
  manganese, 148–150
  molybdenum, 155–157
  nickel, 160–161
  nutritional functions of, 118–120
  phosphorus, 128–130
  selenium, 146–148
  silicon, 158–160
  sodium, 133–134
  sulfur, 136–139
  toxicity of, 121–122
  vanadium, 162–163
  zinc, 144–146
MIOs, see Mixed-function oxidases
Mitochondria, in the ETS, 228
Mixed-function oxidases (MIOs), 285
Molybdenum, 155
  absorption, 157
  deficiency, 156
Monoamine oxidase inhibitors, 280
Monoglycerides, 24, 185, 192
Mononucleotides, 258
Monosaccharides, 9
Monosodium glutamate (MSG), 42
Morning sickness, 95
MSC, see Maximum substrate concentration
MSG, see Monosodium glutamate
MSUD, see Maple syrup urine disease
Multivitamin preparation, 94
Muscle
  contraction, 13, 125

loss, 91
weakness, 111
Myoglobin, 140, 310
Myristic acid, 25

N

Nematodes, 147
Neomycin, 280
Niacin, 83
  deficiency, 91
  discovery of, 88
Nickel, 160
  absorption, 161
  dietary, 161
Nicotinamide, 89, 92
Nicotinic acid, 55
Night blindness, 57, 63
Nitrofurantoin, 280
Nitrogen dioxide, 266
Nondecylic acid, 25
Normoglycemia, maintaining, 11
Nucleases, 179
Nucleic acids, genes, and protein synthesis,
    253–262
  deoxyribonucleic and ribonucleic acid,
    255–258
  genes, codons, anticodons, and tRNAs,
    258–260
  nucleotides, 255
  protein synthesis, 260–262
  purines, 253–254
  pyrimidines, 254–255
Nucleoproteins, 48
Nucleosidases, 179
Nucleotidases, 179
Nutrient absorption, 185–197
  of carbohydrates, 185–187
  of cholesterol, 193–194
  fiber, 187
  of lipids, 188–190
  of lipid-soluble vitamins, 192–193
  low and no calorie fat substitutes, 190–192
  of minerals, 197
  of nutrients, 185
  of protein as amino acids, di- and
    tripeptides, 187–188
  of water-soluble vitamins, 194–197
Nutrient digestion, 173–183
  bile secretion, 177–178

digestion of vitamins and minerals, 181
digestive process, 173–174
feces formation, 183
intestinal mucosal secretions, 181
large intestine, 181–182
mouth, 174–175
pancreatic secretions, 179–181
regulation of digestion, 183
small intestine, 176–177
stomach, 175–176
Nutrient metabolism, dietary
    recommendations and, 287–304
  dietary guidelines for Americans, 297
  dietary reference intakes, 288–297
  Food Guide Pyramid, 297–299
  nutritional labeling, 299–304
  recommended dietary allowances,
    287–288
Nutrition, chemistry and biology concepts of
    importance in, 307–320
  bonding, 309
  coordinate covalent bond, 310
  covalent bond, 309
  energy requirements of enzymatic
    reactions, 314–315
  energy, work, and ATP, 316–318
  enzymology, 312–314
  functional organic groups of nutritionally
    important compounds, 311–312
  ionic bond, 309–310
  molecular weights, 307–309
  other bonding, 310–311
  oxidation–reduction reactions, 315–316
  periodic table, 307
  pH and pOH, 318–319
  polarity and solubility, 319–320
  thermodynamics, 312

O

Olestra, 191
Oligosaccharides, 190
Organ meats, 90, 107
Organophosphates, 129
Orthovanadate, 163
Osteomalacia, 57, 65
Osteoporosis, 126
Ovoflavin, 85
Oxalic acid, 120
Oxaloacetate, 241

Oxidation–reduction reactions, 315
Oxygen utilization, measurement of, 203

P

Palmitic acid, 25, 193, 239
Pancreatic lipases, 180
Pantothenic acid, 56, 109, 223
Parathyroid hormone (PTH0, 67
Parvalbumin, 124, 127
PEA, *see* Primary electron acceptor
Pectins, 14, 187
Pelargonic acid, 25
Pellagra, 57
Penicillamine, 281
Pentadecylic acid, 25
Pentane, 267
Pentanoic acid, 25
Pentoses, 14
Pepsin, 175
Peptide
   bonds, 46, 261
   synthesis, energy requirement for, 262
Periodic table, establishment of 307
Pernicious anemia, 57
Pharmacology, 277
Phenylalanine, 43, 49, 260
Phenylketonuria, (PKU), 44
Phenytoin, 283
Phosphatases, 179
Phosphate transfer, 229
Phosphatides, 112
Phosphatidylcholine, 24
Phosphatidylethanolamine, 24
Phosphatidylserine, 24
Phosphoenolpyruvate, 241
Phospholipids, 30
Phosphorus, dietary reference intake values
   for, 292
Photophobia, 86
Photosynthesis, energy transfer and, 321–330
   Calvin cycle, 326–330
   dark reactions, 326
   light reactions, 323–326
   photosynthesis, 322–323
   plant respiration, 330
Phytic acid, 120
PKU, *see* Phenylketonuria
Plants, elements required by, 6
Plasma membrane, 209

Plasmologens, 24
Platelet aggregation, 71
Polyhydroxyaldehydes, 9
Polyhydroxyketones, 9
Polyunsaturated fatty acid (PUFA), 233
Poppyseed oil, 36
Potential energy, 316
Prealbumin, 50
Precancerous polyps, 20
Premenstrual syndrome, 95
Primary electron acceptor (PEA), 323
Primordial atmosphere, composition of, 3
Proline, 49, 260
Proprionic acid, 25
Prostaglandin(s), 24, 38
   immediate precursor for, 37
   metabolism, 71
Prostanoic acid, 38
Protein(s), 41–52
   amino acid classification, 41–45
   catabolism, 51
   classification of amino acids by function,
      48–49
   consumption habits, 52
   deficiency, 63
   -energy malnutrition, 51–52
   excessive protein intakes, 52
   functions of proteins in body, 50–51
   quality, 49–50
   status, 50
   structure, 45–48
PTH, *see* Parathyroid hormone
PUFA, *see* Polyunsaturated fatty acid
Pyrazinamide, 281
Pyridoxine hydrochloride, 94
Pyrimidines, 254
Pyruvate, 243
   carboxylase, 150
   kinase, 131
   phosphokinase, 132

R

Radiation sickness, 95
Ranitidine, 281
RBP, *see* Retinol-binding protein
RDA, *see* Recommended dietary allowance
Recommended dietary allowance (RDA),
   130, 287, 289
Redox reactions, 153

Resting energy expenditure, 205
Retinoids, 59
Retinol-binding protein (RBP), 60
Retinyl esterases, 180
Riboflavin, 181
  deficiency, 88
  function of, 92
  in multivitamin supplement, 56
  rich food sources of, 86
Ribonucleic acid (RNA), 1, 211, 255
Rickets
  prevention of, 65
  vitamin D and, 57
RNA, *see* Ribonucleic acid
Rubedoxins, 141
Ruminants, calories derived by, 14

S

Salatrim, 191
Scurvy, 57, 77
Secretory glands, 167
Selenocysteine, 260
Serine, 49, 260
Serotonin, 93
Shortenings, 27
Silicon, 159, 160
Silicones, 1
Skin disorders, 65
Slipped tendon disease, 149
Small intestine, 178
SOD, *see* Superoxide dismutase
Sodium, 133
  pumps, 134
  retention, 134
Somatotrophin, 50
Sphingolipids, 24
Sphingomyelins, 112
Squalene, 248
Starch
  hydrolysis of, 173, 178
  synthesis of, 12
Stearic acid, 25
Steroids, 210
Sucralfate, 281
Sucrase, 181
Sucrose, 10
Sulfasalazine, 281
Sulfates, 16
Sulfite oxidase, 141

Sulfur metabolism, 139
Superoxide
  anion, 266
  dismutase (SOD), 150, 154, 274
  formation of, 265

T

Taurine, 93
Taurocholate, synthesis of, 137
TCA cycle, *see* Tricarboxylic acid cycle
Tetracyclines, 281
Tetrahydrofolic acid (THFA), 278
Tetrapyrroles, 122
TG, *see* Thyroglobulin
Theophylline, 281
Thermodynamics, 312
THFA, *see* Tetrahydrofolic acid
Thiamin
  deficiency of, 81
  in multivitamin supplement, 56
  pyrophosphate (TPP), 82, 255
Thiazides, 281
Thiolase, 148
Threonine, 49, 260
Thrombocytopenia, 103
Thromboplastin, 75
Thromboxanes, 38
Thymine, 254
Thyroglobulin (TG), 151
Thyroid-stimulating hormone (TSH), 46
Thyroxine, 50
Tocopherol, 71
Total parenteral nutrition (TPN), 108, 115
TPN, *see* Total parenteral nutrition
TPP, *see* Thiamin pyrophosphate
Trace minerals, 118
Transferrin, 141
Triamteren, 281
Tricarboxylic acid cycle, 108, 202, 223
Triglyceride(s)
  classification of, 24
  hydrolysis of, 173
  importance of, 23
  synthesis, 244
Tripeptides, 188
Tryptophan, 49, 91, 93
TSH, *see* Thyroid-stimulating hormone
Tyrosinase, 154
Tyrosine, 49, 260

U

Ulcers, 20
Ultraviolet radiation, 266
Undecylic acid, 25
Universe, major elements of, 5
Uracil, 254, 258
Uric acid, 271
Uronic acid, 14

V

Valine, 42, 49, 260
Valproic acid, 281
Vanadium, 162, 163
van der Waals forces, 310
Vasopressin, 46
Vegetable oils, hydrogenated, 27
Very low-density lipoprotein (VLDL), 21,
    194
Vitamins, 55–116
  biotin, 104–108
    deficiency, 107–108
    dietary recommendations, 107
    food sources, 107
    form, 105
    function, 105–107
    pharmacological doses, 108
    toxicity, 108
  fat-soluble, 23
  fat-soluble and water-soluble vitamins,
      57–58
  folic acid, 95–100
    deficiency, 99
    dietary recommendations, 98–99
    food sources, 98
    forms, 96
    functions, 96–98
    pharmacologic doses, 99
    toxicity, 99–100
  niacin, 88–92
    deficiency, 91
    dietary recommendations, 91
    food sources, 90–91
    forms, 89
    functions, 89–90
    pharmacologic doses, 91–92
    toxicity, 92
  pantothenic acid, 108–111
    deficiency, 110–111

  dietary recommendations,
      110
    food sources, 109
    form, 108
    function, 108–109
    pharmacologic doses, 111
  riboflavin, 84–88
    deficiency, 86–88
    dietary recommendations, 86
    food sources, 86
    forms, 85–86
    functions, 86
    pharmacologic doses, 88
    toxicity, 88
  substances in foods having characteristics
      of vitamins, 111
    carnitine, 114–115
    choline, 111–113
    myo-inositol, 115–116
    taurine, 113–114
  thiamin, 81–84
    deficiency, 84
    dietary recommendations, 84
    food sources, 83
    forms, 81–82
    functions, 82–83
    pharmacologic doses, 84
    toxicity, 84
  vitamin A, 59–65
    deficiency, 63
    dietary recommendations, 63
    food sources, 63
    forms, 60
    functions, 60–62
    pharmacologic doses, 63–65
    toxicity, 65
  vitamin B$_6$, 92–95
    deficiency, 95
    dietary recommendations, 94
    food sources, 93–94
    forms, 92
    function, 03
    pharmacologic doses, 95
    toxicity, 95
  vitamin B$_{12}$, 100–104
    deficiency, 103–104
    dietary recommendations, 103
    food sources, 102–103
    forms, 100–102
    function, 102

pharmacologic doses, 104
toxicity, 104
vitamin C, 76–81
  deficiency, 81
  dietary recommendations, 80
  food sources, 78–80
  forms, 77–78
  function, 78
  pharmacologic doses, 81
  toxicity, 81
vitamin D, 65–69
  deficiency, 68
  dietary recommendations, 68
  food sources, 68
  forms, 66–67
  function, 67–68
  pharmacologic doses, 68–69
  toxicity, 69
vitamin E, 69–72
  deficiency, 72
  dietary recommendation, 71
  food sources, 71
  forms, 69–70
  function, 70–71
  pharmacologic doses, 72
  toxicity, 72
vitamin K, 72–76
  deficiency, 75–76
  dietary recommendations, 74–75
  food sources, 74
  forms, 73–74

function, 74
pharmacologic doses, 76
toxicity, 76
vitamins as coenzymes, 58–59
VLDL, *see* Very low-density lipoprotein

W

Warfarin, 73
Water, 167–170
  balance, 168–169
  body distribution, 167
  dietary recommendations, 170
  function, 167–168
  molecular, 168
Waxes, 24
Western American diet, 219
Wheat germ, 71
Wilson's disease, 155

X

Xanthine dehydrogenase, 148
Xerophthalmia, 57

Z

Zinc
  metalloproteins and, 48
  supplements, 145, 146
  in terrestrial plants, 144